Ultrasonography of the Female Reproductive System

Springer Nature More Media App

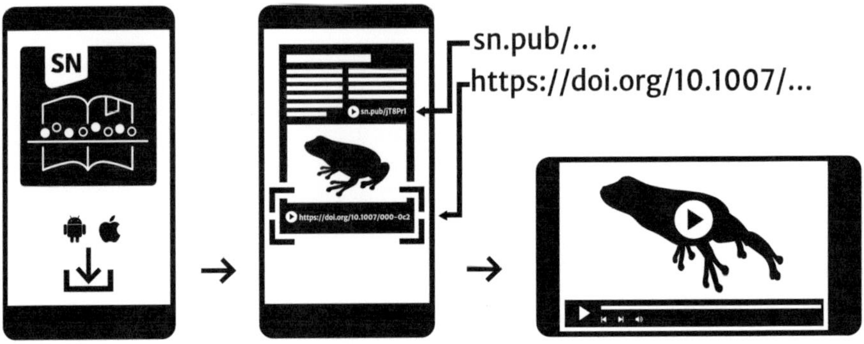

1. Download → **2. Scan Link** → **3. Enjoy Video**

Support: customerservice@springernature.com

Da Li • Zhijing Na • Xinlu Wang • Na Zuo
Editors

Ultrasonography of the Female Reproductive System

Springer

Science Press
Beijing

Editors
Da Li
Center of Reproductive Medicine
Shengjing Hospital of China Medical University
Shenyang, China

Zhijing Na
Center of Reproductive Medicine
Shengjing Hospital of China Medical University
Shenyang, China

Xinlu Wang
Department of Ultrasound
Shengjing Hospital of China Medical University
Shenyang, China

Na Zuo
Center of Reproductive Medicine
Shengjing Hospital of China Medical University
Shenyang, China

This work contains media enhancements, which are displayed with a "play" icon. Material in the print book can be viewed on a mobile device by downloading the Springer Nature "More Media" app available in the major app stores. The media enhancements in the online version of the work can be accessed directly by authorized users.

ISBN 978-981-95-1372-7 ISBN 978-981-95-1373-4 (eBook)
https://doi.org/10.1007/978-981-95-1373-4

Jointly published with Science Press
The print edition is not for sale in China (Mainland). Customers from China (Mainland) please order the print book from: Science Press.

This Springer imprint is published by the registered company Springer Nature Singapore Pte Ltd.
The registered company address is: 152 Beach Road, #21-01/04 Gateway East, Singapore 189721, Singapore

Preface

Diagnostic ultrasound is one of the three primary medical imaging techniques and has been widely used in clinical settings for decades. With increasing diagnostic and treatment needs and technological advancements, the imaging capabilities of ultrasound equipment have significantly improved. Over time, diagnostic ultrasound has evolved from A-mode and M-mode ultrasound to B-mode, Doppler, and 3D ultrasound techniques. These advancements have expanded its clinical applications and underscored its value in diagnosis and treatment.

The female reproductive organs, including the uterus, ovaries, fallopian tubes, and vagina, are located deep in the pelvis, making early diagnosis and dynamic monitoring during the reproductive cycle challenging. With its noninvasive nature, absence of radiation, high resolution, real-time imaging, and ease of use, ultrasound has become indispensable in female reproductive medicine. The rapid progress of ultrasound technology has profoundly impacted assisted reproductive medicine, gynecological diagnostics, and pregnancy monitoring. The improved resolution of ultrasound now allows diagnostic results for gynecological conditions to approach the accuracy of postoperative histopathological diagnosis. Furthermore, ultrasound contrast technology has enabled accurate, noninvasive, and repeatable assessments of intrauterine lesions and tubal patency. Techniques such as 3D ultrasound imaging and advanced image analysis have also become integral in diagnosing complex obstetric and gynecological conditions. These advancements enhance diagnostic accuracy and efficiency, enabling more individualized patient care.

The book *Ultrasonography of the Female Reproductive System* comprises eight chapters, beginning with the basic anatomy and physiology of the female reproductive system and the fundamental principles of gynecological ultrasound. It introduces transvaginal gynecological ultrasound and progresses to the clinical applications of ultrasound in reproductive medicine, including its role in assisted reproductive technologies and the evaluation of physiological and pathological conditions.

This book provides comprehensive and systematic coverage, integrating female reproductive medicine with ultrasound technology. It covers routine ultrasound examinations, common reproductive diseases, standardized examination techniques, and essential clinical knowledge. Additionally, it includes illustrative cases and ultrasound images tied to critical concepts. Bridging foundational knowledge with clinical applications, this book offers a step-by-step approach to deriving valuable clinical insights from challenging ultrasound examinations in reproductive medicine.

Emphasizing practicality, the book presents over 540 representative ultrasound images and 29 digital videos, incorporating unique image collages and schematic diagrams that outline anatomical structures in ultrasound images. This comparative layout enhances information retention while maximizing clarity and accessibility for readers.

We hope this book reflects the current landscape and advances in fertility ultrasound while serving as a practical clinical reference for professionals. Our aim is to contribute to improving diagnostic techniques and training in fertility ultrasound. Despite extensive editing and expert review, there may be some omissions or inaccuracies. We sincerely welcome feedback and suggestions from our readers.

Shenyang, China

Da Li
Zhijing Na
Xinlu Wang
Na Zuo

Acknowledgment

We sincerely thank the clinicians, researchers, and institutions whose expertise and collaboration shaped this work. Special gratitude to colleagues who contributed clinical cases, images, and technical insights, as well as the editorial team for refining complex concepts into accessible content. We are indebted to reviewers for their critical feedback and to our families for their unwavering support. Finally, we acknowledge the global medical community's role in advancing reproductive ultrasound—may this book inspire continued innovation in patient care.

Contents

1 Anatomy and Physiology of the Female Reproductive System

Da Li and Zhijing Na

1.1 Anatomy of the Female Reproductive System

The female reproductive organs include the internal and external reproductive organs. The external reproductive organs are the parts of the reproductive organs exposed to the outside, and the internal reproductive organs are located in the pelvis. Female reproductive organs have both endocrine and reproductive functions [1].

1.1.1 External Genitalia

The external female reproductive organs are also known as the vulva. It includes the mons pubis, labia majora (outer lips of the vagina), labia minora (inner lips of the vagina), clitoris, and the vaginal vestibule, which are bordered by the pubic symphysis in front, the perineum in back, and are located between the medial femurs, on either side (Fig. 1.1).

1. Mons pubis: It is an elevated structure in front of the pubic symphysis and is rich in adipose tissue. Pubic hair begins to sprout on the mons pubis at puberty and is distributed in an inverted triangular shape.
2. Labia majora: They are a pair of folds of skin located along the inner side of the two thighs, starting from the mons pubis and ending at the perineum. The outer side of the labia majora is skin, with pigmentation, containing sebaceous glands and sweat glands, while the inner side is mucosa-like. The subcutaneous tissue of labia majora is loose and rich in blood vessels, nerves, and lymphatic vessels, making it prone to posttrauma hematoma.

D. Li (✉) · Z. Na
Shengjing Hospital of China Medical University, Shenyang, China

D. Li et al. (eds.), *Ultrasonography of the Female Reproductive System*,
https://doi.org/10.1007/978-981-95-1373-4_1

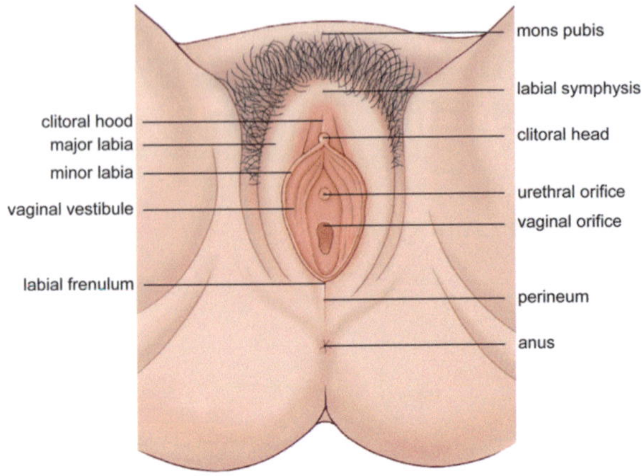

Fig. 1.1 Female external genital organs

3. Labia minora: These are a pair of thin skin folds on the inner side of the labia majora, fused at the anterior end and then divided into two lobes. The anterior lobe forms the clitoral prepuce, and the posterior lobe forms the clitoral girdle. The labia majora and minora converge at the posterior end to form the frenulum labium pudendal. The labia minora skin is moist, brown in color, rich in nerve endings, and very sensitive.
4. Clitoris: Located just below the tip (junction) of the labia minora, the clitoris consists of erectile tissue and can, therefore, swell in size. The clitoris is divided into three parts: the clitoral head in front, which is exposed to the vulva and sensitive to stimulation; the clitoral body in the middle; and the two clitoral pedicles in the posterior, which are attached to the left and right pubic bone.
5. Vaginal vestibule: It refers to the diamond-shaped area between the two lips of the labia minora, posterior to the clitoris and anterior to the labial girdle. Between the vaginal opening and the frenulum labium pudendal, there is a shallow fossa called the navicular fossa, also known as the fossa of the vestibule of the vagina, which disappears in multipara (a woman who has had multiple births).
   (a) Urethral opening (meatus): This round opening has folded closed edges below the clitoris. The posterior wall on either side of the external urethral opening is lined with paraurethral glands, which have tiny openings and are prone to harboring bacteria.
   (b) Vestibular bulbs: Also known as bulbs of the vestibule or clitoral bulbs, they are located on either side of the vaginal opening and consist of venous plexus with erectile properties. Their anterior end is attached to the clitoral head and posterior end to the Bartholin's glands, with the surface covered by bulbocavernosus muscle.
   (c) Bartholin's glands (or greater vestibular glands): They are a pair of soybean-sized glands covered by bulbocavernosus muscle in the posterior part of the labia majora. The ducts of these glands open in the groove between the labia minora and the hymen at the back of the vaginal vestibule, where they secrete mucus. These glands are not noticeable or palpable under normal

circumstances, but occlusion of the duct(s) may result in cyst(s) or abscess(es) in these glands.

(d) Vaginal opening: It is located posterior to the urethral opening and is rimmed by folds of mucous membranes called the hymen, which are lined with connective tissue, blood vessels, and nerves. In typical cases, there is a hole (or multiple holes in rare cases) in the center of the hymen, the size of which varies greatly. In pathological cases, this hole can be closed or absent, which requires a surgical incision, enabling normal menstrual discharge. The hymen can be ruptured by sexual intercourse or by strenuous physical activity and remains only as a hymenal scar after vaginal delivery.

1.1.2 Internal Genitalia

The female internal reproductive organs include the vagina, uterus, fallopian tubes, and ovaries (Fig. 1.2).

1. Vagina: It is an upwardly wide and downwardly narrow muscular canal located centrally in the lower part of the pelvic cavity (the true pelvis). The front wall of the vagina is 7–9 cm in length, and the back wall is 10–12 cm in length. The vagina is not only an organ for sexual intercourse but also a channel for menstrual blood to be discharged and for the fetus to be delivered.
   (a) Location: The anterior wall of the vagina is adjacent to the bladder and urethra; the posterior wall is close to the rectum. Its upper end wraps around the cervix, and the lower end opens into the vaginal vestibule. The crypt between the cervix and the vagina is called the vaginal fornix (vaginal vault, vault of vagina), which is divided into four parts: anterior, posterior, and lateral (left and right). The posterior component of the fornix is adjacent to the recto-

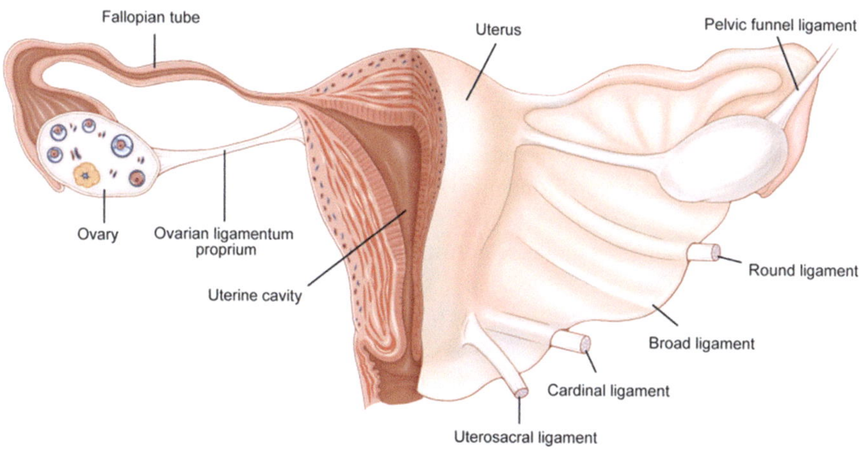

Fig. 1.2 Female internal reproductive organs (back view)

uterine recess (the lowest point of the pelvis). In clinical practice, this anatomical cavity is often the puncture site for (blood and/or pus) drainage.

(b) Tissue structure: The vaginal wall is composed of mucous membrane layer, muscular layer, and fibrous tissue layer from inside to outside. The mucous membrane layer is covered by nonkeratinized stratified squamous epithelium without glands, which is highly extensible due to multiple folds. The mucous membrane layer in the upper 1/3 of the vagina is subject to periodic changes influenced by sex hormones. The muscular layer consists of two layers of smooth muscle, that is, the inner circular and outer longitudinal layers, and is covered by a layer of fibrous tissue. The vaginal wall is rich in venous plexus, making it prone to bleeding or hematoma formation after injury.

2. Uterus (or womb): It is a thick-walled muscular organ with a cavity and is the organ that bears the fetus and generates menstrual blood. The uterus is an inverted pear-shaped organ with a slightly flattened front and back, consisting of the corpus uteri (body of the uterus) and the cervix uteri. The ratio of the corpus uteri and the cervix varies with age and ovarian function, with the ratio being 1:2 before puberty, 2:1 in women of childbearing age (~15–49 years old), and 1:1 after menopause. The uterus weighs about 50 g–70 g, is 7 cm–8 cm long, 4 cm–5 cm wide, 2 cm–3 cm thick, and has a capacity (volume) of about 5 mL. The top end of the corpus uteri is defined as the fundus of the uterus, with the cornua uteri (horns of the uterus) on either side of it. The narrowest section connecting the body of the uterus and the cervix is called the isthmus of the uterus, with the upper end termed the anatomical introitus due to its anatomical narrowness and the lower end termed the histological introitus due to the transition of the endometrium into the mucous membrane of the cervix. The isthmus of the uterus lengthens during pregnancy. It can extend to 7–10 cm at the end of gestation, forming a part of the soft delivery canal, and is commonly used as the incision site for cesarean delivery. The uterine cavity is triangular in shape, wide at the top and narrow at the bottom, connected to the fallopian tubes on both sides and the cervical canal at the bottom. The cervical canal of the uterus is a pike-shaped cavity (~3 cm long in adult women), the lower end of which is the external opening of the cervix to the vagina. The cervix of the uterus is divided into the lower part (the portio vaginalis or ectocervix), which protrudes into the vagina, and the upper supravaginal part (or endocervix). The external opening of the cervix is round before vaginal delivery but develops a transverse cleft after transvaginal childbirth, dividing the cervix into an anterior and a posterior lip.

(a) Location: The uterus is located in the center of the pelvis, with the fundus of the uterus below the level of the pelvic inlet and the external opening of the cervix slightly above the level of the sciatic spine. It is posterior to the bladder, anterior to the rectum, connected to the vagina at its lower end, and the fallopian tubes and ovaries on either side. When the bladder is empty, the normal uterus of an adult woman is in a mildly anteriorly tilted and forward-flexed position.

(b) Tissue structure: The body of the uterus consists of three layers from the inside out: the endometrium (mucosa), myometrium (muscularis), and peritoneum (serosa). The endometrium is subdivided into stratum compactum, stratum spongiosum, and stratum basalis. Of these, 2/3 of the interior surface is the functional layer (stratum compactum + stratum spongiosum), which is periodically regulated by ovarian hormones. The stratum basalis, that is, the basal layer, is the other 1/3 of the endometrium adjacent to the myometrium, which is not affected by hormones and does not undergo periodic changes. Myometrium consists of a large amount of smooth muscle tissue, a few elastic fibers, and collagen fibers. The peritoneum covers the uterine fundus and its anterior and posterior portions. The peritoneum of the anterior isthmus of the uterus is forwardly reflexed to form the vesicouterine pouch. In contrast, the peritoneum of the posterior cervix and posterior fornix of the vagina is backwardly reflexed at the back of the uterus to form the recto-uterine pouch, also known as the Douglas pouch. The cervix mainly comprises connective tissue with a small amount of smooth muscle, elastic fibers, and blood vessels. The mucosa of the cervical canal consists of a single layer of high columnar epithelium, with glands secreting alkaline mucus to form mucus plugs, which are subject to periodic changes as influenced by sex hormones. The vaginal part of the cervix is covered by stratified squamous cells. The junction of columnar and squamous epithelium is the most susceptible site for cervical cancer.

(c) Ligaments of the uterus: There are four pairs of ligaments of the uterus.

The broad ligaments are a pair of wing-like, double-layered folds of peritoneum that extend from the anterior and posterior walls of the uterus to connect the two sides of the uterus to the pelvic wall, which restrict the uterus from tilting to the sides. The broad ligament on each side is divided into anterior and posterior lobes with free upper ends. Its medial 2/3 wraps around the fallopian tubes, and its lateral 1/3 wraps around the ovarian arteries and veins, forming the infundibulopelvic ligament, also known as the suspensory ligament of the ovary (the fimbriae of the fallopian tube tubes is not covered by the peritoneum). The broad ligament between the medial side of the ovary and the uterine horn is slightly thickened and is called the proper ligament of the ovary (or utero-ovarian ligament, ovarian ligament). The broad ligaments flanking the body of the uterus are rich in blood vessels, nerves, lymphatic vessels, and loose connective tissue, which are termed paracervical tissues. The uterine arteries, veins, and bilateral ureters pass through the base of the broad ligaments.

The round ligaments are a pair of cord-like, smooth muscle and connective tissue bands. On each side, the round ligament arises from slightly below the proximal end of the fallopian tube in front of the horn of the uterus, travels forward and outward under the anterior lobe of the broad ligament, reaches the lateral pelvic wall, and then stops at the anterior end of the labia majora via the inguinal canal. The round ligaments are about 12–14 cm long and uphold the anteriorly tilted position of the uterus.

The cardinal ligaments, also known as the transverse cervical ligaments, are a pair of tough tissue bundles of smooth muscle and connective tissue fibers that run transversely between both sides of the cervix and the pelvic wall along the lower part of the broad ligaments. The cardinal ligaments hold the cervix in place and prevent uterine prolapse.

The uterosacral ligaments (covered by the peritoneum) consist of smooth muscle, connective tissue, and nerves governing the bladder. They originate from behind and superior to the junction of the corpus uteri and the cervix uteri and run laterally around the rectum to the front of the second and third sacral vertebrae. The uterosacral ligaments draw the cervix backward and upward, maintaining the uterus in an anteriorly tilted position.

3. Fallopian tubes (or uterine tubes, oviducts): They are a pair of muscular ducts (8–14 cm in length) close to the ovaries that serve as a venue for sperm to couple with the egg and transport the fertilized egg. They are wrapped by the free upper edges of the broad ligaments, connected to the horns of the uterus on the medial side, and are free and umbrella-shaped (fimbriae) on the lateral side.
   (a) Morphology: The fallopian tubes are divided into four sections from medial to lateral: the interstitial part (or interstitium) is located in the uterine wall, with the narrowest lumen, about 1cm in length; the isthmus is lateral to the interstitial part, which is fine and relevantly straight, about 2–3 cm in length; the ampulla is lateral to the isthmus, characterized by a thin wall and a wide and curved lumen, with abundant folds, about 5–8 cm in length, in which fertilization often happens; the infundibulum is about 1–1.5 cm long, is the most lateral part of the fallopian tube, which is funnel-shaped and with many finger-like protrusions (known as fimbriae) at the opening of the tube, enabling it to "pick up the egg."
   (b) Tissue structure: The tubal tissue is divided into the mucosae, the smooth muscle layer, and the serosa layer from inner to outer. The mucous layer is covered by a single layer of columnar epithelium. These epithelial cells are divided into ciliated columnar, secretory, and peg cells. Of these, ciliated cells assist in the transport of fertilized eggs. Contraction of the muscles of the muscularis mucosa assists in egg pickup and transport of fertilized eggs and, to some extent, prevents retrograde flow of menstrual blood and the spread of infection from the uterine cavity into the abdominal cavity. Muscle contractions and mucosal epithelial cells are periodically influenced by sex hormones.
4. Ovaries: They are a pair of flat oval gonads that vary in size and shape with age. The surface of the ovary is smooth before puberty and gradually becomes uneven following ovulation. The ovary size in women during the fertile period is about 4 cm × 3 cm × 1 cm, weighing about 5 g to 6 g and grayish-white in color, while the ovary gradually atrophies and stiffens after menopause (Fig. 1.3).
   (a) Location: On each side, the ovary is attached to the infundibulopelvic ligament on the lateral side and the proper ligament of the ovary on the medial side, suspended between the uterus and the pelvic wall, and connected to the

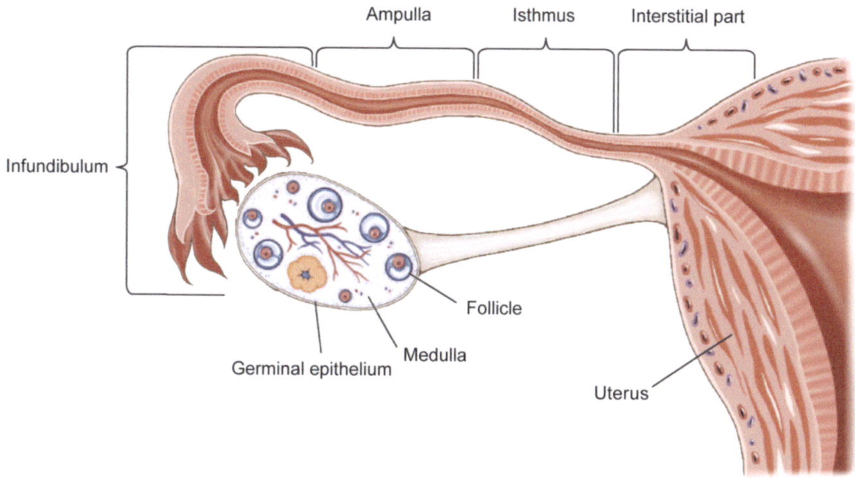

Fig. 1.3 Fallopian tube and ovary

broad ligament by the mesovarium. In the middle of the ovary's anterior margin is the ovary's hilum, where nerves and blood vessels enter and leave the ovary by passing through the pelvic funnel ligament. Meanwhile, the posterior edge of the ovary is free.

(b) Tissue structure: The surface of the ovary is not covered by the peritoneum but a single layer of cuboidal epithelium known as the germinal epithelium. Underneath the germinal epithelium is a layer of dense fibrous tissue known as the tunica albuginea. Further inward is the ovarian substance, further divided into an outer cortical layer (cortex) and an inner medullary layer (medulla). The cortex is the main body of the ovary, consisting of developing follicles of various sizes, the corpus luteum, the remnants resulting from the degeneration of the corpus luteum, and interstitial tissue. The medulla is connected with the hilum of the ovary and consists of loose connective tissue, abundant blood vessels, nerves, lymphatic vessels, and a small number of smooth muscle fibers.

1.1.3 Blood Vessels and Lymphatic Vessels

The blood vessels supplying the female reproductive organs are accompanied by lymphatic vessels. The female reproductive organs and pelvis are supported by abundant lymphatic nodes and lymphatic drainage, with veins and lymphatic vessels coinciding in clusters and networks between the organs.

1. Arteries: The blood supply to the female internal and external genital organs mainly comes from the ovarian artery, uterine artery, vaginal artery, and internal pudendal artery (Fig. 1.4).

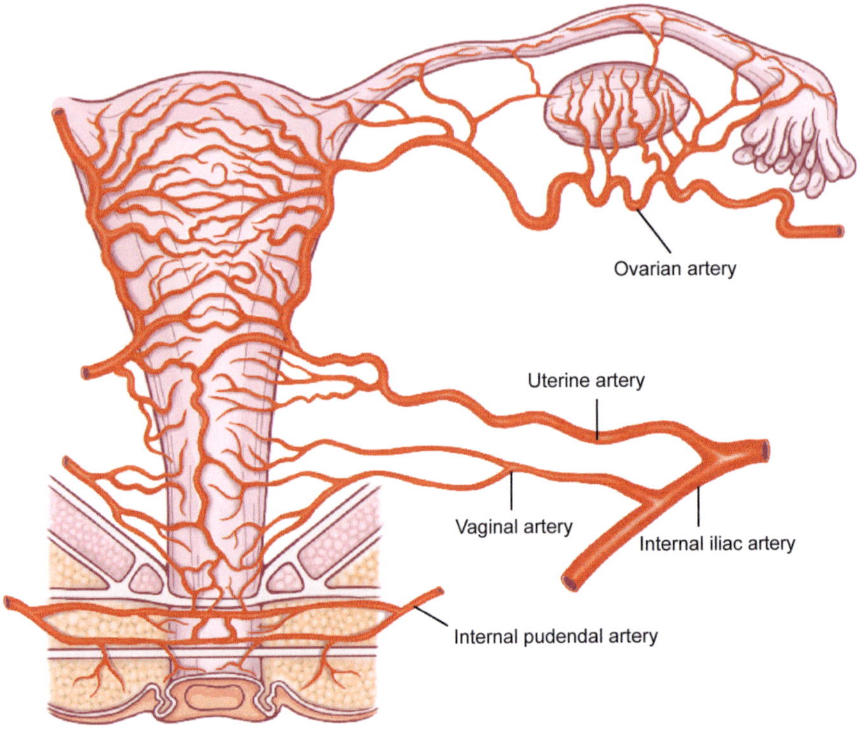

Fig. 1.4 Female pelvic arteries

(a) Ovarian artery: It emanates from the abdominal aorta, travels anteriorly along the psoas major muscle in the retroperitoneum, descends outward to the pelvic rim, crosses the ureter and the lower part of the common iliac artery, transverses inwardly across the infundibulopelvic ligament, and then crosses backwardly through the mesovarium, branching off to enter the ovary through the ovarian hilum. Before entering the ovary, the ovarian artery gives off some branches that travel within the mesosalpinx to supply the fallopian tube, and its ending coincides with the ascending ovarian branch of the uterine artery near the uterine horn.

(b) Uterine artery: It branches from the anterior trunk of the internal iliac artery, travels behind the peritoneum along the lateral pelvic wall downward and forward, passes through the base of the broad ligament and the para-uterine tissues to reach the lateral side of the uterus (approximately at 2 cm horizontally outward from the internal cervical orifice), and traverses the ureter to the lateral border of the uterus, where it splits into the upper and lower branches. The upper branch of the uterine artery is thicker and meanders upward along the lateral border of the uterus, which is known as the uterine branch and further splits into the branches to the fundus, the branches to the fallopian tube, and the branches to the ovary at the uterine horn. The lower branch is thinner, with its small subordinate branches supplying the cervix and the upper part of the vagina, and is known as the cervical-vaginal branch.

(c) Vaginal artery: It branches from the anterior trunk of the internal iliac artery, with its subordinate branches supplying the anterior and posterior walls of the lower and intermediate parts of the vagina, the bladder dome, and the bladder neck. The vaginal artery coincides with the cervical-vaginal branch and branches of the internal pudendal artery. The arterial blood supply to the vagina can therefore be summed up as follows: the upper section is supplied by the cervical-vaginal branch of the uterine artery; the middle section is supplied by the vaginal artery; and the lower section is supplied mainly by the internal pudendal artery and the middle hemorrhoidal artery.

(d) Internal pudendal artery: It is the terminal branch of the anterior trunk of the internal iliac artery, which passes out of the pelvic cavity through the inferior foramen of the pyriformis muscle at the greater sciatic foramen, encircles the dorsal surface of the sciatic spine, reaches the ischiorectal fossa through the lesser sciatic foramen, and splits into four branches: the inferior hemorrhoidal artery, supplies the lower part of the rectum and anus; the perineal artery, supplies the superficial part of the perineum; the vulvar labial artery, supplies the labia majora and minora; the clitoral artery, supplies the clitoris and vestibular bulb.

2. Veins: The pelvic veins are accompanied by the eponymous arteries. They are more numerous than the arteries and constitute venous plexuses, interconnecting with each other and facilitating the spread of pelvic vein infections when they occur. For example, the ovarian vein runs alongside the ovarian artery and joins the inferior vena cava to the right and the left renal vein to the left. Therefore, injury to these vessels should be avoided when reaching the renal vein level when performing para-aortic lymphadenectomy. In addition, varicose veins are more common in the left pelvis because the renal veins are quite thin, making blood flow easily impeded.

3. Lymphatic system: Female internal and external genital organs and the pelvis are endowed with abundant lymphatic supplies, with lymph nodes usually arranged along the corresponding blood vessels, distributed in clusters or strings. The number and location of these lymph nodes vary greatly. In cases of infections or cancerous tumors in internal or external genital organs, they can spread or metastasize via the lymphatic ducts to various parts of the body (Fig. 1.5).

(a) Lymph nodes of the external genitalia: They are divided into superficial and deep lymph nodes, namely, the superficial inguinal lymph nodes and the deep inguinal lymph nodes.

(b) Pelvic lymph nodes: These include the iliac, presacral, and lumbar lymph nodes (para-abdominal aortic lymph nodes). The iliac lymph nodes consist of the obturator, internal, external, and common iliac lymph nodes.

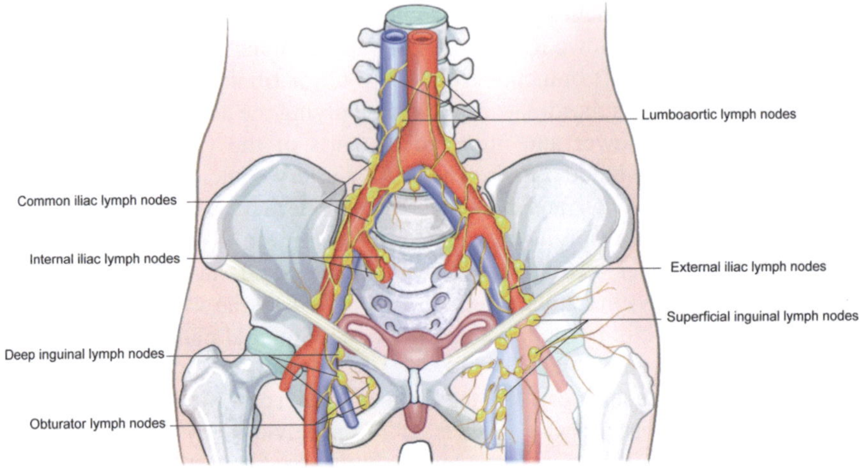

Fig. 1.5 Lymphatic distribution in the female genitalia

1.2 Ovarian Cycle and Ovulation

The ovary is a female genital gland with both reproductive and endocrine functions. At different stages of a woman's life (from puberty to menopause), the (cyclical) function and morphology of her ovaries change considerably [2].

1.2.1 Development and Regulation of Follicles Before Puberty

At 6 weeks to 8 weeks of the embryonic stage, the primordial germ cells undergo continuous mitotic divisions, which result in more cells with increasing size, referred to as oogonia, approximately 600,000 in number. From the 11th–12th week of embryonic development, the oogonia enter the first meiosis and rests in the prediplotene stage. At this time, they are called primary oocytes, and their number reaches a peak at 16 to 20 weeks of embryonic development, with the two ovaries containing a total of 6 to 7 million germ cells, of which 1/3 are oogonia, and 2/3 are primary oocytes. Between the 16th week of embryonic development and 6 months after birth, a monolayer of spindle-shaped pregranulosa cells surrounds a primary oocyte that rests in the diplotene stage of meiosis to form a primordial follicle, which is the basic female reproductive unit and the only form of oocyte reserve. Follicles continue to atresia during fetal life, with about 2 million remaining at birth. Subsequently, most follicles degenerate during childhood, leaving only about 300,000 by puberty.

1.2.2 Development and Maturation of Follicles After Puberty

From puberty until menopause, the ovary undergoes cyclic changes in morphology and function, known as the ovarian cycle. The process of follicular development from autonomous to regular maturation relies on gonadotropin regulation. A batch of follicles (3–11) will develop for women entering their reproductive years every month. After recruitment and selection, only one dominant follicle will reach full maturity and be discharged as an egg. Meanwhile, the rest of the follicles will deteriorate independently through the apoptosis mechanism called follicular atresia. In a woman's lifetime, typically, only 400 to 500 follicles will develop to maturity and be released as eggs, representing only about 0.1% of their total number.

1. Primordial follicle: The transformation of the primordial follicle into a primary follicle is the starting point of follicular development. The primordial follicle, which can lie dormant in the ovary for decades, consists of a primary oocyte surrounded by a single layer of spindle-shaped pregranulosa cells. It takes more than 9 months for a primordial follicle to develop into a preantral follicle, 85 days for a preantral follicle to develop into a mature follicle that undergoes a sustained growth phase (grade 1 to grade 4 follicles), and an exponential growth phase (grade 5 to grade 8 follicles).
2. Preantral follicle: As the body grows and develops, the function of the adrenal glands gradually perfects, and the androgens produced by the reticular zones and adipose tissue in the adrenal cortex gradually increase, so that androgens in the blood are at a high level. The primordial follicle begins to develop autonomously in response to androgens, with the granulosa cells within the follicle generating follicle-stimulating hormone (FSH) receptors, estrogen (E) receptors, and androgen (A) receptors, and the thecal cell generating luteinizing hormone (LH) receptors. These receptors equip the granulosa cells and thecal cells to be responsive to the above hormones. However, the number of receptors produced at this time is relatively small. The above development is a long process—after 270 days or more of development, the primordial follicle becomes a preantral follicle, also known as a class 1 secondary follicle.
3. Antral follicle: Under the continuous action of FSH, the granulosa cells of the preantral follicle produce a small amount of estrogen. Under the combined effect of estrogen and FSH, follicular fluid generated between the granulosa cells increases. Meanwhile, the follicle enlarges up to 500 μm in diameter, called the antral follicle. In response to androgen stimulation, FSH receptors on granulosa cells and LH receptors on thecal cells in the antral follicle constantly increase, resulting in enhanced sensitivity of these cells to signals. With more receptors and cells, more FSH ligands are required to support follicular growth and development. However, due to the underdevelopment of the hypothalamus before puberty, the hypothalamic-pituitary-ovarian (HPO) axis remains suppressed long-term, resulting in a relatively stable and low level of FSH and LH. With low FSH levels, the antral follicle can only develop into a class 4 follicle, which takes about 60 days.

4. Preovulatory follicle: Upon reaching puberty, as the hypothalamus develops toward maturity, gonadotropin-releasing hormone (GnRH) production progressively increases. In response to GnRH, FSH and LH produced by the pituitary gland continue to increase. When the blood FSH level exceeds a certain threshold, a batch of class 4 follicles (3–11 follicles) begin to develop simultaneously a "recruitment" process. FSH acts on its receptors on the surface of granulosa cells, causing them to produce estrogen. Sensing the estrogen concentration, the hypothalamus and pituitary gland mildly inhibit FSH production by negative feedback. Only one follicle with the lowest threshold (the most sensitive, with the most receptors) can continue to grow and develop properly under low FSH levels and eventually become the dominant follicle. Meanwhile, the remaining follicles stop developing and then degenerate (atresia). This process described above is called "selection". The dominant follicle continues to develop in response to FSH stimulation. Concurrently, its granulosa cells generate LH and prolactin receptors in preparation for generating the corpus luteum and luteinization. Eventually, after about 25 days, the class 4 follicle develops into a preovulatory follicle (class 8 follicle) characterized by increased follicular fluid, enlarged follicular cavity, and a significant increase in follicular volume, with a diameter of up to 18 mm to 23 mm (Fig. 1.6).

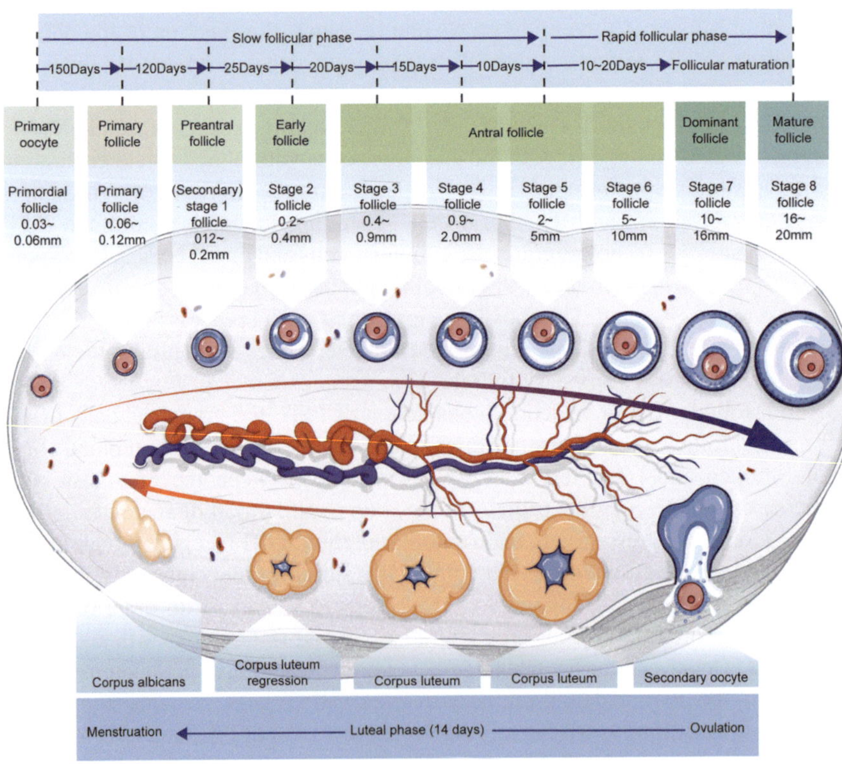

Fig. 1.6 Development and maturation of the follicle

1.2.3 Ovulation

Ovulation is the oocyte expelled from the ovary with its external oocyte-corona-cumulus complex (consisting of the zona pellucida, the corona radiata, and the cumulus oophorus). This process involves the completion of the first meiotic division of the oocyte, the breakdown of the collagen layer of the follicular membrane, and the expulsion of the ovum (egg cell) following the formation of the stigma (a small hole in the follicle) [3]. Ovulation most often occurs about 14 days before the next menstrual period. The egg may be discharged alternately from both ovaries or continuously from one ovary.

The peak secretion of estradiol by the mature follicular cell before ovulation (E2 ≥200 pg/mL) exerts a positive feedback effect on the hypothalamus, prompting a massive release of GnRH from the hypothalamus, which induces the release of gonadotropins from the pituitary gland, resulting in an LH/FSH peak. The LH peak appears 36 hours before the follicle rupture and is a reliable sign of impending ovulation. Before ovulation, the follicle luteinizes and produces a small amount of progesterone. The LH/FSH peak acts synergistically with progesterone to activate the proteolytic enzyme in the follicular fluid, causing the follicular collagen to digest and form a small pore known as the stigma. The significant increase of prostaglandins in the follicular fluid before ovulation promotes the release of proteolytic enzymes from the follicular wall and also enhances the contraction of smooth muscle in the ovary, which facilitates ovulation.

1.2.4 Formation and Degeneration of Corpus Luteum

After ovulation, the follicular fluid flows out, the pressure in the follicular cavity decreases, and the follicular wall collapses, forming many folds. Meanwhile, the follicular granulosa cells and thecal cells within the follicular wall intrude inward, which are enveloped by the theca of the ovarian follicle—together, they constitute the corpus luteum. The follicular granulosa cells and thecal cells further luteinize in response to the LH peak, forming granulosa lutein cells and theca-lutein cells, respectively. The diameter of the corpus luteum increases from 12 μm–14 μm to 35 μm–50 μm. On the 7th to 8th day after ovulation, which corresponds to approximately the 22nd day of the menstrual cycle, the corpus luteum peaks in size and function, with a diameter of 1–2 cm and a yellowish appearance.

If the discharged egg is fertilized, the corpus luteum enlarges under the action of chorionic gonadotropin secreted by the trophoblast cells and transforms into the corpus luteum of pregnancy (or corpus luteum graviditatis), which degenerates at the end of the first trimester of gestation. After that, the placenta is developed and secretes steroid hormones to maintain the pregnancy.

If the egg is not fertilized, the function of the corpus luteum is limited to 14 days, and it begins to degenerate on the 9th to 10th day after ovulation. When the corpus luteum degenerates, its cells progressively become smaller and shriveled, with the surrounding connective tissue and fibroblasts intruding into the corpus luteum. This process leads to fibrosis of the corpus luteum tissue and a whitish appearance, at which point the corpus luteum turns into a corpus albicans. After the degeneration of the corpus luteum, menstruation takes place, new follicles begin to develop, and a new cycle is initiated.

1.3 Endometrium and Menstruation

1.3.1 Cyclic Changes of the Endometrium

The endometrium is morphologically divided into the functional layer and the basal layer. The functional layer is subject to cyclical changes regulated by hormonal fluctuations. Based on the histological changes in the functional layer, the menstrual cycle can be divided into three phases: proliferative, secretory, and menstrual. The basal layer is close to the myometrium, does not undergo exfoliation, and is not regulated by hormonal changes. The basal layer can regenerate and repair endometrial wounds, regenerating the functional layer.

The physiologic characteristics of the proliferative, secretory, and menstrual phases are described in detail below, using a normal 28-day menstrual cycle as an example (Fig. 1.7).

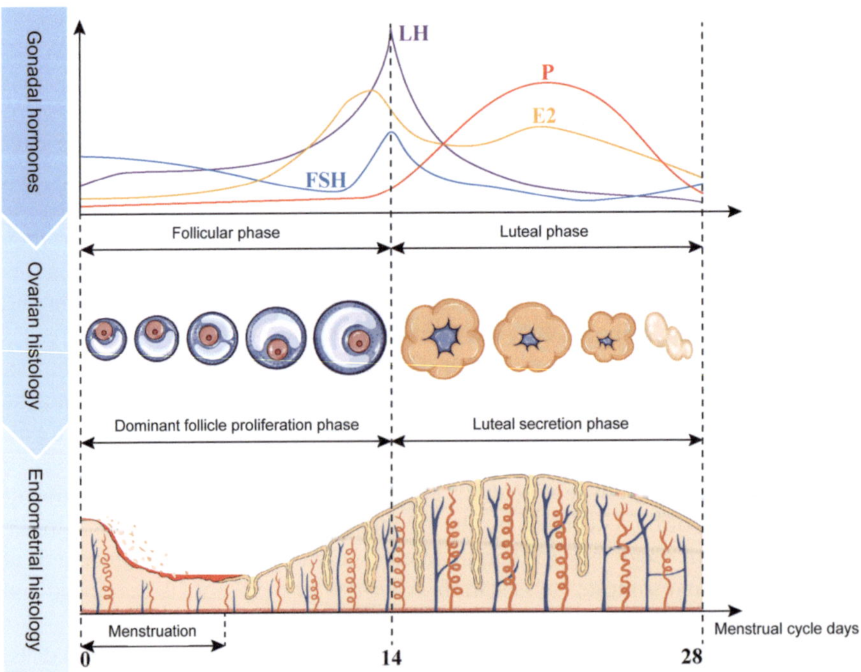

Fig. 1.7 Cyclic changes of the endometrium and hormone secretion

Table 1.1 Physiological characteristics of the proliferative phase

	Days of the menstrual cycle	Characteristics
Early proliferative phase	Day 5–7	During this period, the endometrium is thin, only 1–2 mm. The endometrial glands are short, straight, thin, and sparse. The glandular epithelial cells are cuboidal or low pillar-shaped. The interstitial tissue is dense, with stellate interstitial cells. The small arteries in the interstitial tissue are relatively straight and thin-walled
Middle proliferative phase	Day 8–10	In this phase, the endometrial glands increase in number, elongate, and become slightly curved. The glandular epithelial cells proliferate actively, are columnar in shape, and begin to have mitotic figures. Interstitial edema is most obvious during this period. Spiral arterioles gradually develop, and their walls become thicker
Late proliferative phase	Day 11–14	The endothelium thickens to 3–5 mm in this phase, with an uneven and slightly wavy surface. The glandular epithelium cells turn into high columnar in shape and proliferate into pseudostratified epithelium, with an increase in nuclear mitotic figures. The glands become longer and curved. Stellate interstitial cells incorporate into a meshwork. Tissue edema is quite pronounced. Small arteries proliferate with enlarged, curved lumens

1. Proliferative phase: It refers to the 5th–14th day of the menstrual cycle—corresponds to the follicular phase of the ovarian cycle. In this phase, the thickness of the endometrium increases from 0.5 mm to 3–5 mm under the action of estrogen, and the surface epithelium, glands, mesenchyme, and blood vessels of the endometrium exhibit proliferative changes. An important change in glandular cells during the proliferative phase is increased ciliated and microvillous cells. The proliferative phase can be subdivided into early, middle, and late phases (Table 1.1).
2. Secretory phase: The secretory phase lasts from the 15th to the 28th day of the menstrual cycle and corresponds to the luteal phase of the ovarian cycle. Estrogen and progesterone secreted by the corpus luteum lead to continued thickening of the endometrium, further growth and curvature of glands and blood vessels, initiation of secretion, and interstitial laxity and edema. During this phase, the endometrium is thick, loose, soft, and rich in nutrients, favoring the development of a fertilized egg. The secretory phase is also subdivided into three phases: early, middle, and late (Table 1.2).
3. Menstrual phase: The first to the fourth day of the menstrual cycle is the period when the functional layer of the endometrium disintegrates and falls off from the basal layer, which is the final result of the unfertilized egg, degeneration of the corpus luteum in the ovary, and the sudden drop in estrogen and progesterone levels. Twenty-four hours before menstruation, the endometrial spiral arterioles rhythmically contract and diastole. This is followed by gradually intensified vasospastic contraction, resulting in ischemic necrosis and exfoliation of distal vascular walls and tissues. The shed endometrial fragments, together with blood, flow out of the vagina, which is the onset of menstruation.

Table 1.2 Physiological characteristics of the secretory phase

	Days of the menstrual cycle	Characteristics
Early secretory phase	Day 15–19	In this phase, the endothelial glands grow longer and curve more significantly. The glandular epithelial cells begin to exhibit glycogen-containing subnuclear vacuoles, a histologic feature of this phase. The interstitium of the endothelium remains edematous, and the spiral arterioles continue to proliferate and curve
Middle secretory phase	Day 20–23	In this phase, the endometrium becomes thicker and saw-toothed than before. The interstitium becomes even more lax and edematous. The spiral arterioles further proliferate and coil. At this point, the secretory epithelial cells within the glands rupture from the apical cell membrane, allowing the intracellular glycogen to escape into the glands, a process known as apocrine secretion. The secretory activities in the endometrium also involve the exudation of plasma, after which immunoglobulins bind to binding proteins secreted by the epithelial cells and enter the endometrial cavity. Such secretory activities peak on the seventh day after the mid-menstrual LH peak and are synchronized with blastocyst implantation
Late secretory phase	Day 24–28	This phase is premenstrual, corresponding to the corpus luteum's degradation. The endometrium in this period is spongy and up to 10 mm thick. The endometrial glands have openings toward the uterine cavity, with discharges of glycogen and other secretions. The interstitium during this time is even more lax and edematous. The interstitial matrix beneath the surface epithelial cells differentiates into hypertrophic predecidual cells and small round granular cells with lobulated nuclei and rosette granules. During this phase, the spiral arterioles grow rapidly beyond the thickness of the endometrium, become more coiled, and their lumens are also dilated

1.3.2 Normal Menstruation

Menstruation refers to the periodic shedding of the endometrium and bleeding accompanying the cyclical changes of the ovaries. Regular menstrual cycles are an important sign of reproductive maturity. The age of first menstruation is related to nutrition, heredity, physical condition, and other factors, and is mostly at 13–15 years old. With better nutritional conditions, the age of first menstruation tends to move earlier, which may be as early as 11–12 years old. Clinical concern should be aroused if menstruation has not yet begun after 16 years of age.

Menstrual blood is dark red and contains, in addition to blood, fragments of endometrium, inflammatory cells, cervical mucus, and shed vaginal epithelial cells. Moreover, menstrual blood contains prostaglandins and large amounts of fibrinolytic enzymes derived from the endometrium. It is because of the dissolving effect of these fibrinolytic enzymes on fibrin that menstrual blood does not coagulate. However, clots may result when there is a high volume of menstrual blood or when the bleeding is too fast.

Normal menstruation is cyclical and self-limiting. The first day of bleeding is the beginning of the menstrual cycle, and the interval between the first days of two menstrual periods is one menstrual cycle, which typically ranges from 21 to 35 days, with an average of 28 days. Each menstrual period is usually 2 to 8 days, with an average of 4 to 6 days. The menstrual volume is the total blood loss during a menstrual period, which is normally 20 mL–60 mL, with more than 80 mL being considered heavy menstrual bleeding (hypermenorrhea or menorrhagia). Menstruation is a physiological phenomenon and generally has no special symptoms. However, due to pelvic congestion and the effects of prostaglandins, some women experience lower abdominal pain and lumbosacral discomfort or uterine contraction pain during menstruation and may also suffer from headaches and mild neurological instability.

1.3.3 Regulation of the Menstrual Cycle

The menstrual cycle regulation is a complex process that primarily involves the hypothalamus, pituitary gland, and ovaries. The hypothalamus secretes GnRH, which regulates ovarian function by modulating gonadotropin secretion by the pituitary gland. Sex hormones secreted by the ovaries, in turn, have feedback effects on the hypothalamus and pituitary gland. The hypothalamus, pituitary gland, and ovaries regulate and interact with each other to form a coherent and coordinated neuroendocrine system known as the HPO axis [4]. The neuroendocrine activities of the HPO axis are governed by the higher centers in the brain. In addition to the reciprocal regulation of hormones produced by the hypothalamus, pituitary gland, and ovaries, the inhibin-activin-follistatin system and some other endocrine glands also participate in the regulation of the menstrual cycle.

GnRH is a decapeptide secreted by neuronal cells in the arcuate nucleus of the hypothalamus, which is transported to the adenohypophysis through the pituitary portal system to regulate the synthesis and secretion of pituitary gonadotropins. The secretion of GnRH is characterized by a pulsatile release with a frequency of one release per 60 min to 120 min, which is related to the temporal phase of the menstrual cycle. Physiologic and pathologic changes in the menstrual cycle are accompanied by corresponding changes in the pulsatile secretion pattern of GnRH. The pulsatile release of GnRH regulates the LH/FSH ratio.

1. Pituitary reproductive hormones: These include gonadotropins and prolactin, of which gonadotropins refer to FSH and LH secreted by gonadotropin cells of the pituitary gland. They respond to pulsatile stimulation by GnRH, are also secreted in a pulsatile pattern, and are also regulated by follicular sex hormones and inhibin.
2. The regulation process of the menstrual cycle
   (a) Follicular phase: The length of the menstrual cycle depends on the duration of the follicular phase. After atrophy of the corpus luteum, estrogen, progesterone, and inhibin A levels are minimized, which relieves their inhibitory

effects on the hypothalamus and pituitary gland, resulting in the restart of GnRH secretion by the hypothalamus and an increase in FSH secretion by the pituitary gland. These secretory activities promote follicular development, which leads to estrogen secretion by the follicles and proliferative phase changes in the endometrium. The gradually increasing estrogen inhibits GnRH secretion from the hypothalamus and decreases FSH secretion from the pituitary gland. As the follicles develop, the estrogen secreted by the follicles peaks and lasts for more than 48 h, generating positive feedback on the hypothalamus and pituitary gland, resulting in LH and FSH peaks and promoting ovulation.

(b) Luteal phase: LH and FSH levels decrease dramatically after ovulation, accompanied by corpus luteum formation and maturation. The progesterone secreted by the corpus luteum causes the endometrium to undergo secretory phase changes. The progesterone level peaks on the seventh to eighth day after ovulation, and the estrogen level hits a second small peak. The combined negative feedback of estrogen, progesterone, and inhibin decreases LH and FSH secretion by the pituitary gland so that the corpus luteum begins to atrophy, and the secretion of estrogen and progesterone decreases. The endometrium then loses its hormonal support, resulting in the peeling of its functional layer and the onset of menstruation. The reduction in estrogen, progesterone, and inhibin levels releases their negative feedback on the hypothalamus and pituitary gland, which leads to an increase in FSH secretion and the beginning of follicular development and a new menstrual cycle.

References

1. Roy A, Matzuk MM. Reproductive tract function and dysfunction in women. Nat Rev Endocrinol. 2011;7(9):517–25.
2. Grin L, Vo KCT, Sato Y, et al. Ageing and chronic disease-related changes in the morphometric characteristics of ovarian follicles in cynomolgus monkeys (Macaca fascicularis). Hum Reprod. 2021;36(10):2732–42.
3. Duffy DM, Ko C, Jo M, et al. Ovulation: parallels with inflammatory processes. Endocr Rev. 2019;40(2):369–416.
4. Ruohonen ST, Poutanen M, Tena-Sempere M. Role of kisspeptins in the control of the hypothalamic-pituitary-ovarian axis: old dogmas and new challenges. Fertil Steril. 2020;114(3):465–74.

Fundamentals of Ultrasonic Diagnosis and Common Ultrasound Techniques in Female Reproduction

2

Da Li and Xinlu Wang

2.1 Fundamentals of Ultrasonic Diagnosis

Ultrasound imaging has been one of the fastest-evolving medical imaging modalities over the past half-century. Diagnostic ultrasound offers several advantages, including safety, noninvasiveness, portability, ease of use, affordability, and the ability to provide real-time imaging. This section will outline the fundamentals of ultrasound technology and its applications in gynecology, focusing on female reproductive health.

2.1.1 Ultrasound

Ultrasound refers to mechanical vibration waves generated by an object, classified as sound waves with a frequency exceeding 20 kHz. In medicine, ultrasound leverages its unique physical properties—specifically the acoustic characteristics of ultrasonic waves as they propagate through human tissues and organs—for diagnostic and therapeutic purposes.

When ultrasound waves travel through human tissues, they primarily manifest as longitudinal waves with very high frequencies and short wavelengths, capable of transmitting in a specific direction. As these waves propagate, they undergo various physical phenomena, including reflection, refraction, scattering, and diffraction. These processes form the foundation of clinical ultrasound imaging.

D. Li (✉) · X. Wang
Shengjing Hospital of China Medical University, Shenyang, China
e-mail: wangxl1@sj-hospital.org

D. Li et al. (eds.), *Ultrasonography of the Female Reproductive System*,
https://doi.org/10.1007/978-981-95-1373-4_2

2.1.2 Ultrasonic Probe

The ultrasonic probe, also known as the ultrasound transducer, is the most critical component of any ultrasound diagnostic system. The basic principle of probe operation is as follows: the core element of the transducer, a piezoelectric wafer, converts alternating current into short ultrasonic pulses through the inverse piezoelectric effect. These pulses propagate through the body, where they encounter tissue interfaces and are reflected as echoes.

As the sound waves travel deeper into the tissue, each reflective interface generates echoes that sequentially return to the probe. The transducer then processes these returning echoes using the positive piezoelectric effect, converting them into electrical signals. These signals are ultimately processed and displayed as ultrasound images on the monitor (Fig. 2.1). This process enables the sequential capture of echoes from superficial layers to deeper structures, allowing for the visualization of internal anatomy.

An ultrasonic probe must exhibit both acoustic and functional characteristics. The appropriate probe is selected depending on the scanning site and the specific purpose of the examination in clinical practice. Therefore, it is essential to understand the features and applications of commonly used ultrasonic probes.

The following is an overview of the types of ultrasonic probes frequently utilized in the Department of Reproductive Medicine.

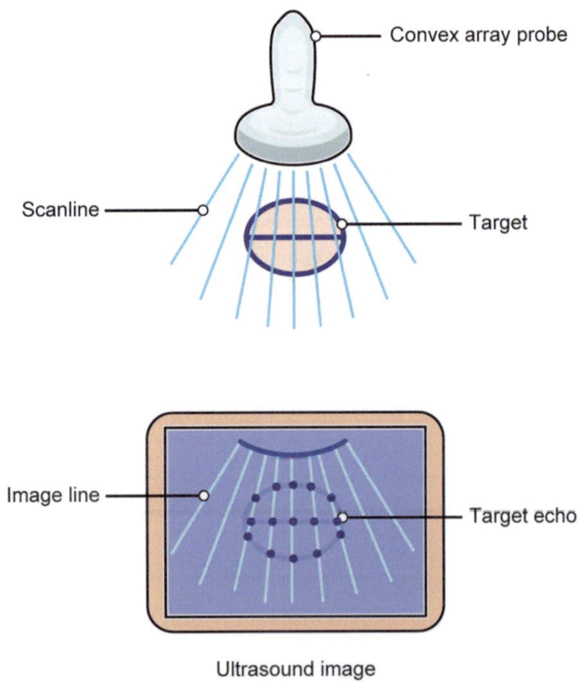

Fig. 2.1 Principles of imaging with an ultrasonic probe

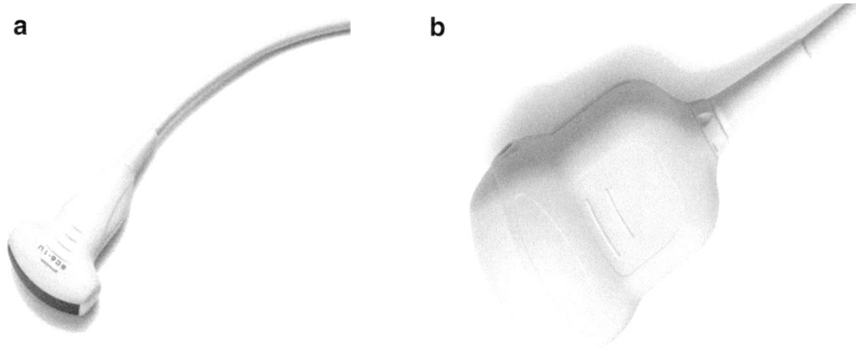

Fig. 2.2 Abdominal ultrasonic probes. Image (**a**) is an abdominal 2D ultrasonic probe; image (**b**) is an abdominal volume probe

1. Abdominal ultrasonic probes

   Most abdominal ultrasonic probes (or transducers) operate at frequencies between 3.5 and 6.0 MHz. They can be classified into two main types: two-dimensional (2D) probes and volume probes (Fig. 2.2). Volume probes are equipped with an internal electronic chip that enables automatic sweeping. During scanning, a volume probe remains stationary while its acoustic beams automatically adjust their direction to capture comprehensive volume data within the area of interest. After computerized reconstruction, the collected three-dimensional (3D) data generates a 3D image of the scanned region.

   The key characteristics of abdominal probes include a small contact surface with the body, a narrow near-field view, a wide far-field view, an extended imaging range of up to 90°, and a fan-shaped imaging pattern (Fig. 2.3). These probes are primarily employed for abdominal ultrasound examinations and obstetric and gynecological (O&G) assessments. In the Department of Reproductive Medicine, abdominal ultrasonic probes are predominantly utilized for ultrasound-guided embryo implantation procedures.
2. Intracavitary ultrasonic probes

   Intracavitary ultrasonic probes (or transducers) operate at frequencies ranging from 2 to 11 MHz and are available in two types: two-dimensional (2D) and volume probes (Fig. 2.4). Key characteristics of intracavitary probes include a small contact surface with the body, a narrow near-field view, a wide far-field view, an extended imaging range of up to 230°, and a fan-shaped imaging profile (Fig. 2.5).

   These probes are designed for intracavitary scanning, either transvaginally or transrectally. In reproductive medicine, intracavitary probes are commonly employed for routine uterine and adnexal assessments, follicle monitoring, and other diagnostic purposes.
3. Interventional ultrasonic probes

   Interventional ultrasonic probes can be classified into specialized puncture probes and interventional probes equipped with a puncture guide rack. A

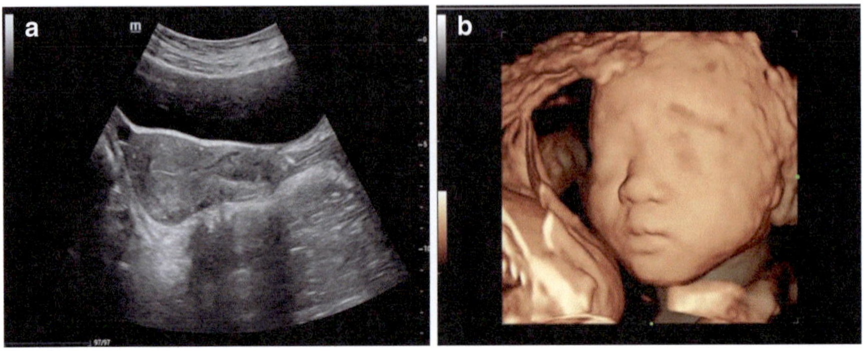

Fig. 2.3 (**a**) An abdominal 2D ultrasound image showing a longitudinal view of the uterus was obtained via transabdominal scanning. (**b**) Transabdominal volume ultrasound scan image displaying a fetal facial volume in surface mode

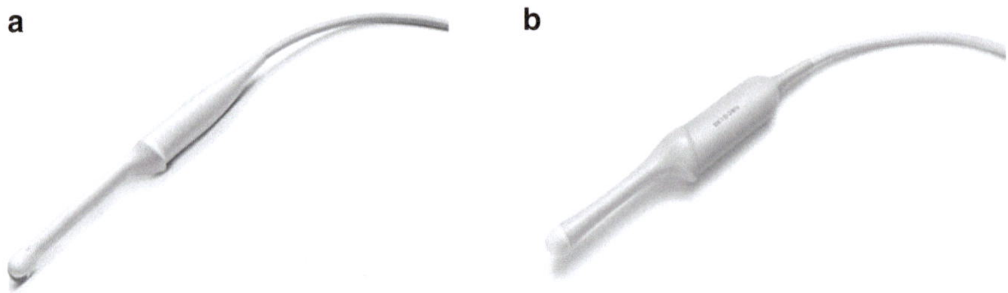

Fig. 2.4 Intracavitary ultrasonic probes. Image (**a**) is an intracavitary 2D ultrasonic probe; image (**b**) is an intracavitary volume probe

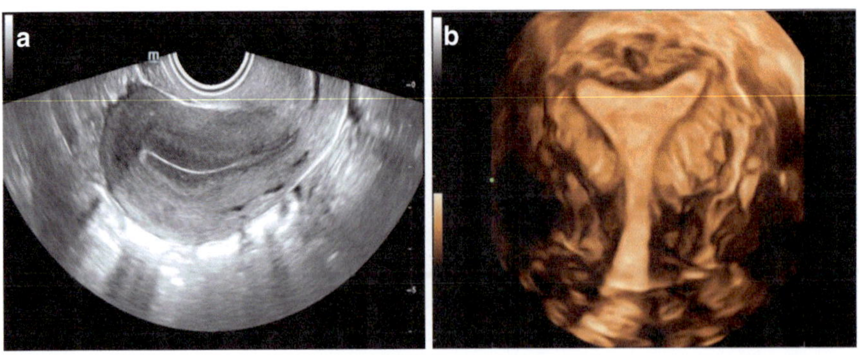

Fig. 2.5 (**a**) Intracavitary 2D ultrasound image showing the midsagittal plane of the uterus. (**b**) Intracavitary volume ultrasound image displaying a 3D view of the uterus in the coronal plane

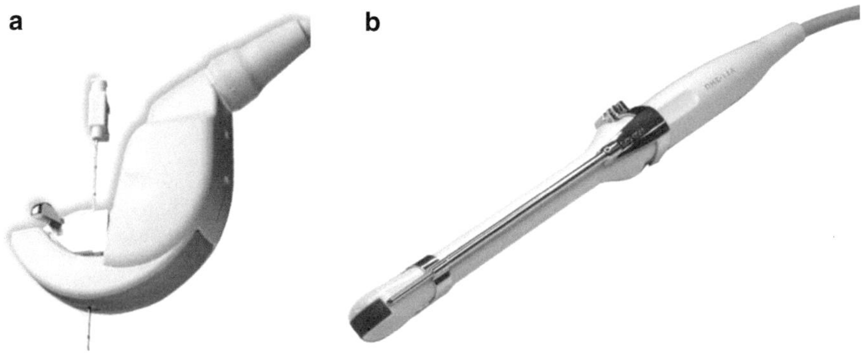

Fig. 2.6 Interventional ultrasonic probes. Image (**a**) is a specialized puncture probe; image (**b**) is an interventional ultrasonic probe with a puncture rack

specialized puncture probe may consist of either a hollow circular single-crystal transducer or a multiarray transducer (multiple crystals arranged in arrays), often featuring a wedge-shaped groove (Fig. 2.6a). Alternatively, a puncture guide rack may be attached to the probe's left (or right) side, serving as a guiding device (Fig. 2.6b). This rack marks the trajectory of the puncture needle as it enters the tissue, which is displayed on the screen to assist with accurate positioning.

The main clinical applications of interventional ultrasound include ultrasound-guided puncture biopsy, aspiration, and ablation therapy. In reproductive medicine, interventional ultrasonic probes are primarily used for ultrasound-guided egg retrieval and fetal reduction procedures.

2.1.3 Ultrasound System/Equipment

A brightness-mode (B-mode) ultrasound system consists primarily of a probe, a transmitter/receiver unit, a digital scanning converter, an external control device, and a power supply [1].

Advances in computer technology have led to the development of computer-based ultrasound systems, also known as computerized diagnostic ultrasound systems. The computerization of ultrasound instruments enhances the system's functionality, enabling video playback, image processing, archive management, and image transmission. Operating a diagnostic ultrasound system is akin to working with a "mainframe computer," so familiarizing physicians with the system's operation can significantly improve productivity.

While the control panel of a diagnostic ultrasound console may appear complicated (Fig. 2.7), instructions for using the buttons can be accessed through the Quick Action Card (Fig. 2.8) integrated within the system. Alternatively, technical guidance is available from the manufacturer to help train users in operating the system and understanding the unique features of the equipment.

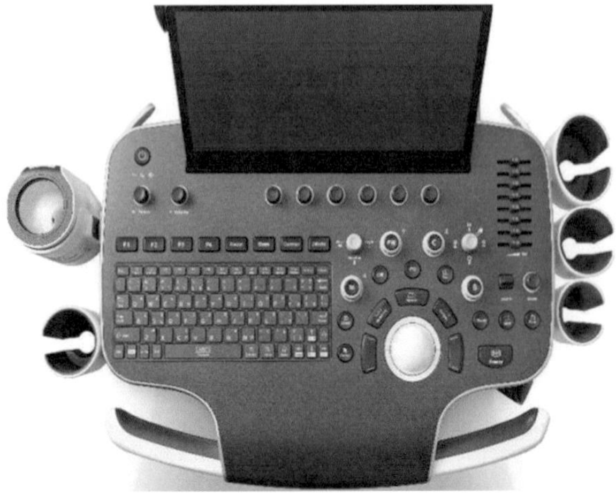

Fig. 2.7 Control panel of an ultrasound system

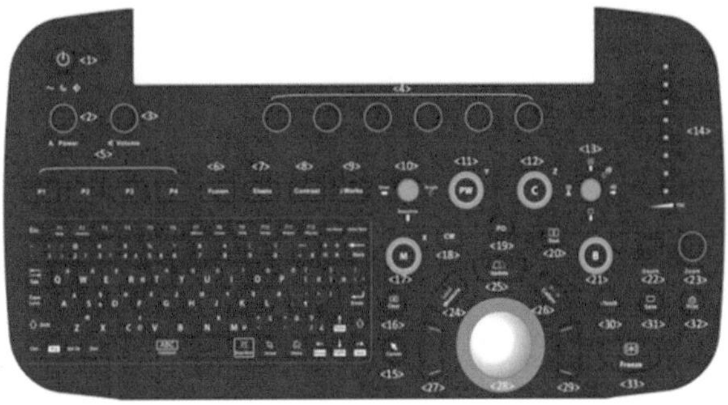

Fig. 2.8 Quick action card integrated within an ultrasound system

2.2 Common Ultrasound Techniques

2.2.1 Principles and Applications of 2D Ultrasound Imaging

2D ultrasound is based on displaying the echo signal's strength as brightness or luminance. A series of scattered and reflected signals generated by individual interfaces encountered by a single acoustic beam as it propagates are visualized as varying levels of brightness or luminance along the scan line. Therefore, the distribution of echo signals along the scan line represents the structure of the sound beam in one linear direction [2]. The time required to acquire each scan line is directly related to the number of scan lines and the depth of the image, which in turn determines the time needed to capture a complete image frame.

Diagnosis based on B-mode ultrasound is achieved by analyzing the sectioned sonograms. Different tissues in the human body have distinct echo intensities and varying degrees of acoustic attenuation, which form the basis for interpreting B-mode ultrasound images. Additionally, other imaging modalities,

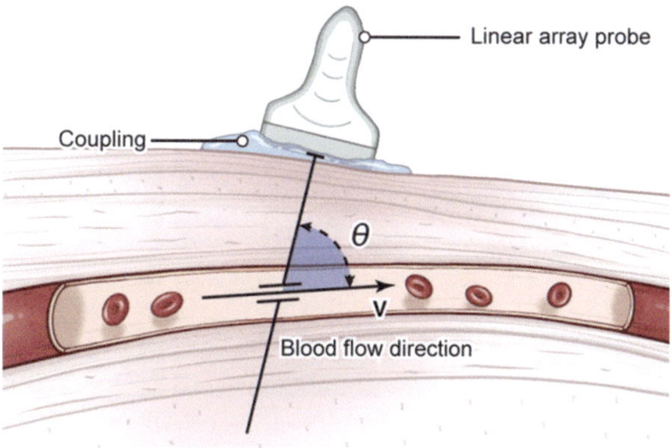

Fig. 2.9 Schematic diagram of the Doppler effect

such as color Doppler, spectral Doppler, and 3D imaging, are derived from B-mode ultrasound images, making the acquisition of high-quality 2D images a key focus in clinical practice.

2.2.2 Principles and Applications of Doppler Ultrasound Imaging

When the vibration source (sound wave source) and the observer move closer together, the frequency of the sound wave increases. Conversely, when they move apart, the frequency decreases. This change in frequency is called the Doppler shift, and the phenomenon is known as the Doppler effect (Fig. 2.9).

In Doppler ultrasound, the angle between the sound beam and the direction of blood flow can affect the accuracy of the blood flow velocity measurement when observing the movement of human red blood cells. To minimize error, the angle between the sound beam and blood flow direction should generally be kept within 30° when possible.

The Doppler signals acquired by the probe are processed in various ways and displayed differently in clinical settings. Spectral displays are referred to as spectral Doppler, while color displays include color Doppler flow imaging and color Doppler power mapping.

1. Spectral Doppler

   Blood flow measurement methods based on Doppler include continuous wave Doppler (CW), pulsed wave Doppler (PW), and high pulsed repetition frequency Doppler (HPRF).

   (a) Continuous wave Doppler

   A continuous wave Doppler unit typically consists of two transducers: one continuously transmits ultrasound, while the other continuously receives it.

   The advantage of continuous wave Doppler is that it can display blood flow signals at different depths within the same spectrum without being lim-

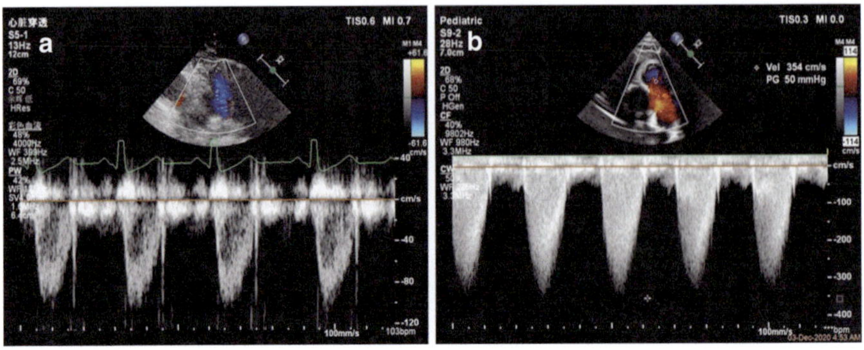

Fig. 2.10 (**a**) Pulsed wave Doppler spectrum of a normal pulmonary valve orifice. (**b**) Continuous wave Doppler spectrum of pulmonary valvular stenosis

ited by high-speed blood flow. The disadvantage, however, is that it cannot identify the exact location of the signal source. Continuous wave Doppler systems are commonly used in clinical practice to detect high-speed blood flow, particularly in the heart (Fig. 2.10).

(b) Pulsed wave Doppler

The underlying principle of pulsed wave Doppler involves the intermittent emission of pulse waves, a distance-selective technique (which selects blood flow at a specific depth for analysis), and the selective reception of back-scattered signals for processing localized signals. The probe emits a series of pulse waves, which travel to the sampling volume and return to the transducer after a certain period of time.

Several factors affect the efficacy of a pulsed wave Doppler system, primarily the pulse repetition frequency (PRF), sampling depth, and transducer frequency.

PRF refers to the number of pulse wave sets emitted per unit of time, which is inversely proportional to the time interval between two pulse sets. In other words, the higher the PRF, the shorter the time interval. One-half of the PRF is known as the Nyquist limit frequency. When the frequency shift exceeds the Nyquist limit, aliasing occurs, leading to a failure to display the correct or complete spectral pattern or to identify the direction and size of the spectrum.

In clinical practice, PRF limits the maximum velocity that can be detected (typically between 1 and 2 m/s). This makes it unsuitable for measuring high-speed blood flow, especially in conditions like cardiovascular diseases where blood velocities may exceed 5–6 m/s. Since the sampling depth is inversely proportional to the PRF, the greater the sampling depth, the lower the maximum blood flow velocity that can be detected for a given transducer frequency.

In reproductive medicine, pulsed wave Doppler is mainly used to measure uterine arterial blood flow, endometrial arterial blood velocity, and

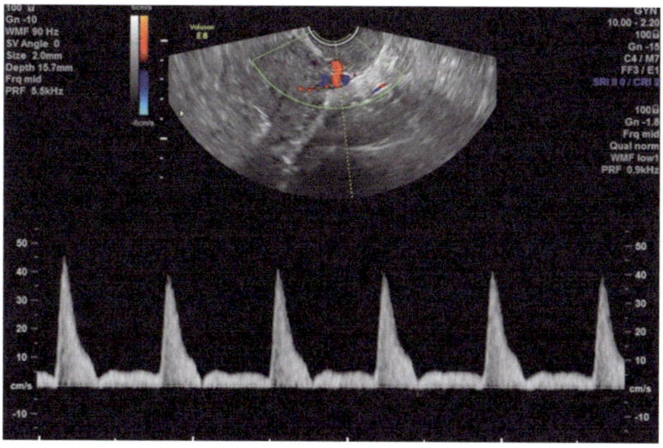

Fig. 2.11 Doppler spectrum of uterine artery blood flow in a nonpregnant woman

other related parameters. Below, we will use the uterine artery (Fig. 2.11) as an example to briefly demonstrate how Doppler spectrum analysis is conducted:

The direction of the spectrum represents the direction of blood flow. Under routine settings, blood flow toward the probe is displayed as positive, corresponding to the portion of the spectrum above the baseline (the red and blue bars in the image indicate the direction of blood flow, with red representing flow toward the probe and blue indicating flow away from the probe). The baseline is typically positioned in the center of the spectral scale but can be adjusted up or down to align with the magnitude of the measured velocity. For example, the figure shows that the uterine artery blood flow spectrum is positive. The baseline can be lowered so that the spectral waveform aligns with the mid-position.

The uterine artery in nonpregnant women typically has a high-resistance flow, and its spectrum is divided into systolic and diastolic phases. The systolic phase shows a sharp peak, while the diastolic phase displays a hump-like peak and a visible early diastolic notch. The highest point of the systolic spike represents the peak velocity of blood flow, usually measured in cm/s.

The spectral morphology of blood flow varies across different parts of the body. For instance, the spectral pattern of blood flow at the normal pulmonary valve orifice in Fig. 2.10a differs from that of the uterine artery. Additionally, the grayscale of the spectrum reflects the number of erythrocytes at the same velocity in the sampling volume—the darker the color, the greater the number of erythrocytes at that speed, and vice versa. Turbulence in the blood flow can be detected by coarse noise in the audio accompanying the spectrum.

2. Color Doppler

Color Doppler flow imaging (CDFI), developed from pulsed wave Doppler, is the first noninvasive, real-time technique capable of visualizing blood flow in the heart and blood vessels. Its imaging mechanism is similar to that of spectral Doppler, but it presents the distribution and direction of blood flow on a 2D

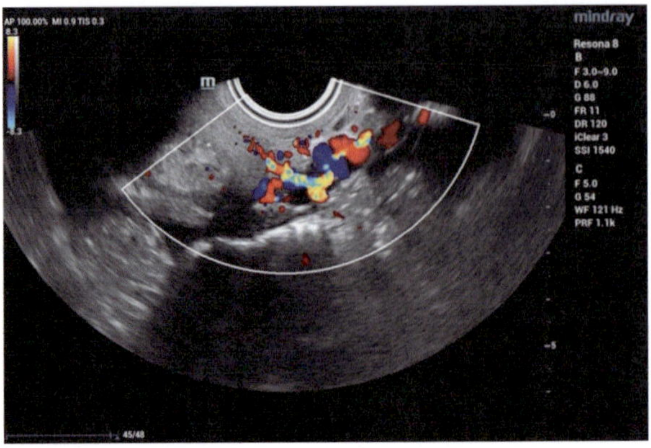

Fig. 2.12 Color Doppler image of the uterine arteries in a nonpregnant woman

image. It displays information about the magnitudes and directions of blood flow by transforming the extracted signals into red, blue, and green colors for visualization.

The main factors that affect color Doppler imaging are temporal resolution, velocity resolution, and spatial resolution. Temporal resolution refers to the ability to display blood flow in real time. A color frame rate that is too low can impair the display of structures and blood flow. Velocity resolution refers to the ability to distinguish blood flows at different speeds in real time. When the velocity exceeds the Nyquist limit frequency, color aliasing may occur. Spatial resolution refers to the ability to accurately display the directionality of blood flow in real-time, primarily shown by the width of the colored blood flow.

Figure 2.12 shows a color flow image of normal uterine arteries in a nonpregnant woman. The white fan-shaped box represents the sampling frame, and its size setting can affect the display of color flows. Generally, the size of this box should be set to encompass only the observation area. The different colors within the sampling frame represent the directions of blood flow, with the routine setting of red for flow toward the probe and blue for flow away from the probe. The brightness of the color indicates the speed of the blood flow: the brighter the color, the faster the blood flow, and vice versa.

Additionally, it is important to adjust the appropriate speed scale and color gain based on the blood flow speed at the observation site. For detecting low-speed blood flow, the speed scale should be lowered to improve detection; conversely, the speed scale should be increased for high-speed blood flow to prevent color aliasing. The color gain (i.e., color brightness) should also be adjusted according to the detected blood flow speed. Excessive gain results in diffuse, flickering color spots, and the gain should be gradually reduced until the color spots disappear.

3. Power Doppler

Power Doppler ultrasonography, also known as Power Doppler Imaging (PDI), utilizes the intensity or energy distribution of red blood cells in the bloodstream for imaging (Fig. 2.13). While CDFI reflects the velocity, direction, and speed changes of blood flow, PDI focuses on the power of the Doppler signals,

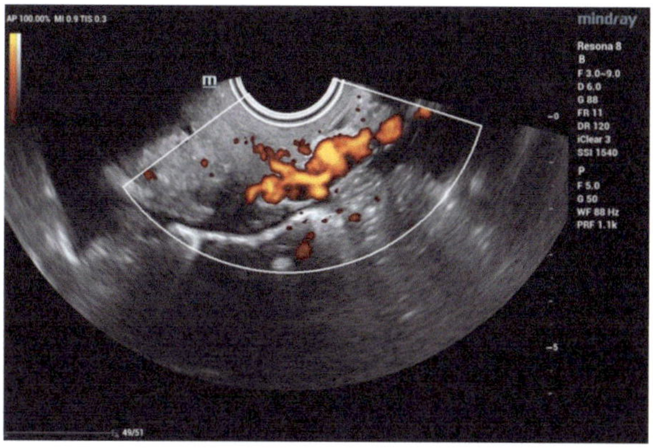

Fig. 2.13 Power Doppler image of the uterine arteries in a nonpregnant woman

making it particularly sensitive to low-velocity blood flows. PDI offers several advantages over CDFI:

(a) Increased sensitivity to low-velocity blood flow, allowing for the detection of blood flow signals across a broader range of velocities.
(b) The ability to display blood flow patterns that are relatively unaffected by the angle of view, facilitating the visualization of blood flow distributions and perfusion patterns in different regions.
(c) It avoids the color mosaics that can occur in CDFI when velocities exceed the Nyquist limit.

2.2.3 Principles and Applications of 3D Ultrasound Imaging

3D ultrasound technology addresses the limited spatial visualization of 2D ultrasound, making it an important complement to traditional imaging techniques.

1. Principles of 3D Imaging

3D ultrasound builds upon 2D ultrasound imaging, meaning high-quality 3D images can only be obtained if the 2D images are of sufficient quality. 3D imaging techniques are divided into static 3D imaging and real-time 3D imaging. In static 3D ultrasound, the probe is placed at a fixed position during scanning and cannot be moved, resulting in a series of static images. In contrast, real-time 3D imaging extends static 3D by incorporating a time variable, enabling continuous volume acquisition and simultaneous reconstruction. This method allows both the target of observation and the probe to move.

Typically, 3D ultrasound imaging involves the following steps: data acquisition, 3D reconstruction, image display, and 3D image slicing/analysis.

(a) Data acquisition

Data acquisition refers to the process by which a diagnostic ultrasound system collects a series of 2D images from multiple locations within an area of interest in the body. Data acquisition methods include mechanical positioning scanning, free-hand scanning, 2D array transducer scanning, and matrix array transducer scanning (the approach most commonly used by ultrasound systems today) [2].

Since 3D ultrasound imaging relies on reconstructing 2D images, its temporal and spatial resolution is typically lower than that of conventional 2D ultrasound. Additionally, the speed of 3D ultrasound imaging remains a bottleneck that limits the development of real-time 3D imaging. However, the quality of real-time 3D ultrasound images involves a trade-off between the fan angle of the scan and the number of frame captured per second. Optimizing image quality for a specific clinical application requires balancing these two parameters.

(b) 3D reconstruction

3D reconstruction methods include stereo-geometric construction (GCS) modeling, surface contour extraction, and voxel modeling. Volume reconstruction is most commonly used and typically realized through voxel-based algorithms. Each voxel is projected into its corresponding 3D position within the volume to create a voxel-based volume model in this approach.

(c) 3D image display and the cutting and analyzing of images

Among the various image display modes in 3D ultrasound, the most suitable mode should be selected based on the target organ, site, and nature of the lesion. Common display modes include 3D rendering mode, three-plane mode, Tomographic Ultrasound Imaging (TUI), OmniView technology, and volume contrast imaging (VCI).

Stereoscopic rendering modes are categorized into surface, perspective, and HDlive modes. By adjusting the mixing ratio of the two modes, different rendering effects can be achieved, such as surface mode, maximum mode, X-ray mode, minimum mode, and HDlive mode. Different observational results can be obtained using various modes for the same lesion site (Fig. 2.14). For example, surface mode is commonly used to visualize the endometrium, early pregnancy fetus, and tubal contrast imaging; maximal mode is typically employed to visualize the fetal skeleton; X-ray mode is often used for viewing intracranial structures of the fetus, intrauterine devices, and the endometrium; and HDlive mode can provide more detailed and three-dimensional images depending on the direction of the light source.

TUI displays volumetric data in multiple parallel planes, resembling the imaging techniques used in computerized tomography (CT) or magnetic resonance imaging (MRI). The parameters of the image planes, such as the number of layers, layer spacing, position, and tilt, can be adjusted to suit the target area and the specific purpose of the observation (Fig. 2.15).

Fig. 2.14 (**a**) HDLive mode. (**b**) Image of the same fetal face in iLive mode with a different light source position. (**c**) Image of the same fetal face in iLive mode with a different light source position. (**d**) Image of the same fetal face in iLive mode with a different light source position. (**e**) Image of the same fetal face in iLive mode with a different light source position. (**f**) Fetal spine shown in maximum mode. (**g**) Fetal spine shown in X-ray mode. (**h**) Endometrium shown in X-ray mode

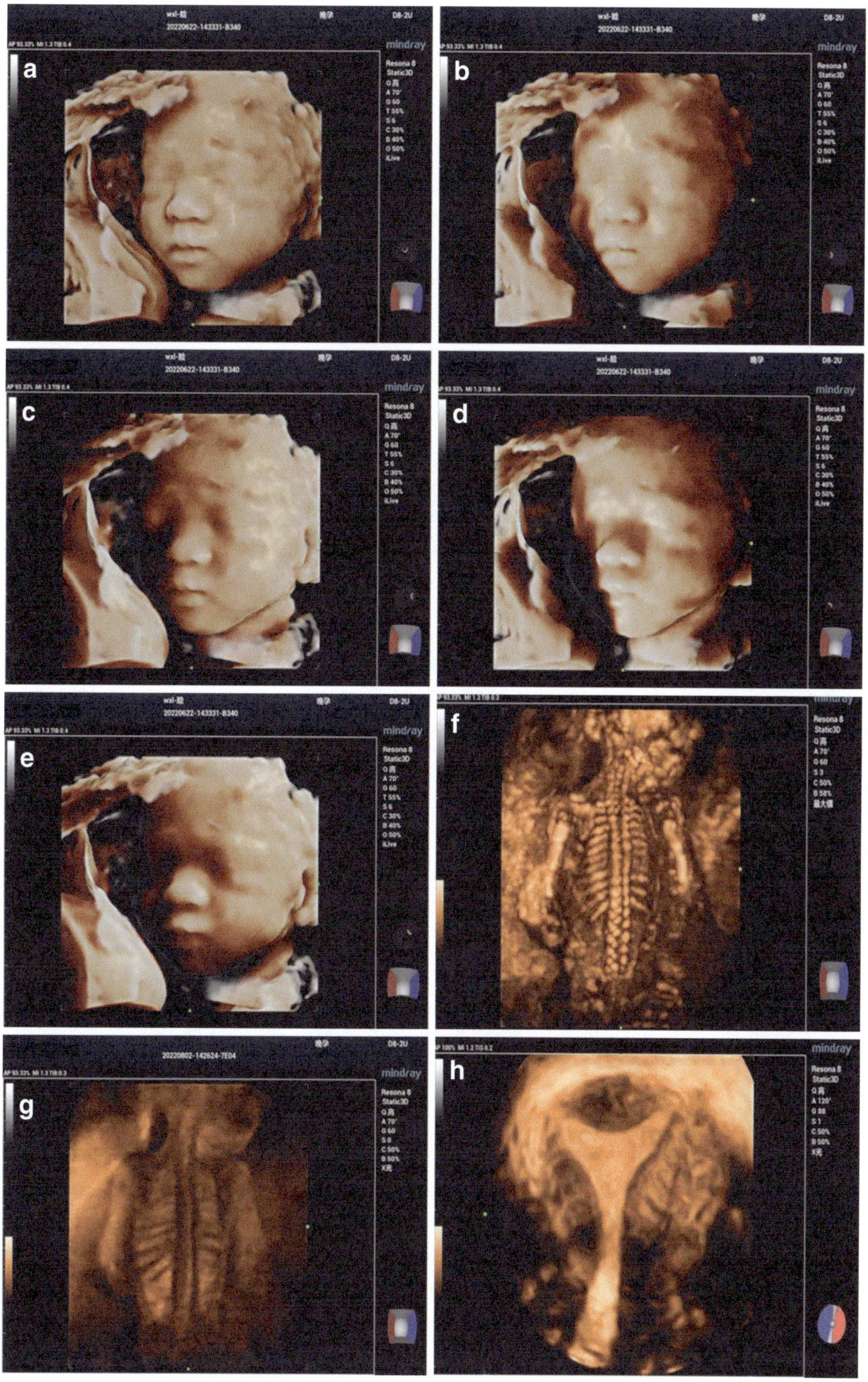
a
b
c
d
e
f
g
h

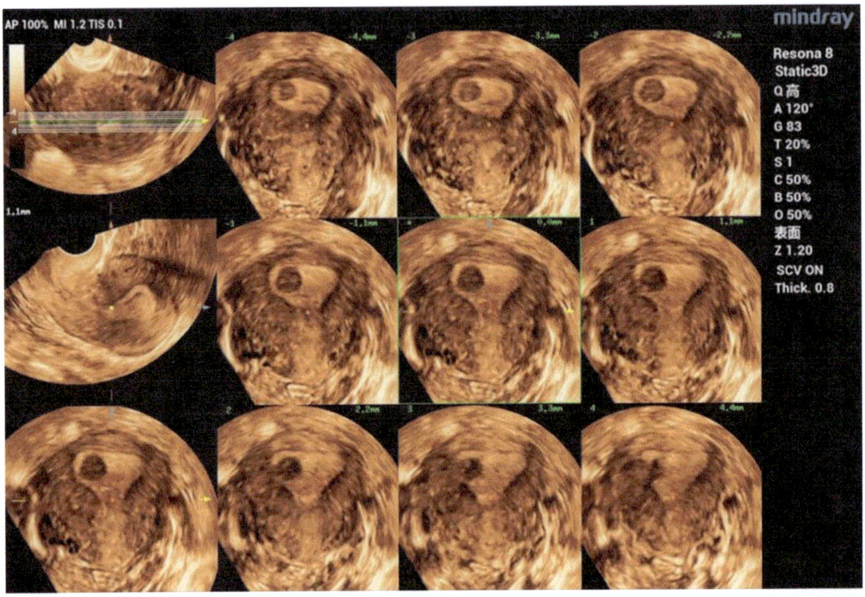

Fig. 2.15 Relationship of the submucosal fibroid to the uterine cavity and myometrium shown in iPage mode

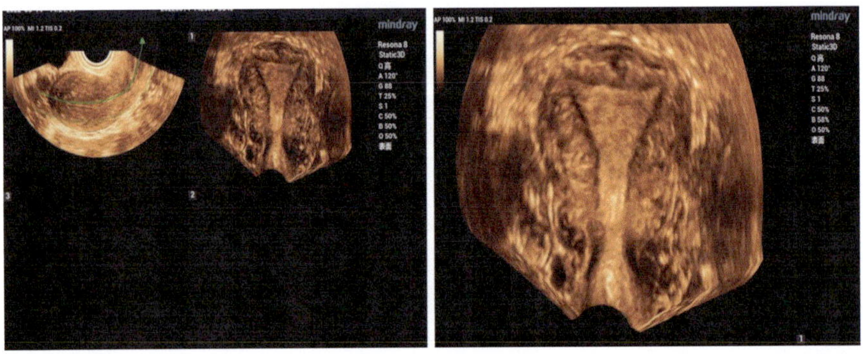

Fig. 2.16 Coronal image of the endometrium displayed in OmniView mode

The OmniView mode offers curved sectioning that allows for customized sectioning, adapting to the shape of the area being observed. For example, when evaluating uterine malformations in a 3D coronal view, an anterior or posterior inclination of the uterus can cause the endometrium to not align in the same plane, hindering the complete visualization of all relevant information (Fig. 2.16). In contrast, the free-cutting feature allows imaging that follows the direction of the endometrium, providing a full coronal view of the entire uterus.

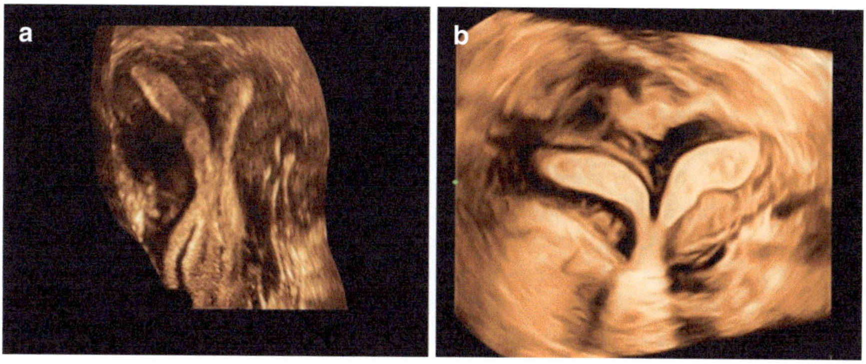

Fig. 2.17 (**a**) A complete septate uterus. (**b**) A bicornuate uterus

2. 3D ultrasound in reproductive medicine
   (a) 3D ultrasound-assisted diagnosis of uterine anomalies

There are several diagnostic techniques available for detecting female genital malformations, including hysteroscopy, laparoscopy, MRI, hysterosalpingography, and ultrasonography. Hysteroscopy and hysterosalpingography are helpful for revealing the morphology of the uterine cavity and endometrium but cannot show the complete contour of the uterus. Additionally, hysteroscopy is invasive, and hysterosalpingography involves radiation exposure, which may have some health risks. While MRI provides high-resolution imaging of soft tissues and superior diagnostic accuracy, it is expensive and only sometimes feasible for routine use. Laparoscopy, though effective for visualizing the uterus, often requires hysteroscopy to fully assess the uterine cavity and endometrium.

Ultrasonography is the most commonly used diagnostic method for uterine malformations in clinical practice (Fig. 2.17). Transvaginal 2D ultrasound can identify certain abnormal developments of the uterus, but it lacks the ability to comprehensively and accurately display the coronal image of the uterus. This limitation increases the risk of misdiagnosis and overlooked details, especially in cases of complex uterine malformations. In contrast, 3D ultrasound provides a more intuitive and stereoscopic view of the uterine contour, the uterine fundus notch, endometrial morphology, and the longitudinal and transverse dimensions of the uterine cavity. Furthermore, 3D ultrasound allows easy switching between multiple planes—sagittal, horizontal, and coronal—improving diagnostic accuracy.

Since 1995 [3], several studies have investigated the accuracy of 3D ultrasound for diagnosing uterine malformations. One study compared the diagnostic accuracy of MRI and 3D ultrasound using the classification system of Müllerian duct anomalies from the American Fertility Society (AFS) (1988). This study showed good concordance between the two methods, with a kappa index of 0.880 (95% CI, 0.769–0.993) [4]. Similarly, Graupera et al. compared MRI and 3D ultrasound using the ESHRE/ESGE classification system for female genital anomalies. Their results indicated high agreement between the two techniques in identifying a normal uterus and differentiating between hemi-uterus (unicornuate uterus), septate uterus, and bicornuate uterus [5].

Kougioumtsidou et al. [6] compared 3D ultrasound with hysteroscopy and laparoscopy for diagnosing uterine malformations using the ESHRE/ESGE classification system. They found that 3D ultrasound exhibited excellent diagnostic accuracy, with sensitivity, specificity, positive predictive value, and negative predictive value for diagnosing septate uterus being 100%, 92.3%, 98%, and 100%, respectively (kappa index 0.950). For bicornuate uterus and hemi-uterus (unicornuate uterus), these values were all 100% (kappa index 1.0). These findings suggest that 3D ultrasound is a reliable and accurate method for diagnosing uterine malformations, making it suitable for routine clinical use.

In practical applications, the use of 3D ultrasound for diagnosing uterine malformations comes with the following tips:

(i) Image Quality and Acquisition:

The acquisition of high-quality 2D images is the cornerstone of obtaining accurate 3D images. Therefore, ensuring clear 2D images is essential for producing precise 3D results. To improve image quality, the examination should ideally be conducted during the proliferative phase of the endometrium. This phase provides better contrast between the endometrium and the myometrium, aiding in clearer visualization. For uteruses that are over-flexed or positioned horizontally, the position can be adjusted by applying gentle pressure, improving the ability to acquire accurate 3D images. In terms of ultrasound technique, transvaginal ultrasound generally provides superior image resolution and clearer 3D images compared to transabdominal ultrasound. Additionally, transrectal ultrasound can be an effective alternative for improving diagnostic accuracy in women who have not yet been sexually active.

(ii) Optimizing 3D Imaging Display:

Enhancing the display settings of the 3D ultrasound system can further improve the clarity of the images. For example, the free-cutting mode allows for arbitrary slicing of the 3D data, making it easier to visualize the uterus in different planes. This mode reduces the likelihood of diagnostic errors that may arise when the uterus is not aligned in the same plane as the cervix, such as in cases where the uterus is flexed or tilted.

(b) 3D ultrasound-assisted diagnosis of polycystic ovaries

Polycystic ovary syndrome (PCOS) is a condition characterized by hyperandrogenemia, ovulatory dysfunction, and polycystic ovaries, affecting approximately 8%–13% of women of reproductive age [7]; the National Institutes of Health (NIH) criteria from 1990 were widely used to diagnose PCOS. However, it was not until 2003 that the European Society of Human Reproduction and Embryology (ESHRE) and the American Society for

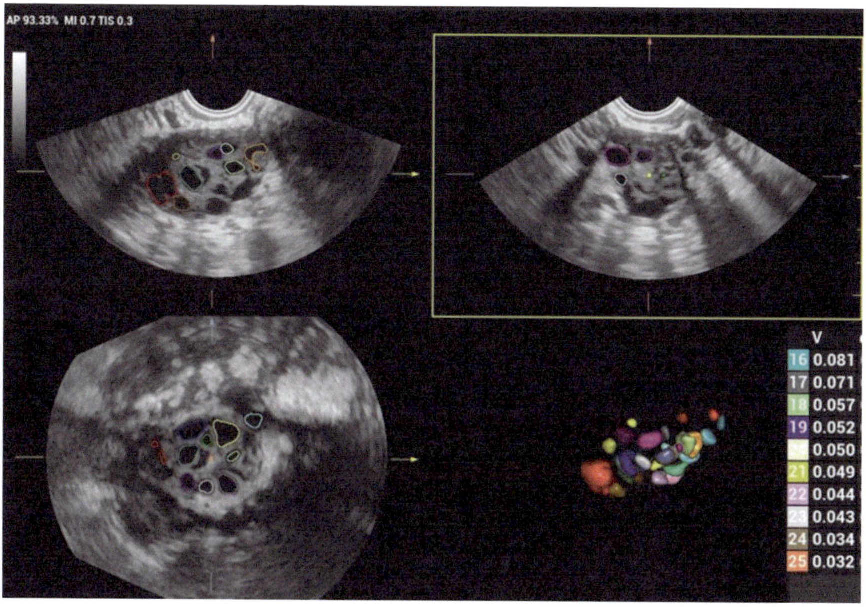

Fig. 2.18 Automatic measurement of follicle counts and follicle diameters in the ovary with the Smart FLC function of a 3D ultrasonography system

Reproductive Medicine (ASRM) expanded the diagnostic criteria to include imaging evaluation of the ovaries [8].

Ultrasonography has long been the primary tool for evaluating polycystic ovarian morphology (PCOM). However, determining the presence of polycystic ovaries through 2D ultrasound is inherently subjective. In contrast, 3D ultrasound provides more accurate and objective assessments by offering automatic measurement and quantification of the number and mean diameter of antral follicles and the ovarian volume (Fig. 2.18). This technology can enhance the evaluation of the ovaries, allowing for more precise measurements compared to traditional 2D methods.

Furthermore, when combined with power Doppler, 3D ultrasound allows for the quantification of ovarian blood flow indices, such as the vascularization index, blood flow index, and vascular blood flow index of the ovarian interstitial arteries. These indices provide additional insight into ovarian health and can aid in better understanding the vascularization of polycystic ovaries [9–11].

Despite these advantages, some studies have suggested that 3D ultrasonography may overestimate or underestimate the number of antral follicles compared with 2D ultrasound. This discrepancy is likely due to the lack of a universally accepted standard for measuring relevant parameters by ultrasound [12]. As a result, while 3D ultrasounds show promising diagnoses of PCOS, further research is needed to standardize techniques and improve the accuracy of these measurements.

(c) Endometrial receptivity

Embryo implantation is the most critical step in achieving a successful pregnancy, representing a complex process of embryo-endometrial interaction. According to the literature, embryo quality issues account for one-third of implantation failures, while suboptimal endometrial receptivity (ER) and altered embryo-endometrial responses account for the remaining two-thirds [13]. ER refers to the ability of the endometrium to support the localization, adhesion, invasion, and, ultimately, embryo implantation. Successful implantation and pregnancy are only possible when the embryo encounters a receptive endometrium. The "window of implantation" (WOI) is defined as the optimal period when the endometrium is sufficiently receptive to allow the implantation of the blastocyst and subsequent pregnancy. This window typically occurs between day 20 and day 24 of a normal menstrual cycle [14].

Endometrial biopsy and ultrasonography are commonly used to assess ER. Endometrial biopsy specimens can be evaluated for morphological features, molecular markers, and proteomic profiles. However, as an invasive procedure that does not provide real-time results, the clinical application of endometrial biopsy is limited. In contrast, ultrasonography is the most commonly used noninvasive method for assessing ER, offering real-time evaluation.

Ultrasonographic evaluation of ER is primarily based on the assessment of the endometrial morphological profile (thickness, volume, and type of endometrium), endometrial blood flow profile (including uterine artery and spiral artery blood flow indices), and endometrial peristalsis. Three-dimensional ultrasound allows for more accurate measurements of endometrial volume and, when combined with power Doppler, provides visualization of blood flow patterns and vascularization within the endometrium. Several studies have investigated the utility of 3D ultrasound in assessing ER [15–17]. However, despite its advantages, the assessment of ER by ultrasound still suffers from low specificity (though high sensitivity) and poor predictive value. Moreover, there is a lack of large, randomized controlled trials to validate its efficacy, and no standardized scoring system for evaluating ER exists. The details and significance of ultrasound-based ER assessment will be covered in Chap. 6.

(d) Application of 3D ultrasound in the diagnosis of other gynecological diseases

Since the introduction of 3D ultrasonography, the ability to obtain the coronal plane of the uterus has provided valuable additional information for the diagnosis of various gynecological diseases [18]. Uterine conditions such as submucosal fibroids, endometrial polyps, and uterine adhesions can impede embryo implantation, potentially leading to infertility. The coronal plane view offered by 3D ultrasound allows clinicians to assess the extent of fibroid protrusion into the uterine cavity, as well as the size, number, and location of endometrial polyps and intrauterine adhesions, all of which are crucial for

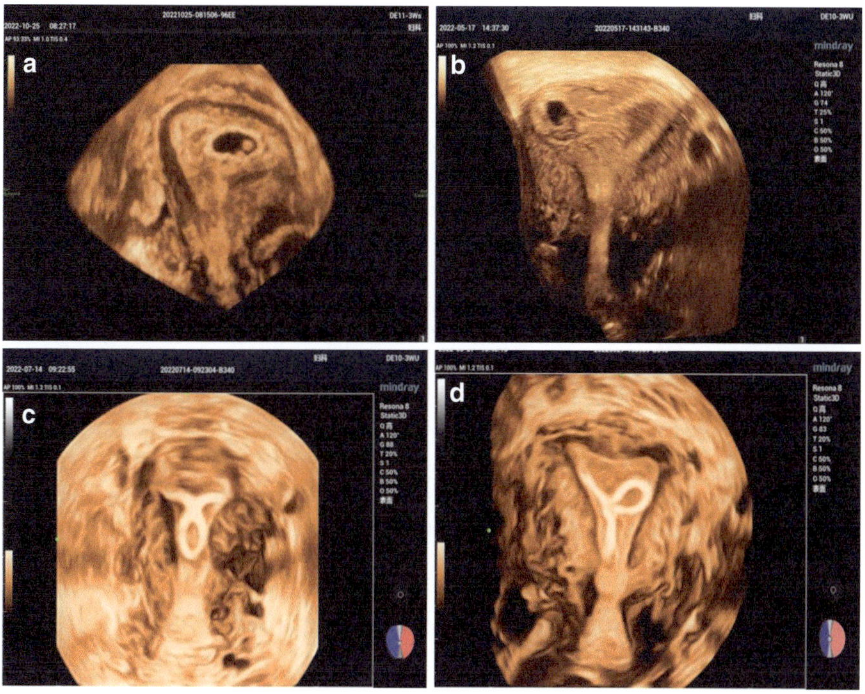

Fig. 2.19 (**a**) Normal early pregnancy. (**b**) A gestational sac in the uterine horn (indicated by the arrow). (**c**) An IUD in a normal position. (**d**) An IUD has rotated within the uterine cavity

planning hysteroscopic surgery [19]. This detailed preoperative assessment provides essential diagnostic information for clinical management.

Three-dimensional ultrasonography is also valuable in early pregnancy, particularly in determining the location of the gestational sac, and it aids in identifying cornual and interstitial pregnancies [20]. Additionally, 3D ultrasound is instrumental in evaluating the morphology and position of intrauterine devices (IUDs), helping to determine whether the IUD is displaced, embedded, or deeply embedded within the uterine myometrium [21, 22] (Fig. 2.19).

The uterine junctional zone (JZ) is the area connecting the myometrium and the endometrium, first described by Hricak et al. in 1983 [23]. Both the JZ and the endometrium originate from the Müllerian duct during embryonic development, whereas the outer myometrium is derived from the mesenchyme. This results in distinct histologic characteristics of the JZ compared to the outer myometrium [24]. On MRI T2-weighted imaging, the JZ often appears as a low-signal, band-like region located between the high-signal endometrium and medium-signal myometrium [25].

The JZ expresses both estrogen and progesterone receptors, and, like the endometrium, its thickness undergoes cyclic changes influenced by hormonal fluctuations [24]. The normal thickness of the JZ ranges from 5 to 8 mm, with a thickened JZ being associated with infertility and miscarriage, as reported in the literature [26–28]. Uterine contractions originate from the JZ, and altered peristaltic contractions in the JZ may lead to reproductive abnormalities and adverse pregnancy outcomes [29, 30].

The primary imaging methods used to assess the JZ are MRI and 3D ultrasonography. While MRI remains the gold standard for JZ evaluation, JZ measurement in the coronal plane using 3D ultrasound has demonstrated good interobserver and intraobserver consistency [31]. Several studies have measured JZ thickness in the coronal plane using 3D ultrasound, suggesting that altered JZ thickness is linked to recurrent miscarriage and can help to predict the outcomes of assisted reproductive technologies (ARTs) such as artificial fertilization [29, 32, 33]. However, there needs to be standardized criteria for acquiring the coronal plane to measure JZ in 3D ultrasound, as well as uncertainty about the optimal timing for measurement and the most reliable measurement method. Further research is needed to address these issues.

2.2.4 Contrast Agents and Ultrasound Imaging Techniques

Due to blood's low reflectivity to ultrasound signals, conventional Doppler ultrasound often yields suboptimal image quality when detecting deep vessels or low-velocity blood flow within lesions. In response to such issues, the contrast-enhanced ultrasound (CEUS) technique has been developed to improve diagnostic accuracy. CEUS involves the injection of an ultrasound contrast agent (UCA), which enhances the detection of blood perfusion in tissues, allowing for more precise visualization of the delicate vascular structures in both normal and diseased tissues.

1. The principle of contrast-enhanced ultrasound

   The physical basis of contrast-enhanced ultrasound lies in the acquisition of contrast-enhanced images by utilizing the nonlinear effects and strong backscattering of ultrasound contrast agents within the blood when exposed to ultrasound waves in the acoustic field.
2. Commonly used UCAs

   An ideal UCA should possess several favorable attributes: size and properties similar to those of human red blood cells, biological inertness, no interference with human hemodynamics, and stable passage through the pulmonary circulation after intravenous injection. UCAs consist of two main components: a gaseous core and an outer shell. Based on the type of core and shell, UCAs are classified into three generations: the first generation has an air-based core, the second generation has an inert gas core, and the third generation is still under development. Below are a few examples of commonly used UCAs:

(a) Levovist

Levovist (Schering AG, Berlin, Germany) is a sugar-based Doppler signal-enhancing agent composed of 99.9% D-galactose and 0.1% palmitic acid. When mixed with water, it produces microbubbles. More than 99% of these microbubbles are less than 8 μm in diameter (average 1–3 μm), enabling them to circulate through the body via the pulmonary circulation and enhance the echogenic intensity of blood flow signals in 2D images [34].

(b) Optison

Optison (GE Healthcare) is a second-generation contrast agent developed by Molecular Biosystems. It consists of perflutren-containing microspheres made from heat-treated human albumin. Optison (suspension) is available at a concentration of (5–8) × 10^8 microspheres/mL, with the diameter of these microspheres ranging from 3.0 to 4.5 μm [35]. It is used for left ventricular visualization as well as for myocardial perfusion assessment following intravenous injection [36].

(c) Definity

Definity (North Billerica, MA, USA) is a second-generation contrast agent with an octafluoropropane core encapsulated in a phospholipid shell that requires activation by mechanical vibration before use. Like Optison, it is FDA-approved for left heart visualization and is also approved for liver and kidney visualization in Canada and Australia [35].

(d) Sonovue

Sonovue (Bracco, Italy) is a second-generation UCA approved for marketing in most countries worldwide. It contains an inert sulfur hexafluoride core, providing excellent ultrasonic enhancement, and has a single-layer phospholipid shell that offers good stability. Sonovue microspheres, with an average diameter of 2.5 μm, act as blood pool imaging enhancers and do not penetrate into tissues [35]. Sonovue is widely used in China for hysterosalpingo-contrast sonography and contrast-enhanced ultrasonography of veins in gynecology [37, 38].

(e) Sonazoid

Sonazoid (GE Healthcare) microspheres range in diameter from 2 to 3 μm and have a perfluoro-n-butane (PFB) core encapsulated in a phospholipid shell. Sonazoid is more stable than Sonovue and can accumulate in the reticuloendothelial system, such as the liver and spleen—a feature associated with phagocytosis by Kupffer cells in the liver parenchyma [39, 40].

3. Contrast-enhanced ultrasonography in gynecology

(a) Hyterosalpingo-contrast-sonography (HyCoSy)

Tubal factor infertility is the most common cause of female infertility, accounting for 25%–35% of all cases [41]. The patency of the fallopian tubes can be evaluated through hysterosalpingography (HSG), hysterosalpingo-contrast sonography (HyCoSy), and laparoscopic chromoendoscopy, with HyCoSy being the first-line examination for assessing fallopian tube patency [42]. Compared to HSG, HyCoSy offers several advantages: it is free of ionizing radiation, suitable for individuals with iodine allergies, and provides higher sensitivity and specificity. However, the accuracy of HyCoSy depends on the skill of the ultrasonographer, which limits its widespread application and requires further discussion. The details of the HyCoSy examination are covered in Chap. 5.

(b) Intravenous contrast-enhanced ultrasonography in gynecology

The intralesional perfusion profile is crucial for the diagnosis and differential diagnosis of gynecologic diseases. However, the commonly used color Doppler technique has low sensitivity in detecting low-velocity or small intralesional blood flows, limiting its application.

Contrast-enhanced ultrasonography (CEUS) of the veins is widely used in gynecology for preoperative diagnosis and differential diagnosis of gynecologic conditions, such as preoperative endometrial or cervical cancer staging and the differential diagnosis of ovarian tumors. It is also valuable for evaluating the effects of nonsurgical treatments, such as assessing interventional therapies for uterine fibroids or uterine adenomyosis [38, 43–46].

Although there are no established diagnostic criteria for intravenous contrast-enhanced ultrasonography in gynecology and a lack of data from multicenter, large-sample studies, the development and integration of molecular biology techniques and ultrasound contrast agents are expected to enhance its role in gynecology in the future.

References

1. Watkin KL. Ultrasound and swallowing. Folia Phoniatr Logop. 1999;51(4–5):183–98.
2. Ren W, Ma C. Basic and clinical application spectrum of ultrasound diagnosis. Chemical Industry Press; 2020.
3. Jurkovic D, Geipel A, Gruboeck K, et al. Three-dimensional ultrasound for the assessment of uterine anatomy and detection of congenital anomalies: a comparison with hysterosalpingography and two-dimensional sonography. Ultrasound Obstet Gynecol. 1995;5(4):233–7.
4. Bermejo C, Martínez TP, Cantarero R, et al. Three-dimensional ultrasound in the diagnosis of Müllerian duct anomalies and concordance with magnetic resonance imaging. Ultrasound Obstet Gynecol. 2010;35(5):593–601.
5. Graupera B, Pascual MA, Hereter L, et al. Accuracy of three-dimensional ultrasound compared with magnetic resonance imaging in diagnosis of Mullerian duct anomalies using ESHRE–ESGE consensus on the classification of congenital anomalies of the female genital tract. Ultrasound Obstet Gynecol. 2015;46(5):616–22.
6. Kougioumtsidou A, Mikos T, Grimbizis GF, et al. Three-dimensional ultrasound in the diagnosis and the classification of congenital uterine anomalies using the ESHRE/ESGE classification: a diagnostic accuracy study. Arch Gynecol Obstet. 2019;299(3):779–89.
7. Teede HJ, Misso ML, Costello MF, et al. Recommendations from the international evidence-based guideline for the assessment and management of polycystic ovary syndrome. Hum Reprod. 2018;33(9):1602–18.
8. Rotterdam ESHRE/ASRM-Sponsored PCOS Consensus Workshop Group. Revised 2003 consensus on diagnostic criteria and long-term health risks related to polycystic ovary syndrome (PCOS). Hum Reprod. 2004;19(1):41–7.

9. Sujata K, Swoyam S. 2D and 3D trans-vaginal sonography to determine cut-offs for ovarian volume and follicle number per ovary for diagnosis of polycystic ovary syndrome in Indian women. J Reprod Infertil. 2018;19(3):146–51.
10. Garg N, Khaira HK, Kaur M, et al. A comparative study on quantitative assessment of blood flow and vascularization in polycystic ovary syndrome patients and normal women using three-dimensional power Doppler ultrasonography. J Obstet Gynaecol India. 2018;68(2):136–41.
11. Bozkurt M, Bozkurt DK, Kurban D, et al. 2-D and 3-D ultrasonographic characteristics of the ovary in women with PCOS and multifollicular ovaries. J Obstet Gynaecol. 2021;41(6):920–6.
12. Brink HV, Pisch AJ, Lujan ME. A comparison of two- and three-dimensional ultrasonographic methods for evaluation of ovarian follicle counts and classification of polycystic ovarian morphology. Fertil Steril. 2021;115(3):761–70.
13. Craciunas L, Gallos I, Chu J, et al. Conventional and modern markers of endometrial receptivity: a systematic review and meta-analysis. Hum Reprod Update. 2019;25(2):202–23.
14. Bergh PA, Navot D. The impact of embryonic development and endometrial maturity on the timing of implantation. Fertil Steril. 1992;58(3):537–42.
15. Tong R, Zhou Y, He Q, et al. Analysis of the guidance value of 3D ultrasound in evaluating endometrial receptivity for frozen-thawed embryo transfer in patients with repeated implantation failure. Ann Transl Med. 2020;8(15):944.
16. Elsokkary M, Eldin AB, Abdelhafez M, et al. The reproducibility of the novel utilization of five-dimensional ultrasound and power Doppler in the prediction of endometrial receptivity in intracytoplasmic sperm-injected women: a pilot prospective clinical study. Arch Gynecol Obstet. 2019;299(2):551–8.
17. Sini I, Handayani N, Harahap A, et al. Role of three-dimensional Doppler ultrasonography and leukemia inhibitory factor from endometrial secretion in predicting endometrial receptivity in IVF treatment: a pilot study. Arch Gynecol Obstet. 2022;306(1):259–65.
18. Grigore M, Popovici R, Himiniuc LM, et al. The added value of three-dimensional ultrasonography in uterine pathology. Exp Ther Med. 2021;22(5):1261.
19. Jiang X, Chen X, Li J, et al. Clinical application of three-dimensional transvaginal ultrasonography in the diagnosis of intrauterine adhesions. J Int Med Res. 2021;49(11):3000605211024520.
20. Durand YG, Capoccia-Brugger R, Vial Y, et al. Diagnostic dilemma between angular and interstitial ectopic pregnancy: 3D ultrasound features. J Ultrasound. 2022;25(4):989–94.
21. Graupera B, Hereter L, Pascual MA, et al. Normal and abnormal images of intrauterine devices: role of three-dimensional sonography. J Clin Ultrasound. 2012;40(7):433–8.
22. Andrade CM, Araujo JE, Torloni MR, et al. Three-dimensional versus two-dimensional ultrasound for assessing levonorgestrel intrauterine device location: a pilot study. J Clin Ultrasound. 2016;44(2):72–7.
23. Hricak H, Alpers C, Crooks LE, et al. Magnetic resonance imaging of the female pelvis: initial experience. AJR Am J Roentgenol. 1983;141(6):1119–28.
24. Tanos V, Lingwood L, Balami S. The importance of the junctional zone of the endometrium in human reproduction. Hum Fertil (Camb). 2022;25(1):4–12.
25. Imaoka I, Nakatsuka T, Araki T, et al. T2* relaxometry mapping of the uterine zones. Acta Radiol. 2012;53(4):473–7.
26. Fusi L, Cloke B, Brosens JJ. The uterine junctional zone. Best Pract Res Clin Obstet Gynaecol. 2006;20(4):479–91.
27. Kunz G, Beil D. Characterization of the uterine junctional zone prior to IVF/ICSI: an observational study. Arch Gynecol Obstet. 2010;281(5):945–53.
28. Meylaerts LJ, Wijnen L, Ombelet W, et al. Uterine junctional zone thickness in infertile women evaluated by MRI. J Magn Reson Imaging. 2017;45(3):926–36.
29. Lazzarin N, Exacoustos C, Vaquero E, et al. Uterine junctional zone at three-dimensional transvaginal ultrasonography in patients with recurrent miscarriage: a new diagnostic tool? Eur J Obstet Gynecol Reprod Biol. 2014;174:128–32.
30. Kim A, Young Lee J, Ji Y, et al. Do endometrial movements affect the achievement of pregnancy during intrauterine insemination? Int J Fertil Steril. 2015;8(4):399–408.

31. Rasmussen CK, Glavind J, Madsen LD, et al. Repeatability of junctional zone measurements using 3-dimensional transvaginal sonography in healthy fertile women. J Ultrasound Med. 2016;35(7):1497–508.
32. Maged AM, Ramzy AM, Ghar MA, et al. 3D ultrasound assessment of endometrial junctional zone anatomy as a predictor of the outcome of ICSI cycles. Eur J Obstet Gynecol Reprod Biol. 2017;212:160–5.
33. Liu Y, Wang L, Wang M, et al. A study on the prediction of reproductive outcomes in frozen embryo transfer cycles by calculating the volume of uterine junctional zone with three-dimensional ultrasound. Ultraschall Med. 2023;44(2):e126–35.
34. Choi BI, Kim AY, Lee JY, et al. Hepatocellular carcinoma: contrast enhancement with Levovist. J Ultrasound Med. 2002;21(1):77–84.
35. Frinking P, Segers T, Luan Y, et al. Three decades of ultrasound contrast agents: a review of the past, present and future improvements. Ultrasound Med Biol. 2020;46(4):892–908.
36. Zhao H, O'Quinn R, Ambrose M, et al. Contrast-enhanced echocardiography has the greatest impact in patients with reduced ejection fractions. J Am Soc Echocardiogr. 2018;31(3):289–96.
37. Wang S. Clinical application and progress of hysterosalpingo-contrast sonography. Chin J Med Ultrasound. 2020;17(2):100–2.
38. Yuan K, Huang YJ, Mao MY, et al. Contrast-enhanced US to improve diagnostic performance of O-RADS US risk stratification system for malignancy. Radiology. 2023;308(2):e223003.
39. Kotopoulis S, Popa M, Mayoral SM, et al. SonoVue® vs. Sonazoid™ vs. Optison™: which bubble is best for low-intensity sonoporation of pancreatic ductal adenocarcinoma? Pharmaceutics. 2022;14(1):98.
40. Sontum PC. Physicochemical characteristics of Sonazoid™, a new contrast agent for ultrasound imaging. Ultrasound Med Biol. 2008;34:824–33.
41. Honoré GM, Holden AE, Schenken RS. Pathophysiology and management of proximal tubal blockage. Fertil Steril. 1999;71(5):785–95.
42. Zamah AM, Power R, Longman RE, et al. Ultrasound and infertility. In: First-trimester ultrasound. Cham: Springer; 2023.
43. Geng J, Tang J. Contrast-enhanced ultrasound in the diagnosis of endometrial carcinoma: a meta-analysis. Exp Ther Med. 2018;16(6):5310–4.
44. Zhang J, Xiang JD, Jia C, et al. Contrast-enhanced ultrasonography for transabdominal and transrectal ultrasound in staging cervical cancer: a reliability study. Ultrasound Med Biol. 2023;49(10):2283–90.
45. Xu C, Tang Y, Zhao Y, et al. Use of contrast-enhanced ultrasound in evaluating the efficacy and application value of microwave ablation for adenomyosis. J Cancer Res Ther. 2020;16(2):365–71.
46. Zhang M, Yin C, Jiang J, et al. Application value of contrast-enhanced ultrasonography in the treatment of uterine fibroids by high-intensity focused ultrasound ablation: a retrospective study. J Clin Ultrasound. 2023;51(1):113–20.

Standardized Protocol for Transvaginal Ultrasound of the Uterus and Adnexa

3

Da Li and Na Zuo

Gynecologic ultrasound examinations can be classified based on the scanning approach into transabdominal, transvaginal, transrectal, and transperineal ultrasounds.

1. Transabdominal ultrasound requires the patient to have a full bladder, which acts as an acoustic window, improving visualization of pelvic structures. However, the image quality may be compromised by subcutaneous fat or intestinal gas. This approach is primarily indicated for patients who are not sexually active, those with vaginal anomalies, or as a complement to transvaginal ultrasound in cases where a broader field of view is needed.
2. Transvaginal ultrasound involves the use of an endoluminal probe inserted into the patient's vagina, providing detailed, high-resolution images of pelvic organs due to the proximity of the probe to the structures being examined. It is the modality of choice for routine gynecologic evaluations in reproductive medicine clinics.
3. Transrectal ultrasound is reserved for cases where transvaginal ultrasound is contraindicated or when transabdominal imaging is inconclusive. Although effective, it is infrequently used in clinical practice.
4. Transperineal ultrasound serves as an alternative approach, particularly for prepubertal patients and older women with conditions such as pelvic organ prolapse.

This chapter focuses on the standardized approach to transvaginal gynecologic ultrasound, a cornerstone diagnostic tool in reproductive medicine.

D. Li (✉) · N. Zuo
Shengjing Hospital of China Medical University, Shenyang, China
e-mail: zuon@sj-hospital.org

D. Li et al. (eds.), *Ultrasonography of the Female Reproductive System*,
https://doi.org/10.1007/978-981-95-1373-4_3

3.1 Preparation and Precautions Before Transvaginal Ultrasound Examination

3.1.1 Patient Selection

Transvaginal gynecologic ultrasound is typically performed on females with a history of sexual activity, as it involves the insertion of a probe into the vaginal canal. Most patients seen in fertility clinics fall into this category, as they are generally sexually active.

However, there are instances where the procedure may be considered for patients who are nonsexually active, such as adolescents or women with unique circumstances. In such cases, ensuring the patient is fully informed about the procedure is crucial. Explicit informed consent must be obtained before proceeding. This is especially important when considering transvaginal ultrasound for women with atypical sexual histories, such as those whose male partners have erectile dysfunction or other conditions affecting sexual activity. Comprehensive counseling should precede the procedure to ensure the patient's comfort and understanding.

3.1.2 Patient Positioning and Precautions

During the examination, the patient should be positioned in the lithotomy position to facilitate optimal access and imaging. A small cushion or the patient's clenched fists may be placed under the hips for added comfort and better visualization. Conducting the transvaginal ultrasound on a gynecologic examination table enables easier manipulation of the transducer and improved visualization from multiple angles.

Privacy is a critical consideration during the procedure. The ultrasound examination should be performed in a secure, private setting to protect the patient's dignity and comfort.

3.1.3 Preparations Before the Ultrasound Scan

1. Equipment setup

The ultrasound machine should be preconfigured before the examination. Settings should aim to minimize ultrasound energy exposure while ensuring diagnostic accuracy. During the scan, the sonographer should adjust key parameters such as scanning depth, gain, and focus based on the real-time images. Enhanced detail can be achieved by using the local zoom function as necessary.

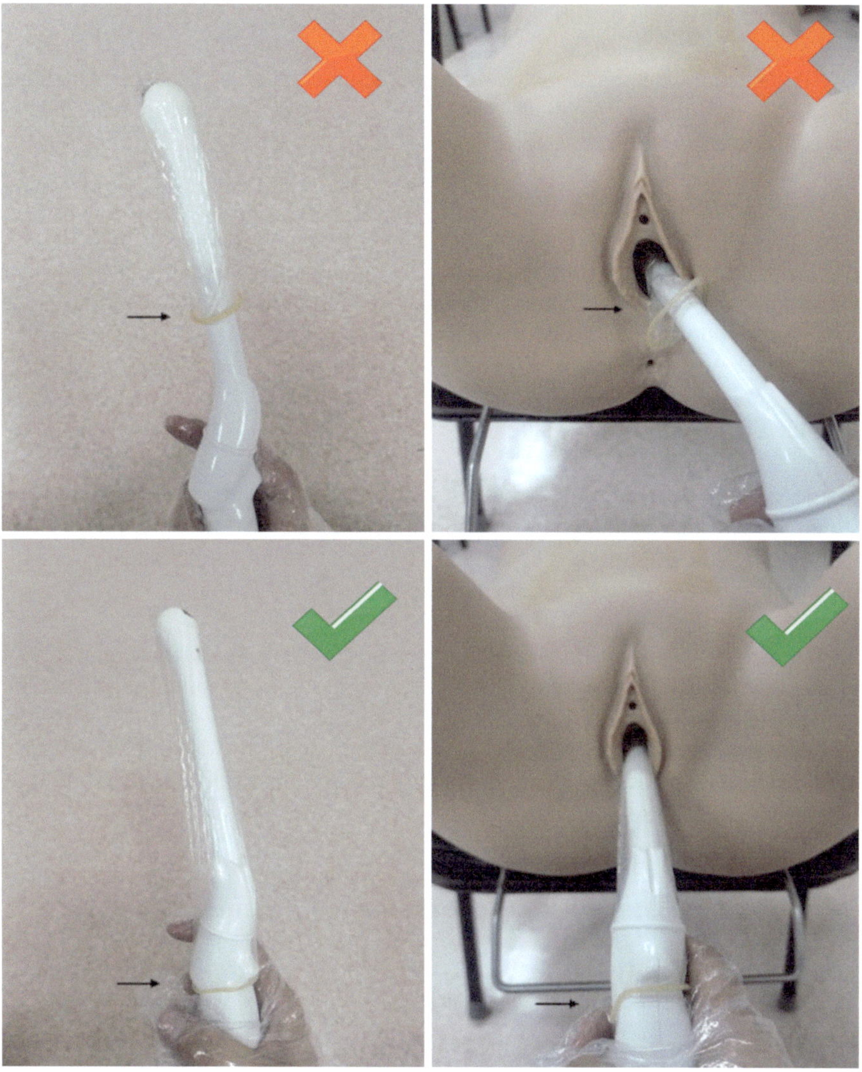

Fig. 3.1 How to apply the transducer cover?

2. Standardized protocol

At our hospital, the following standardized protocol is implemented for transvaginal ultrasound: (a) The sonographer must wear disposable gloves. (b) A single-use drape should be placed on the examination table. (c) One or two disposable covers are applied to the transducer. In cases of menstruation or vaginal bleeding, two covers are used with coupling gel placed between them to prevent leakage. (d) The transducer cover must extend down to the handle to prevent cross-contamination from contact with the patient's vulva during the scan (as illustrated in Fig. 3.1).

3. Patient safety and comfort

All preparatory actions, including equipment setup and transducer handling, should be performed within the patient's view to reassure them and alleviate potential concerns about safety or hygiene.

4. Hygiene and sterilization

Ultrasound probes must undergo regular cleaning and sterilization as per established infection control guidelines. Ensuring proper hygiene protocols reduces the risk of cross-contamination and maintains patient safety.

3.1.4 Storage of Images

Standard views of all relevant pelvic organs should be systematically captured and stored during the examination. Additionally, high-quality positive images and motion clips highlighting key findings should be saved in the ultrasound workstation. Image storage serves multiple purposes:

1. Clinical utility: Stored images allow for postprocessing, detailed review, and comparison with the patient's prior records, aiding in ongoing diagnostic and treatment decisions.
2. Legal documentation: Retaining documented images provides critical evidence in medical disputes, underscoring the importance of meticulous image storage as part of clinical best practices.

3.2 Normal Uterine Images and Measurements

3.2.1 Cervix

The midsagittal plane of the cervix is visualized by advancing the ultrasound probe to the apex of the vaginal canal. The cervix comprises anterior and posterior lips, with the cervical canal spindle-shaped in this view. When mucus is present within the canal, it typically appears as an anechoic (echo-free) region.

When assessing the cervix, its relationship to the uterus and the upper segment of the vagina should be carefully examined. It is also essential to screen for any space-occupying lesions or abnormalities.

Three key cervical dimensions should be recorded during the examination:

1. Longitudinal cervical diameter: Measured from the internal os (internal cervical orifice) to the external os (external cervical orifice). The normal range is 2.5 cm–3 cm.

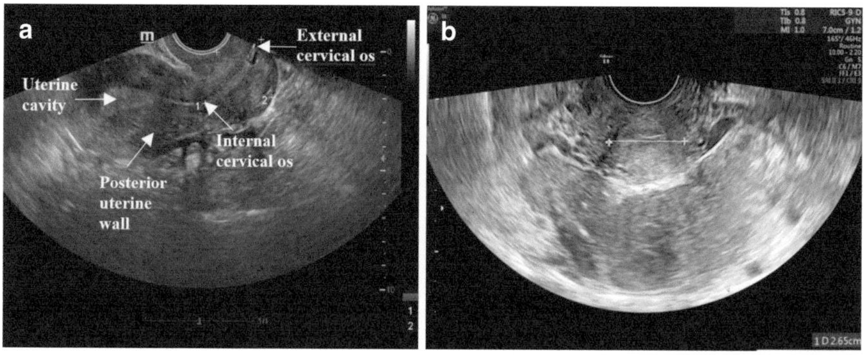

Fig. 3.2 (**a**) The longitudinal and anteroposterior diameter of the cervix. (**b**) The transverse diameter of the cervix

2. Anteroposterior cervical diameter: The maximum distance from the anterior to the posterior aspect of the cervix, measured perpendicular to the longitudinal cervical axis.
3. Transverse cervical diameter: The maximum width of the cervix in the transverse plane.

These measurements help establish normal cervical anatomy and detect deviations that may indicate pathology (Fig. 3.2).

3.2.2 Corpus Uteri (Body of the Uterus)

1. Determining the position of the uterus

   During transvaginal ultrasound, the uterus should be evaluated for its contour, the homogeneity of the myometrium, and the presence of any space-occupying lesions. The uterine position is typically categorized as anteverted, anteverted + anteflexed, retroverted, or retroverted + retroflexed.

   (a) Anteverted vs. retroverted positions:

   Anteverted uterus: The uterus's longitudinal axis is tilted forward, lying anterior to the body's longitudinal axis. On ultrasound, the uterine fundus points toward the bladder (Fig. 3.3a).

   Retroverted uterus: The longitudinal axis of the uterus is tilted backward, lying posterior to the body's longitudinal axis. On ultrasound, the fundus points toward the rectum (Fig. 3.3b).

   (b) Anteflexed vs. retroflexed positions:

   Anteflexed uterus: The angle between the longitudinal axis of the uterus and the cervix is forward-facing (Fig. 3.3c).

   Retroflexed uterus: The angle between the longitudinal axis of the uterus and the cervix is backward-facing (Fig. 3.3d).

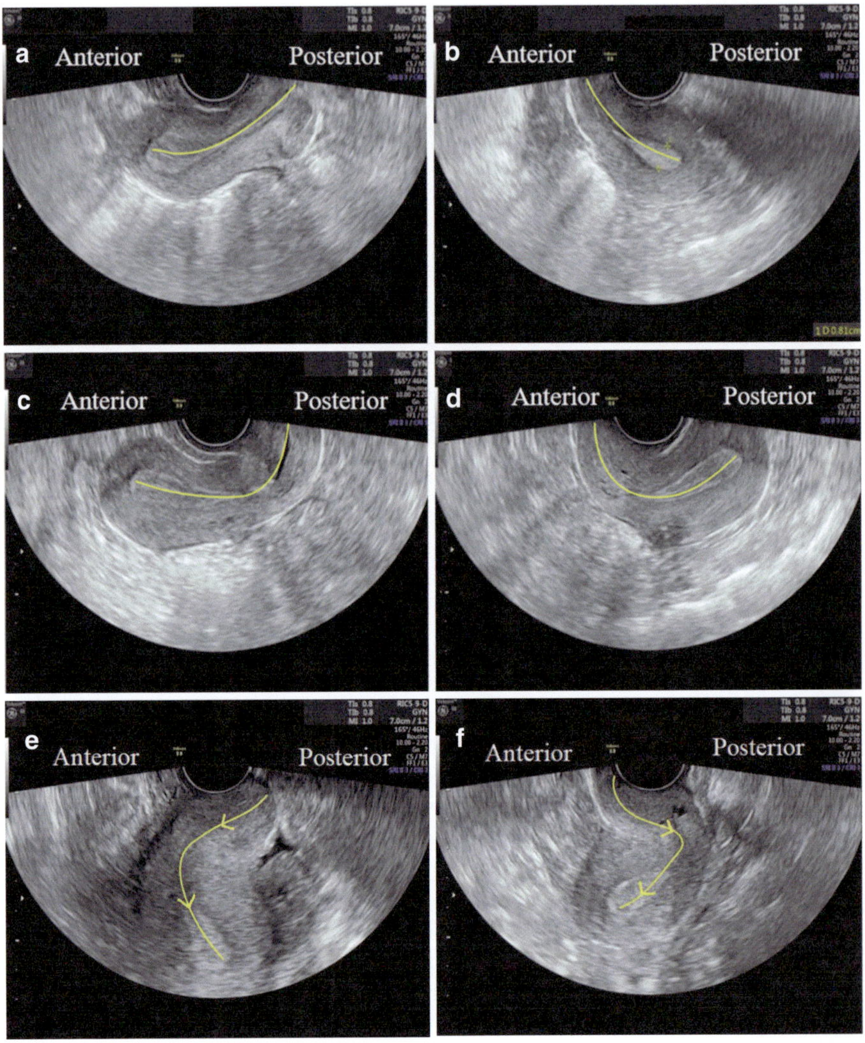

Fig. 3.3 (**a**) An anteverted uterus. (**b**) A retroverted uterus. (**c**) An anteverted and anteflexed uterus. (**d**) A retroverted and retroflexed uterus. (**e**) An anteverted and retroflexed uterus. (**f**) A retroverted and anteflexed uterus

(c) Other, less common uterine positions, while rarely discussed, can significantly impact intrauterine procedures and surgical operations in reproductive medicine. These include the following:
   1. The cervix is angled to the left anteriorly, with the uterine fundus angled posteriorly at a right angle to the cervix (observed in 4.8% of the population). This positioning is depicted in Fig. 3.3e.

   2. The cervix is angled to the right in a retroverted axis, while the uterine body is angled to the left (the rarest position, observed in 0.3% of the population). This positioning is shown in Fig. 3.3f [1].

      A distorted uterine shape or atypical positioning may complicate intrauterine procedures such as placement of a contrast catheter during hysterosalpingography, embryo transfer using a transfer tube, hysteroscopy, or instrument manipulation during abortion procedures.

      These challenges can increase the duration of the procedure and the risk of adjacent tissue injury. To minimize complications, clinicians must thoroughly understand the anatomical characteristics of the uterus and the alignment of the cervical canal and uterine cavity before and during such operations. This understanding is critical for reducing operation time and avoiding inadvertent injuries.

2. Three diameters used for uterine body measurements
   (a) Longitudinal diameter:

      This is the distance from the serosal layer of the uterine fundus to the internal cervical os, measured in the midsagittal plane of the uterus. The normal reference range for women of childbearing age is 5.0 cm–7.5 cm.

   (b) Anteroposterior diameter:

      The maximum distance between the anterior and posterior uterine walls is measured perpendicular to the longitudinal diameter in the same sagittal plane. The normal range for this diameter is 3.0 cm–4.5 cm in women of childbearing age.

   (c) Transverse diameter:

      This is the maximum width of the uterus measured slightly below the uterine horns. To obtain this measurement, the transducer is rotated 90° to visualize the transverse plane of the uterine fundus. The normal reference range for women of childbearing age is 4.5 cm–6.0 cm.

In typical cases, the sum of these three measurements is less than 15.0 cm [2] (Fig. 3.4).

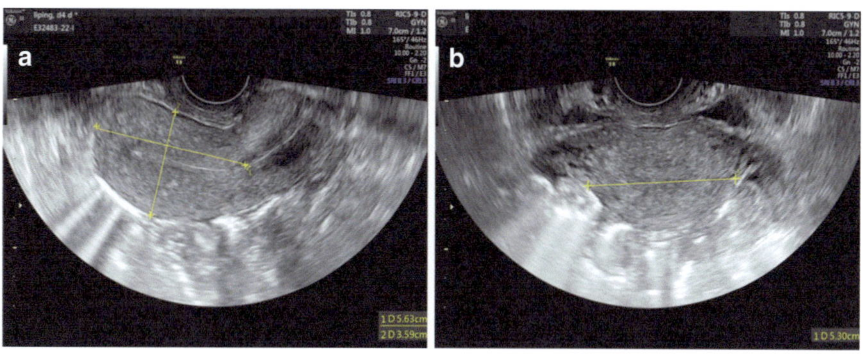

Fig. 3.4 (**a**) The longitudinal and anteroposterior diameters of the uterus. (**b**) The transverse diameter of the uterus

3.2.3 Endometrium

1. Measurement of endometrial thickness

Endometrial thickness is measured in the midsagittal plane of the uterus at the thickest point of the endometrium. A line is drawn perpendicular to the midline of the endometrium, with the measurement point located at the junction between the endometrium and the myometrium. Both the basal laminae on each side of the junction should be included in the measurement [3] (Fig. 3.5).

If fluid is present within the uterine cavity, the thickness of the endometrium on the anterior and posterior walls should be measured separately (Fig. 3.6).

Normal endometrial thickness at various phases of the menstrual cycle: (a) Menstruation: The endometrium is shed, and its thickness ranges from 2 mm to 3 mm. (b) Early proliferation (days 5–7 of the menstrual cycle): The endometrium

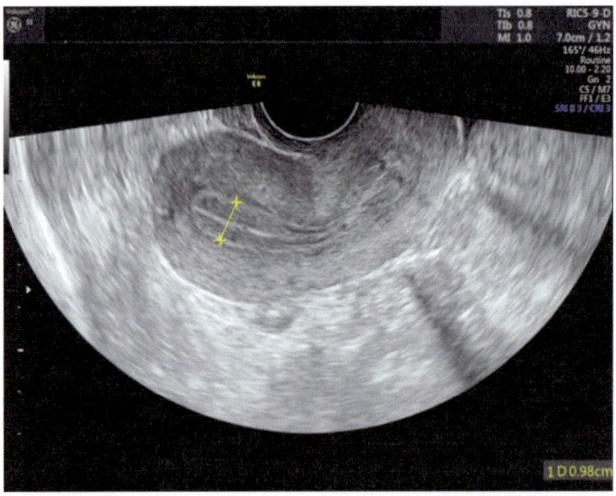

Fig. 3.5 Measurement of endometrial thickness

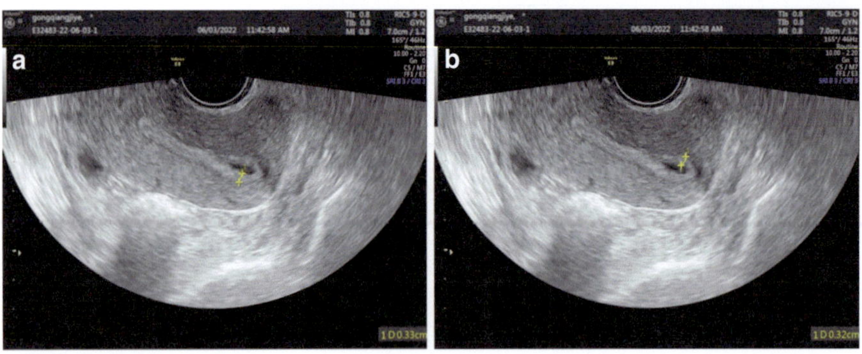

Fig. 3.6 (**a**) Endometrial thickness at the anterior wall. (**b**) Endometrial thickness at the posterior wall

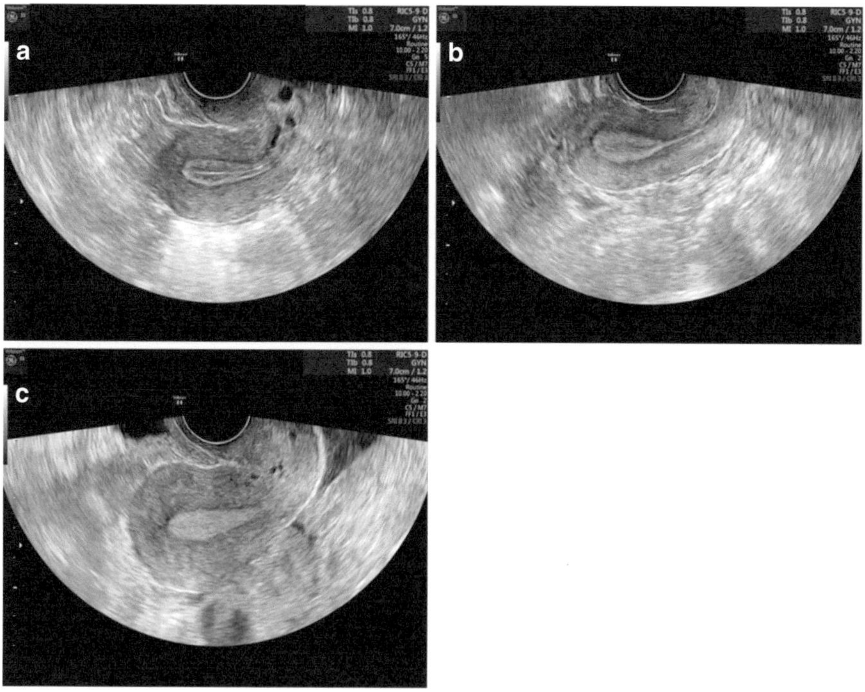

Fig. 3.7 (**a**) Triple line endometrium. (**b**) Isoechogenic endometrium. (**c**) Homogeneous hyperechogenic endometrium

measures 5 mm–6 mm. (c) Mid proliferation (days 8–10 of the menstrual cycle): The endometrium thickens to 7 mm–8 mm. (d) Late proliferation (days 11–14 of the menstrual cycle): The endometrium is 9 mm–10 mm thick. (e) Secretory phase: The endometrium reaches its thickest point, measuring up to 12mm, and in some cases, it can reach up to 15 mm [2].

2. Evaluation of endometrial morphology

The endometrium undergoes cyclic changes in response to hormones secreted by the ovaries. As ovarian follicles mature and estrogen secretion increases, the endometrium progressively thickens, a process primarily driven by estrogen. This phase is referred to as the proliferative phase of the endometrium, which corresponds to the follicular phase of the ovarian cycle.

On ultrasound, the proliferative phase endometrium is characterized by: (a) strong echogenicity in the basal layer; (b) low echogenicity in the functional layer; (c) strong-echo intrauterine midline (Fig. 3.7).

After ovulation, both estrogen and progesterone influence the endometrium, stimulating the secretion activity of endometrial glands and the proliferation of blood vessels. This phase is known as the secretory phase of the endometrium, corresponding to the luteal phase of the ovarian cycle.

On ultrasound, the secretory phase endometrium is characterized by the following: (a) increased echogenicity in the functional layer; (b) decreased clarity of the intrauterine midline; (c) in the late secretory phase, all layers of the endometrium show homogeneous, medium-strength echogenicity.

Endometrial patterns can be categorized into three types: (a) Triple line: Hypoechoic with well-defined outer walls and a central echogenic line. (b) Isoechogenic: Isoechoic with a poorly defined central echogenic line. (c) Homogeneous hyperechogenic: Hyperechoic with no visible central line [4] (Fig. 3.7).

3.3 Normal Ovarian Images and Measurements

3.3.1 Ovary

To visualize the ovary, the ultrasound probe should be positioned on the parietal side of the uterus, allowing the normal ovary to be seen anterior to the iliac vessels. Both bilateral ovaries and adnexal areas should be carefully examined for any space-occupying lesions.

For ovarian measurements, the longitudinal and anteroposterior diameters of the ovary should be measured in the plane showing the ovary's maximal long axis. The ultrasound probe is then rotated 90° to obtain a section perpendicular to the previous one, which allows for the measurement of the transverse diameter of the ovary [3] (Fig. 3.8). The normal size of an ovary is approximately 4 cm × 3 cm × 1 cm.

3.3.2 Measurement of Follicles

There is no universal consensus or standardized guideline for measuring follicle size [5].

A common clinical practice for regularly shaped follicles is to measure two diameters perpendicular to each other in the largest section of the follicle and then

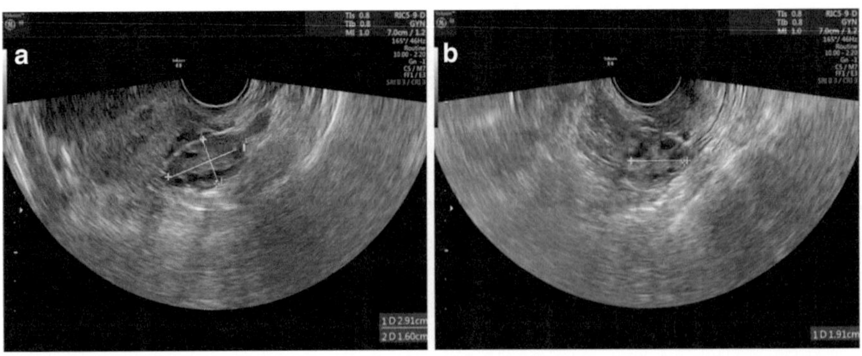

Fig. 3.8 (**a**) Measurement of the longitudinal and anteroposterior diameters of the ovary. (**b**) Measurement of the transverse diameter of the ovary

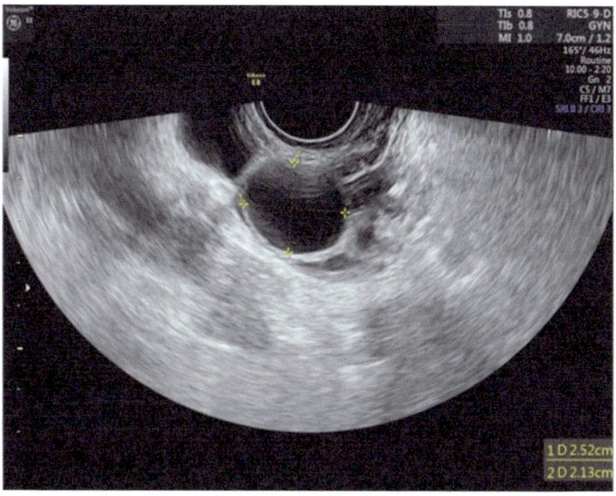

Fig. 3.9 Measurement of follicle size

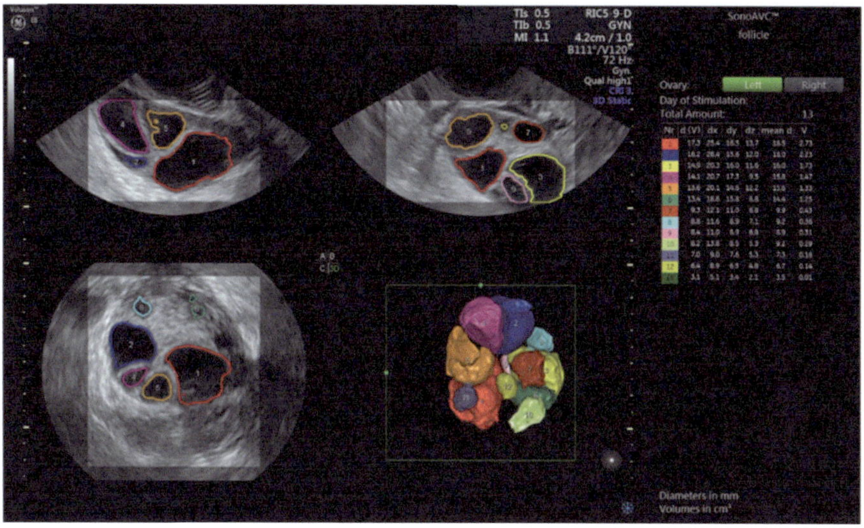

Fig. 3.10 Measurement of follicular volume

average these values to represent its size (Fig. 3.9). Mature follicles typically range from 18 mm to 25 mm in diameter. However, follicles are three-dimensional and often have irregular shapes, which reduces the reliability of measurements, especially when multiple large follicles are developing simultaneously during superovulation [6, 7].

Follicular volume is considered the most accurate method for assessing follicle size [7] (Fig. 3.10). However, this technique requires high-quality imaging and accurate measurements can fail in 5% of patients. In 15% of patients, image post-processing is necessary to obtain reliable values [5]. As a result, follicular volume is not routinely used in clinical practice.

For irregularly shaped follicles, the sonographer must carefully search for the dominant follicle and select the most representative diameters for measurement. During this process, avoiding selecting overly large or small sections is crucial. Additionally, measurements should consider the patient's menstrual phase, endometrial thickness, endometrial morphology, and blood hormone levels to evaluate the follicle's developmental stage and maturity comprehensively.

3.3.3 Criteria for Antral Follicle Count

Antral follicles are identified by ultrasonography on the second to fourth day of the menstrual cycle. Follicles measuring between 2 mm and 10 mm in size are considered antral follicles. Nonechoic areas within the ovary that are pinpoint-sized or smaller than 2 mm cannot be classified as antral follicles.

The total number of antral follicles in both ovaries is an important indicator of ovarian reserve and helps to predict the ovarian response to gonadotropins [8]. This count plays a crucial role in selecting an appropriate ovulation regimen and determining the correct dose of gonadotropins [9] (see Sect. 6.4 in Chap. 6 for more details).

3.4 Normative Writing of Reports

A well-standardized ultrasound report should include the following elements: (a) basic patient information; (b) representative images of organs or lesions; (c) description of findings during the examination; (d) ultrasonographic diagnosis and any relevant recommendations.

The report must be written using specialized and standardized terminology, ensuring that all descriptions are purposeful, clear, and objective. It should detail the major findings and provide appropriate context for any subfindings, facilitating accurate communication of results and clinical decision-making.

3.4.1 Description of Findings on Ultrasound

1. Uterus

   Body of the uterus: Describe the position, size, and echogenicity of the uterus. Note the presence or absence of any space-occupying lesions, and provide detailed descriptions of any lesions, including their location, size, margins, echogenicity, and anatomical relationship to the myometrium or endometrium.

   Cervix: Include the size of the cervix, the presence or absence of space-occupying lesions, and a description of the characteristics of any lesions observed.

Endothelium: Measure endometrial thickness and describe its morphological patterns. Note the presence or absence of any space-occupying lesions and describe their characteristics.

2. Ovaries

Describe the bilateral ovarian size, the size of the dominant follicle, the number of antral follicles in both ovaries, and the morphological profile of any space-occupying lesions, if present.

3. Fallopian tubes

Normal fallopian tubes are generally not clearly visualized on ultrasound without contrast enhancement. However, abnormalities such as hydrosalpinx or pyosalpinx can be detected. If such abnormalities are present, describe the size, morphology, and echogenic characteristics of the affected fallopian tube(s).

4. Pelvic cavity

Document the presence or absence of pelvic effusion. If present, provide details on the echogenic nature, width, and depth of the effusion. Also, note the presence or absence of any space-occupying lesions in the pelvic cavity and provide descriptions of any such lesions. Finally, assess and document the mobility of pelvic organs.

3.4.2 Ultrasonic Diagnosis and Recommendations

Ultrasonic diagnosis consists of four major components: (a) anatomical localization; (b) physical diagnosis; (c) diagnosis of possible diseases; (d) clinical recommendations.

The diagnostic process begins by identifying the presence and nature of any lesions: (a) Direct ultrasonic diagnosis can be made for cases where the exact disease is identifiable (e.g., uterine anomalies, adenomyosis). (b) For cases where a definitive diagnosis cannot be made, but a probable diagnosis is suspected, the most likely condition can be suggested based on clinical experience (e.g., "Consider high probability of…"). (c) For cases where a definitive diagnosis cannot be given, it is important to characterize the physical nature of the lesion (e.g., solid echogenicity, cystic-solid mixed echogenicity, nonechogenicity, high echogenicity, and low-moderate mixed echogenicity).

Finally, based on the findings, appropriate clinical recommendations should be provided. For instance: (a) If uterine echogenicity is unclear, a hysteroscopy may be recommended. (b) For heterogeneous endometrial echogenicity prior to menstruation, repeat ultrasonography after menstruation could be advised.

References

1. Sanders RC, Parsons AK. Anteverted retroflexed uterus: a common consequence of cesarean delivery. AJR Am J Roentgenol. 2014;203(1):117–24.
2. Chinese Ultrasound Doctors Association. Chinese gynecological ultrasound examination guidelines. Bei Jing: People's Medical Publishing House; 2017. p. 1–192.
3. Abuhamad A, Minton KK, Benson CB, et al. Obstetric and gynecologic ultrasound curriculum and competency assessment in residency training programs: consensus report. J Ultrasound Med. 2018;37(1):19–50.
4. Check JH, Dietterich C, Choe JK, et al. Effect of triple line vs isoechogenic endometrial texture on pregnancy outcome following embryo transfer according to use of controlled ovarian stimulation (COH) or estrogen/progesterone replacement. Clin Exp Obstet Gynecol. 2013;40(1):37–9.
5. Rodríguez-Fuentes A, Hernández J, García-Guzman R, et al. Prospective evaluation of automated follicle monitoring in 58 in vitro fertilization cycles: follicular volume as a new indicator of oocyte maturity. Fertil Steril. 2010;93(2):616–20.
6. Forman RG, Robinson J, Yudkin P, et al. What is the true follicular diameter: an assessment of the reproducibility of transvaginal ultrasound monitoring in stimulated cycles. Fertil Steril. 1991;56(5):989–92.
7. Ata B, Seyhan A, Reinblatt SL, et al. Comparison of automated and manual follicle monitoring in an unrestricted population of 100 women undergoing controlled ovarian stimulation for IVF. Hum Reprod. 2011;26(1):127–33.
8. Marca AL, Sunkara SK. Individualization of controlled ovarian stimulation in IVF using ovarian reserve markers: from theory to practice. Hum Reprod Update. 2014;20(1):124–40.
9. Hsu A, Arny M, Knee AB, et al. Antral follicle count in clinical practice: analyzing clinical relevance. Fertil Steril. 2011;95(2):474–9.

Ultrasonography in Assisted Reproductive Treatment

4

Da Li, Na Zuo, and Zhijing Na

Ultrasonography is indispensable in reproductive medicine, playing a critical role across various stages of assisted reproductive treatments (ART). Its applications range from assessing the development of the genital organs and evaluating fertility potential to monitoring follicular and endometrial growth during treatment cycles. Ultrasonography also supports key procedural decisions, such as determining the appropriate starting dose of ovulation stimulation medication, guiding oocyte retrieval, facilitating embryo implantation, and assisting in embryo reduction.

Beyond these clinical applications, the fertility specialist relies on ultrasound findings to make informed diagnoses. This involves objectively describing morphological features observed in ultrasound images and integrating these findings with the patient's medical history, menstrual cycle patterns, medication use, and relevant blood test results. Such a comprehensive approach ensures accurate clinical evaluations and optimizes patient outcomes.

Supplementary Information The online version contains supplementary material available at https://doi.org/10.1007/978-981-95-1373-4_4. The videos can be accessed individually by clicking the DOI link in the accompanying figure caption or by scanning this link with the SN More Media App.

D. Li (✉) · N. Zuo · Z. Na
Shengjing Hospital of China Medical University, Shenyang, China
e-mail: zuon@sj-hospital.org

D. Li et al. (eds.), *Ultrasonography of the Female Reproductive System*,
https://doi.org/10.1007/978-981-95-1373-4_4

4.1 Evaluation of Ovarian Reserve

A woman's fertility encompasses her ability to produce viable oocytes, achieve successful fertilization, and carry a fetus to term. Assessing fertility involves three key dimensions: the ovarian reserve, the structure and function of the reproductive system, and systemic health factors.

Ovarian reserve refers to the number of oocytes remaining in the ovaries, often described as oocyte quantity. This concept is distinct from oocyte quality, which denotes the likelihood of a fertilized oocyte resulting in a live birth. Evaluating ovarian reserve not only aids in estimating reproductive potential but also helps predict ovarian responsiveness to exogenous gonadotropins (GN). Such insights enable fertility specialists to tailor ovulation induction protocols to the individual, enhancing treatment outcomes.

4.1.1 Indicators for the Assessment of Ovarian Reserve

1. Age

A woman's age is the most significant factor in assessing fertility, as ovarian reserve and oocyte quality decline progressively with age due to follicular depletion and atresia. Age serves as the best marker of oocyte quality, with factors such as spindle apparatus disruption, oxidative stress, and mitochondrial damage contributing to reduced oocyte viability. These changes result in fertilization failures and decreased embryo quality [1]. Studies of human embryos demonstrate that the likelihood of aneuploidy is lowest in women aged 26–30. Beyond this range, the risk of aneuploid embryos increases sharply: over 35% by age 36, over 50% by age 39, over 70% by age 42, and over 80% by age 43 [2].

International diagnostic criteria for female infertility identify infertility as the inability to conceive after more than one year of normal, active sexual life. However, guidelines recommend earlier evaluation of ovarian reserve and comprehensive infertility assessments for women aged ≥35 years who fail to conceive after six months of unprotected sexual activity. For women aged ≥40 years, such evaluations should be conducted without delay, and assisted reproductive interventions may be considered to expedite pregnancy [3]. It is important to note that age, while a critical factor, is only a preliminary indicator of ovarian reserve. Comprehensive assessment requires additional tests and analyses to confirm the diagnosis and guide treatment.

2. Endocrine indicators
   (a) Basal follicle-stimulating hormone (bFSH)

   The bFSH level, measured between days 2 and 5 of the menstrual cycle, is a more sensitive predictor of ovarian reserve than age. In women with diminished ovarian reserve (DOR), reduced estradiol levels weaken the negative feedback mechanism on the hypothalamic-pituitary-ovarian axis, resulting in elevated bFSH levels.

However, bFSH levels are subject to significant variability, which limits the predictive value of a single measurement, particularly in younger patients. In clinical practice, a markedly elevated bFSH level is considered a reliable indicator of DOR but must be interpreted in conjunction with other markers for a comprehensive evaluation [4].

(b) Basal estradiol (bE2)

The bE2 level, measured between days 2 and 5 of the menstrual cycle, is useful for identifying patients with DOR who may have normal bFSH levels. In cases of DOR, the early increase in FSH stimulates the premature initiation of new follicular growth, leading to a subsequent rise in estradiol (E2) concentrations.

An early rise in serum E2 is a hallmark of reproductive aging and can lower an otherwise elevated bFSH level into the normal range, potentially leading to a misinterpretation of the test. If the basal FSH concentration is normal but E2 levels are elevated (>60–80 pg/mL), it may indicate ovarian dysfunction related to DOR.

It is important to note that E2 production can be influenced by factors such as ovarian cysts and medications, requiring careful differentiation by clinical practitioners to avoid false conclusions.

(c) Inhibin B (INH-B)

INH-B is a glycoprotein hormone secreted primarily by preantral follicles. Decreased secretion of inhibin B reduces the negative feedback on the pituitary gland, leading to an increase in pituitary FSH secretion and higher FSH concentrations during the late luteal and early follicular phases [5].

A decline in day 3 INH-B level may serve as an early indicator of poor ovarian reserve, often preceding the expected rise in day 3 FSH level. However, some studies do not support its use as a reliable predictive marker in in vitro fertilization (IVF) [6]. As a predictor of ovarian reserve, INH-B is not considered highly sensitive, and its value as a marker of fertility potential remains uncertain [6].

(d) bFSH/Basal luteinizing hormone (bLH) ratio

The bFSH/bLH ratio reflects the dynamics of ovarian reserve. In women with significantly reduced ovarian function, bFSH levels are elevated due to the lack of negative feedback from estrogen, while bLH levels also rise due to the absence of INH-B. However, the increase in bFSH occurs earlier than the rise in bLH, leading to a higher bFSH/bLH ratio. This ratio is valuable for identifying diminished ovarian reserve in women with otherwise normal bFSH levels.

Studies have shown that a bFSH/bLH ratio greater than two may indicate a possible poor ovarian response to gonadotropins [7]. A ratio exceeding 3.6 is more strongly associated with significant DOR [8].

(e) Anti-Müllerian hormone (AMH)

AMH is produced by the granulosa cells of ovarian follicles during the early stages of follicular development. In females, AMH secretion begins during fetal life, peaks around age 18, and then gradually declines, with levels reaching near cessation by around age 50. AMH plays a key role in regulating follicular growth and development. Its secretion is not influenced by the hypothalamic-pituitary-ovarian axis, making it a reliable indicator of the size of the antral follicular pool throughout the menstrual cycle.

AMH is also one of the best predictors of the number of oocytes (eggs) that can be retrieved during ovarian hyperstimulation cycles. Although there are challenges in applying AMH testing—such as variability in testing methods and reagents, relatively high costs, and the time required for testing (which can take hours or more)—it remains one of the most reliable markers of ovarian reserve [9].

3. Antral Follicle Count (AFC)

AMH is expressed by the granulosa cells of growing follicles, and serum AMH levels correlate with the number of antral follicles. AFC by ultrasound quantifies the total number of antral follicles in both ovaries, providing a visual assessment of ovarian reserve and helping predict ovarian responsiveness to ovarian hyperstimulation therapy, as well as the number of oocytes (eggs) that can be retrieved.

AFC has the advantages of being easy to perform, rapid, cost-effective, and highly accurate. These factors make it the preferred method for evaluating ovarian reserve and a routine test for first-time patients in reproductive medicine outpatient clinics. However, AFC cannot predict embryo quality.

It was previously suggested that AFC should be performed during menstruation. However, recent studies have shown that AFC can be reliably performed at any point during the menstrual cycle, maintaining consistent accuracy throughout [10].

It is recommended that all identifiable antral follicles with a diameter between 2 and 10 mm be counted, as this provides the most practical method for assessing AFC in clinical practice. The counting process should begin from the outer ovarian margin of the sweep and continue to the opposite margin. Every round or oval transonic structure within the ovarian margins should be considered a follicle. The number of follicles in each ovary should be combined to obtain the total AFC. Follicles greater than 10 mm in diameter should be excluded from the total follicle count [11].

In our clinical practice, we have observed several conditions that may compromise the identification and counting of antral follicles:

(a) When a large cyst, corpus luteum, or corpus hemorrhagicum is present in the ovary, the antral follicles may be poorly visualized due to compression. However, the antral follicles can be visualized again after cyst fluid is aspirated through a puncture or when a physiological cyst is resorbed during the subsequent menstrual cycle (Fig. 4.1).

(b) Ovarian volume decreases during the luteal phase, leading to the shrinkage of antral follicles, which complicates their observation and counting (Fig. 4.2). Due to this effect, some patients may be misidentified as having diminished ovarian reserve.

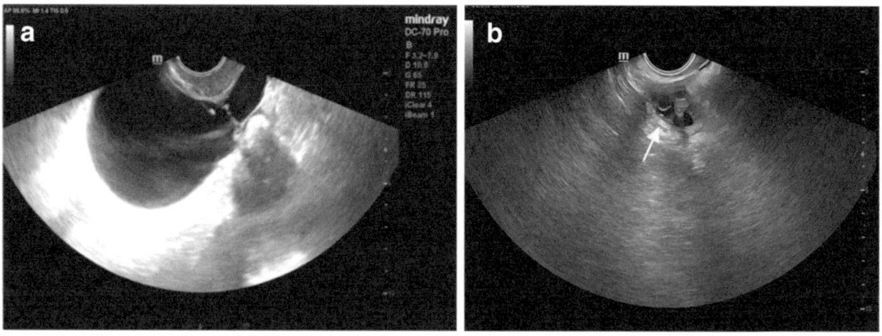

Fig. 4.1 (**a**) Tubal fluid prior to aspiration by puncture, when the ovary and antral follicles were poorly visualized. (**b**) The antral follicles were visible after the fluid has been aspirated by puncture

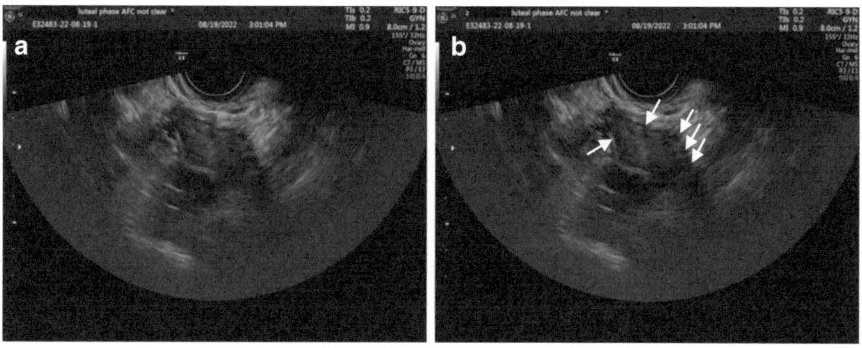

Fig. 4.2 (**a**) Ovarian image during the late luteal phase. (**b**) The arrows indicate the very small antral follicles

(c) In patients receiving long-acting gonadotropin-releasing hormone (GnRH) agonists for GnRH receptor down-regulation, particularly after several months of continuous treatment, the ovaries may become dormant and shrink in size. In some of these patients, only small echogenic areas are visible in the ovaries on ultrasound, making the antral follicles poorly visualized. This can make it inappropriate to diagnose these patients with diminished ovarian reserve. These ovarian and antral follicular changes are typically reversible, as the antral follicles gradually recover following normal menstruation, which facilitates normal ultrasound visualization. Similar changes may also be seen in patients who have been using contraceptives for extended periods (Fig. 4.3).

(d) In hypogonadal patients, ultrasound images often show small ovaries without identifiable antral follicles, which should be differentiated from diminished ovarian reserve or premature ovarian failure. After further testing for sex hormones and AMH levels, if E2 and gonadotropin levels are very low but AMH levels are normal, the abnormal ovarian images can be attributed

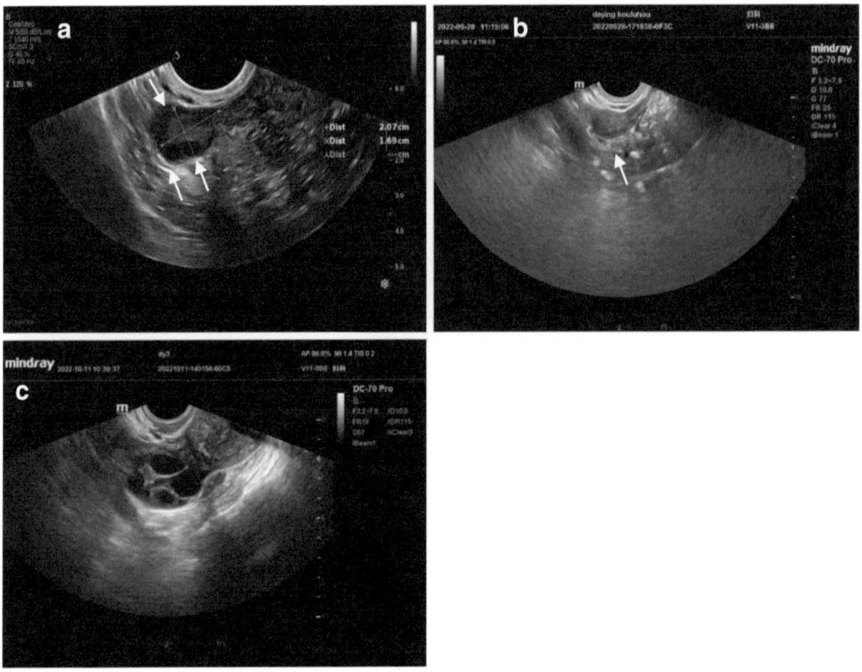

Fig. 4.3 (**a**) Antral follicles in the ovary were clearly visible before oral administration of Diane-35 (ethinylestradiol and cyproterone acetate). (**b**) After one month of oral administration of Diane-35, the ovary appeared generally more solid, with only very small antral follicles visible, which can be easily mistaken for DOR. (**c**) After discontinuing Diane-35 and undergoing ovarian hyperstimulation therapy, multiple follicles developed in the ovary

to a lesion in the superior central nervous system (CNS), while the patient's ovarian reserve remains normal. These patients may require prolonged high-dose gonadotropin therapy to stimulate follicular growth and ovulation. During ovulation stimulation therapy, antral follicles will be visualized on ultrasound as the ovaries gradually increase in size (Fig. 4.4). If one magnifies the pinpoint-sized non-echoic areas in the ovary and mistakes them for antral follicles, the AFC result may be falsely elevated, leading to a missed diagnosis of diminished ovarian reserve.

At present, AFC testing requires standardization of measurement criteria and counting methods to ensure accurate results.

In summary, age, peripheral blood hormone levels, and ultrasound indicators can be used to assess ovarian reserve. AMH levels appear to be a more sensitive marker of ovarian reserve compared to early follicular-phase hormone levels, as AMH tends to decline before bFSH rises. Multiple studies have shown that both AFC and AMH are equally sensitive and specific measures of ovarian reserve. When performed at an experienced center, AFC is a reasonable alternative to AMH [5].

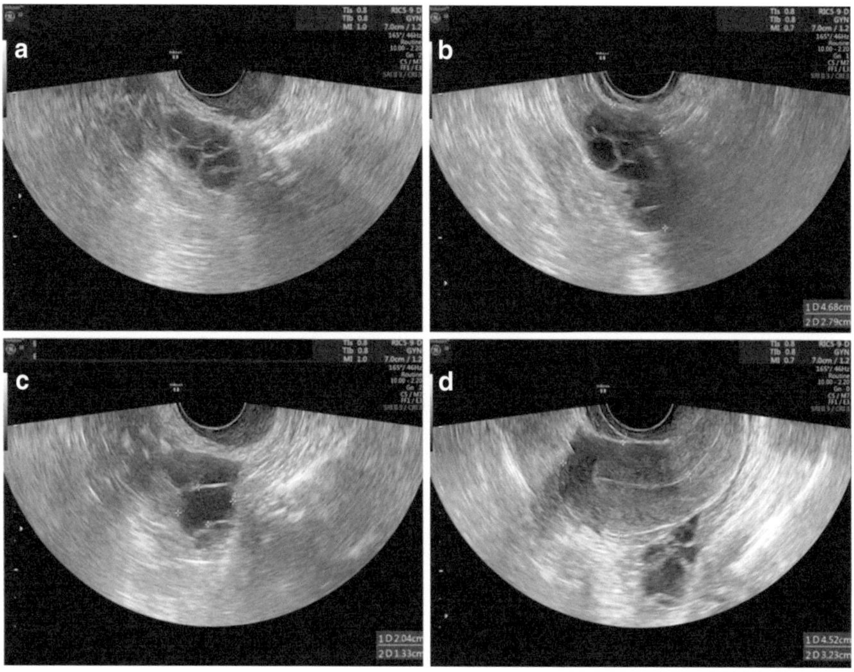

Fig. 4.4 (**a**) The right ovary after 50 days of ovulation stimulation therapy. (**b**) The right ovary after 58 days of ovulation stimulation therapy. (**c**) Mature follicles in the left ovary after 58 days of ovulation stimulation therapy. (**d**) Image of the uterus and uterine body size measurement after 58 days of ovulation stimulation therapy

4.1.2 Commonly Used Terms, Concepts, and Handlings in Assisted Reproductive Medicine Related to Ovarian Reserve

1. Decreased or diminished ovarian reserve (DOR)

DOR is defined as ovarian insufficiency resulting from a decrease in the number of oocytes [12]. It is categorized into physiological DOR (associated with advanced age) and pathological DOR (not age-related) (Fig. 4.5).

Case Presentation:

A 27-year-old female patient was admitted with the chief complaint of "infertility after 7 years of trying to conceive." The patient reported the absence of spontaneous menstrual periods. A gynecologic ultrasound performed seven years earlier at a foreign institution revealed a rudimentary uterus measuring 2.3 cm × 0.9 cm, with no clear images of the bilateral ovaries. The patient received intermittent hormone replacement therapy and underwent a hysterosalpingography, which confirmed that her fallopian tubes were patent. Her husband underwent a semen analysis, which

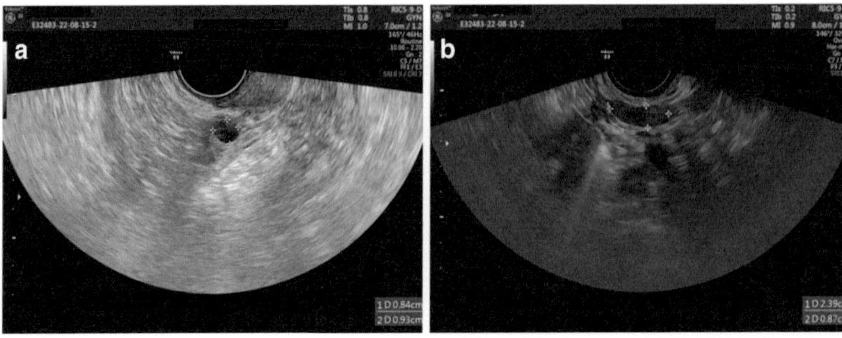

Fig. 4.5 (**a**) A DOR Patient with a small right ovary, in which only one antral follicle was observed. (**b**) The left ovary was small and solid, measuring 2.39 cm × 0.87 cm, with no antral follicles present

yielded normal results. The patient also attempted ovulation stimulation therapy but failed to develop follicles.

An initial ultrasound examination at our clinic indicated significant uterine enlargement compared to the previous exam, with a uterine body size of 3.6 cm × 3.1 cm. The right ovary measured approximately 1.7 cm × 1.2 cm, and the left ovary measured approximately 1.1 cm × 0.7 cm, with no visible antral follicles in either ovary. Sex hormone test results showed E2 <15 pg/mL, FSH 0.53 IU/L, LH <0.2 IU/L, P <0.1 ng/mL, PRL 15 ng/mL, T 0.18 ng/mL, and AMH 4.49 ng/mL.

These results suggested a normal ovarian reserve. Based on the low gonadotropin levels, it was hypothesized that the patient's condition could be related to a lesion in the superior CNS. A head magnetic resonance imaging (MRI) was performed, which revealed an empty sella.

Current Diagnosis: Primary infertility, empty sella syndrome.

Ovulation stimulation therapy was planned to help the patient conceive. Ovulation stimulation therapy for this patient was initiated with a low dose and gradually increased in a stepwise manner. Starting with 75 IU/day, the dose was gradually increased to 450 IU/day, at which point the patient's follicles began to develop. The dose was then reduced to 300 IU/day to prevent the simultaneous development of multiple follicles. The patient underwent ovulation stimulation therapy for a total of 59 days. During this period, the patient's ovaries gradually enlarged, and the AFC increased from zero to multiple antral follicles, with one follicle eventually reaching maturity. At this point, her uterine size was 4.5 cm × 3.2 cm, larger than in the previous scan (Fig. 4.4a–d). The patient was then administered human chorionic gonadotropin (hCG) to induce ovulation and was advised to attempt conception through sexual intercourse.

There is no well-established consensus on the diagnostic criteria for DOR [13]. The American Society for Reproductive Medicine (ASRM) introduced an expert consensus in 2020, which states that AMH and AFC are the most sensitive and reliable markers of ovarian reserve [5]. Although bFSH and bE2 are commonly used biochemical tests in clinical practice, elevated bFSH is not sensitive for diagnosing DOR due to its significant inter- and intracycle variability. Additionally, bE2 should only assist in interpreting a normal bFSH value. When bFSH is normal but bE2 levels rise (>60–80 pg/mL), it suggests a poor ovarian reserve. Commonly used clinical cut-off values for ovarian reserve include AMH (0.7 ng/mL as the lower limit, 8.4 ng/mL as the upper limit) [4, 14] and serum FSH (categorized as <10 or ≥10 mIU/mL) [15]. Low AFC (3–6) has high specificity for predicting poor ovarian reserve [16].

2. Premature Ovarian Insufficiency (POI) and Premature Ovarian Failure (POF)

POI is a clinical syndrome defined by the loss of ovarian activity before the age of 40 years. It is characterized by menstrual disturbances (amenorrhea or oligomenorrhea) along with elevated gonadotropins and low estradiol levels [17]. The diagnosis of POI is based on the presence of menstrual disturbances and biochemical confirmation. The guideline development group recommends the following diagnostic criteria: (a) age <40 years, (b) oligo/amenorrhea for at least four months, (c) an elevated bFSH >25 U/L on two occasions, more than 4 weeks apart [17].

Common etiological factors for POI include hereditary conditions (e.g., Turner's syndrome), medical causes (e.g., ovarian surgery, radiotherapy), immune factors, and environmental influences (e.g., poor lifestyle and environmental factors). In comparison to DOR, POI places greater emphasis on age, etiology, and menstrual status. The early stage of POI is manifested as DOR, while the severe stage of POI is known as POF. POF is characterized by amenorrhea, elevated gonadotropin levels (FSH >40 U/L), decreased estrogen levels, and varying perimenopausal symptoms in women under 40 years of age. POF represents the end stage of POI [18] (Fig. 4.6).

Low levels of serum estrogen may lead to low bone mass and act as a predisposing factor for coronary heart disease, thereby negatively impacting life expectancy. Appropriate physiological estrogen/progestin therapy is considered the standard management for POI. Hormone replacement therapy (HRT) typically consists of administering estrogen for 22 to 28 days, with the addition of progesterone for the

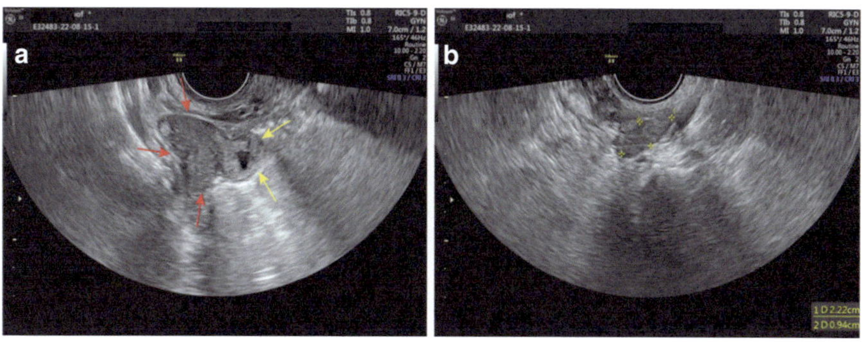

Fig. 4.6 (**a**) The right ovary of a patient with POF (the arrows indicate the ovary). (**b**) The left ovary of a patient with POF

final 10 to 14 days. In this context, 17-β estradiol is preferred over ethinylestradiol or conjugated equine estrogens for estrogen replacement. While there may be advantages to using micronized natural progesterone, the strongest evidence for endometrial protection supports oral cyclical combined treatment [17]. HRT is not recommended for women with a history of breast or ovarian cancer, breastfeeding mothers, or women who have reached the age of 50 years. The decision to stop HRT should be based on individual factors [18].

Case Presentation:
A 28-year-old female patient was admitted to our hospital with the chief complaint of "irregular menstruation for 3 years and difficulty conceiving." The patient had previously experienced regular menstruation with a 30-day cycle but developed irregular periods over the past 3 years, ranging from 5 to 90 days. She had a history of taking oral progesterone for withdrawal bleeding. Her last menstrual period was two months ago, and despite taking oral progesterone due to delayed menstruation, she did not experience withdrawal bleeding. The patient sought fertility guidance at our reproductive center.

The patient had no prior ovulation monitoring or salpingography. Her husband's semen analysis results were normal. A transvaginal ultrasound examination at our clinic revealed that the uterus was normal in size and morphology, with no noticeable space-occupying lesions. The endometrium was 3 mm thick and showed good continuity. The right ovary measured 1.8 cm × 1.1 cm × 0.9 cm, while the left ovary measured 2.1 cm × 0.8 cm × 0.9 cm. Both ovaries appeared solid, and no antral follicles were observed. The preliminary diagnosis was a high probability of POI.

To further define the diagnosis, sex hormones and AMH tests were performed. The results showed E2 <15 pg/mL, FSH 108 IU/L, LH 28 IU/L, P 0.2 ng/mL, PRL 14 ng/mL, T 0.4 ng/mL, and AMH 0.06 ng/mL.

Current Diagnosis: POF.

The patient was informed about her condition and started on Femoston for HRT. Follicular development was monitored during the estradiol phase in the first three treatment cycles, but no dominant follicles were observed.

During the fourth treatment cycle, sex hormone testing was repeated at the time of menstruation, revealing the following results: E2 60 pg/mL, FSH 19.57 IU/L, LH 7.6 IU/L, and P 1.3 ng/mL.

In this cycle, follicular development was not monitored during the estrogen phase. On the 12th day of her menstrual cycle, a self-administered urine LH strip test yielded a strong positive result. The patient returned to the hospital the following morning for an ultrasound examination (as shown in Fig. 4.6a, b). The ultrasonographic findings included the following: (a) Bilateral ovaries appeared solid, with no evident antral follicles. (b) Endometrial thickness of 9 mm, showing a homogeneous hyperechogenic pattern. (c) A thick-walled protrusion (indicated by the yellow arrows) emanating from the right ovary (indicated by the red arrows) was observed, with a small non-echoic area inside.

The imaging features of this protrusion, in conjunction with the patient's medical and menstrual history, suggested a high likelihood of a postovulatory corpus luteum. The patient was instructed to have intercourse as soon as possible and switch her Femoston regimen to estradiol dydrogesterone for the second half of the cycle.

Fourteen days later, a pregnancy test was performed, which returned negative. Femoston therapy was continued for the fifth treatment cycle. On day 8 of estradiol administration, a dominant follicle was detected. Subsequent monitoring showed successful maturation of the follicle, which was then retrieved for IVF. The process resulted in a good-quality embryo for cryopreservation.

3. Resistant Ovary Syndrome (ROS)

ROS is also known as insensitive ovary syndrome (IOS) or Savage syndrome. It occurs when the ovaries are insensitive to both endogenous and exogenous GNs despite having normal follicles. It is a rare cause of hypergonadotropic hypogonadism. The etiology of ROS is typically due to the absence of FSH receptors, defective postreceptor signaling in the ovaries, or the presence of autoimmune abnormalities such as FSH/LH receptor antibodies. These factors can lead to an arrest in ovarian development, a lack of gonadal negative feedback, and elevated circulating FSH and LH levels [19].

Patients with ROS typically present with hypergonadotropic amenorrhea, low or normal estrogen levels (the estrogen is produced by follicles that are partially responsive to gonadotropins), and normal ovarian reserve (as indicated by normal AMH and AFC levels on transvaginal ultrasound). They may also experience poor development of reproductive organs and secondary sexual characteristics in cases of primary amenorrhea, while secondary amenorrhea patients often have normal secondary sexual characteristics. Symptoms of low estrogen, such as hot flashes and vaginal dryness, may also be present.

The diagnostic criteria for ROS include the following: (a) amenorrhea, (b) a normal 46, XX karyotype, (c) elevated FSH levels, usually >40 U/L, elevated or normal LH levels, and low or normal estrogen levels, and (d) normal-sized ovaries with a normal AFC, as shown on ultrasound [21].

It is important to differentiate ROS from POF, as both present with hypergonadotropic amenorrhea and exhibit similar sex hormone profiles and clinical manifestations. However, their ultrasound characteristics differ significantly: ROS typically features normal antral follicles, whereas the absence of antral follicles characterizes POF. Ultrasound assessment of ovarian reserve, alongside AMH testing, provides a reliable means of distinguishing between the two conditions (Fig. 4.7).

That said, the recognition of ROS as a distinct clinical entity has been recently debated. Some researchers propose that ROS may simply represent an early stage in the progression of POF. In one study, FSH receptor gene analysis in 14 women failed to identify a specific mutation unique to either ROS or POF. However, the scope of mutations investigated in that study was limited. With advancements in molecular biology, comprehensive sequencing of the LH receptor and FSH receptor genes has become possible, offering the potential to identify clinically significant anomalies more effectively [19].

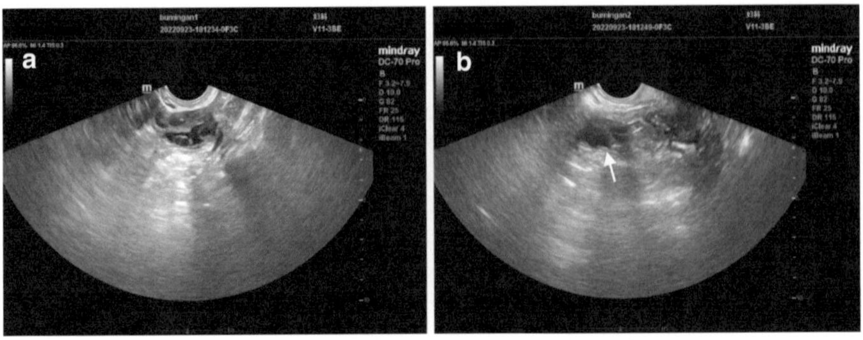

Fig. 4.7 (**a**) The right ovary of a patient with IOS. (**b**) The left ovary of a patient with IOS

The primary treatment for ROS is HRT, which supports the development of sexual characteristics, induces menstruation and protects fertility in adolescent females. In women of childbearing age, HRT also helps maintain sexual characteristics and normal libido, alleviates symptoms associated with low estrogen levels, and reduces the risk of osteoporosis. Additionally, all patients with ROS should take calcium and vitamin D supplements to support bone health and further prevent osteoporosis.

There are no specific or consistently effective treatment regimens for infertility caused by ROS. Estrogen administration suppresses endogenous gonadotropin secretion via negative feedback, activates follicular GN receptors, restores follicular sensitivity to gonadotropins, and facilitates follicular maturation. The first reported case of spontaneous pregnancy in a patient with ROS using estrogen therapy was documented in 1977 [20].

Recent advancements in assisted reproductive technology, particularly the development of pituitary suppression and ovarian stimulation protocols, have significantly improved reproductive outcomes for patients with ROS. Oral contraceptives or GnRH receptor down-regulation therapy with GnRH agonists can suppress endogenous FSH and LH secretion in most patients with ROS. High doses of exogenous GN are then administered to promote ovulation. Once follicular maturation is achieved, hCG is used to trigger ovulation, followed by natural fertilization or IVF-ET.

Despite these advances, the ovaries of ROS patients are often poorly responsive to both endogenous and exogenous GN, especially in those with markedly elevated FSH levels. Such patients may remain unresponsive or hyporesponsive even after extended high-dose exogenous GN therapy.

In vitro maturation (IVM) offers an alternative for ROS patients aiming to achieve pregnancy. This approach involves retrieving immature oocytes from the ovaries, maturing them in vitro, and subsequently performing IVF-ET. Additionally, women with ROS may consider egg donation as an effective option for achieving pregnancy [21].

Case Presentation:
A 35-year-old female patient presented with the chief complaint of "failure to conceive after two years of attempting pregnancy." The patient reported irregular menstrual periods requiring oral progesterone for withdrawal bleeding, with her last menstruation occurring 50 days prior.

Transvaginal ultrasonography revealed a normal uterine size and morphology, the endometrium with a thickness of 5 mm and good continuity, and normal-sized ovaries containing nine antral follicles in the right ovary and five in the left. No obvious space-occupying lesions were observed in the uterus or adnexa. Ovulation monitoring indicated no developing follicles in either ovary, while salpingography confirmed bilaterally patent fallopian tubes. The patient's husband's semen analysis results were normal.

Preliminary Diagnosis: Primary infertility with a normal ovarian reserve and probable ovulatory dysfunction infertility.

Initial Management: The patient was prescribed progesterone to induce withdrawal bleeding and instructed to return on the third day of menstruation for further evaluation and initiation of ovulation induction therapy.

On the third day of menstruation, the patient underwent a detailed assessment:

Sex hormone profile: E2: 28 pg/mL, FSH: 43 IU/L, LH: 9.2 IU/L, P: 0.1 ng/mL, PRL: 11.38 ng/mL, T: 0.46 ng/mL.

Ultrasound findings: Endometrial thickness of 3 mm, with nine antral follicles in the right ovary and five in the left.

Diagnostic Insights: The paradoxical findings of these tests—markedly elevated FSH suggesting diminished ovarian reserve, while the antral follicle count and AMH (3.49 ng/mL, within the normal range) indicated a normal ovarian reserve—pointed to IOS. The diagnosis was updated to primary infertility and IOS.

Treatment Plan: The patient was started on oral Femoston as HRT.

After the first treatment cycle, her sex hormone profile was reassessed during the menstruation: E2 52 pg/mL, FSH 19.41 IU/L, LH 7.12 IU/L, P 0.21 ng/mL, with a significant decrease in FSH level compared to the previous test.

The patient continued with the second cycle of treatment. A repeat sex hormone test during the menstrual period following cessation of the second cycle showed E2 56 pg/mL, FSH 23.07 IU/L, LH 6.65 IU/L, and P 0.46 ng/mL, with a slight increase in FSH level compared to the previous cycle.

To further reduce endogenous FSH levels, the patient was prescribed Diane-35 (a contraceptive) during the subsequent cycle.

After this treatment cycle, another sex hormone test during menstruation showed E2 145 pg/mL, FSH 17.33 IU/L, LH 4.23 IU/L, and P 0.35 ng/mL.

Patient Counseling and Future Management:
The patient was informed of her condition:

Both hormone replacement therapy and contraceptives were utilized to lower endogenous FSH levels and improve ovarian sensitivity in preparation for ovarian stimulation therapy.
However, due to the nature of IOS, the likelihood of dominant follicle development remains low, even with prolonged, high-dose ovarian stimulation therapy.

4. Ovarian Responsiveness to Gonadotropins

Controlled ovarian stimulation (COS) is a process designed to retrieve multiple oocytes within a single menstrual cycle. In clinical practice, the primary parameters used to evaluate the likelihood of success are the patient's age and the number of oocytes retrieved. This has led to the introduction of the concept of ovarian responsiveness to gonadotropins.

Patients classified as high responders (>15 oocytes) demonstrate significantly higher cumulative live birth rates (LBR) compared to poor responders (0–3 oocytes), suboptimal responders (4–9 oocytes), and even normal responders (10–15 oocytes) [22]. However, both insufficient and excessive ovarian responses are associated with increased cycle cancellation rates. In addition, a high ovarian response elevates the risk of ovarian hyperstimulation syndrome (OHSS).

While ovarian responsiveness to gonadotropins is strongly correlated with ovarian reserve, the two concepts are distinct. Ovarian responsiveness focuses on the patient's reaction to ovarian stimulation after treatment, whereas ovarian reserve tests assess the ovaries' pretreatment baseline capacity.

Poor ovarian response (POR) is characterized by a reduced follicular response to maximal stimulation during IVF. This leads to fewer retrieved oocytes, increased cycle cancellation rates, and elevated treatment costs due to the higher drug doses required and the need for repeated treatment cycles. These challenges impose significant emotional, physical, and financial burdens on affected couples [22].

In 2011, the European Society of Human Reproduction and Embryology (ESHRE) introduced the Bologna criteria to define POR [23] (Table 4.1). However, the application of this definition revealed its limitations. The criteria grouped diverse POR populations together, oversimplifying patient categorization and failing to stratify or tailor treatment approaches for different subgroups.

To address these shortcomings, an international group of reproductive medicine experts introduced the Patient-Oriented Strategies Encompassing Individualized Oocyte Number (POSEIDON) criteria in 2016 (Table 4.2) [24]. This updated framework provides a stratified approach to managing POR patients, offering clinicians a practical system to classify infertility patients undergoing ART. The primary goal of the POSEIDON criteria is to enable clinicians to counsel and treat low-prognosis patients more effectively by tailoring interventions to their specific clinical profiles [22].

POSEIDON Groups 1 and 2 are characterized by an unexpected poor ovarian response (≤3 eggs) or a suboptimal response (4–9 eggs) despite normal levels of AMH and AFC. In contrast, poor or suboptimal responses are anticipated outcomes

Table 4.1 Bologna criteria for ovarian hyporesponsiveness (Patients must fulfill at least two of the three following criteria to be classified as having ovarian hyporesponsiveness)

1	Age ≥40 years or presence of risk factors for POR (e.g., hereditary defects or pelvic factors)
2	POR in previous stimulation cycle (≤3 eggs obtained with conventional ovarian stimulation therapy)
3	One abnormal ovarian reserve test result: AFC <5 to 7 or AMH <0.5 to 1.1 ng/mL

Note: In the absence of advanced age and abnormal ovarian reserve test results, POR can be defined by a suboptimal response in two maximal stimulation cycles

Table 4.2 POSEIDON groups for ovarian hyporesponsiveness

POSEIDON group 1 (PG1)	Age <35 years with sufficient prestimulation ovarian reserve parameters (AFC ≥5, AMH ≥1.2 ng/mL) and with an unexpected poor or suboptimal ovarian response. Among these, subgroup 1a, constituted by patients with fewer than four eggs (poor response); subgroup 1b, constituted by patients with 4 to 9 eggs retrieved (suboptimal response) after standard ovarian stimulation
POSEIDON group 2 (PG2)	Age ≥35 years with sufficient prestimulation ovarian reserve parameters (AFC ≥5, AMH ≥1.2 ng/mL) and with an unexpected poor or suboptimal ovarian response. Among them, subgroup 2a, constituted by patients with fewer than four eggs, and subgroup 2b, constituted by patients with 4 to 9 eggs retrieved (suboptimal response) after standard ovarian stimulation
POSEIDON group 3 (PG3)	Age <35 years with poor ovarian reserve prestimulation parameters (AFC <5, AMH <1.2 ng/mL)
POSEIDON group 4 (PG4)	Age ≥35 years with poor ovarian reserve prestimulation parameters (AFC <5, AMH <1.2 ng/mL)

in Groups 3 and 4 due to low ovarian reserve. Importantly, the age-related decline in oocyte quality must be carefully considered and explained across all four groups during ovarian stimulation.

In Groups 1 and 2, the ovarian reserve remains sufficient; however, the challenge lies in the lower-than-expected oocyte yield, which reflects a "hypo-response" to standard GN doses. Adjusting the controlled ovarian hyperstimulation (COH) protocol to address ovarian resistance may effectively increase oocyte numbers. Strategies include using more potent gonadotropin preparations or increasing the follicle-stimulating hormone (FSH) dosage. Additionally, incorporating recombinant luteinizing hormone (rLH) during COH can help mitigate ovarian resistance, particularly in older individuals (Groups 2 and 4).

For Groups 3 and 4, where patients have a poor ovarian reserve, COH regimens, and increased FSH doses may not significantly improve follicle number or quality. In these cases, an alternative strategy such as cycle accumulation—extending the timeframe for oocyte retrieval—can optimize oocyte yield. This approach offers a potential solution for these patients by increasing the pool of retrieved oocytes over multiple cycles [22].

5. Hypogonadotropic Hypogonadism (HH)

Pulsatile secretion of GnRH from the hypothalamus is essential for both the initiation and maintenance of the reproductive axis in humans. Disruption of this episodic GnRH release, or failure of gonadotropin secretion, leads to the clinical syndrome known as HH.

Patients with HH exhibit symptoms related to low estrogen levels, including delayed or absent puberty, underdevelopment of secondary sexual characteristics, amenorrhea, and infertility. HH is categorized into two types: congenital and acquired. Congenital HH is rare and typically results from deficient GnRH secretion, which may occur either independently (known as normosmic congenital hypogonadotropic hypogonadism) or in association with anosmia or hyposmia (as seen in Kallmann syndrome).

Acquired HH, on the other hand, can be caused by a variety of factors, such as tumors in the CNS or pituitary gland, excessive exercise, restrictive dieting and weight loss, and emotional stress or psychological disorders [25].

The diagnosis of HH requires a thorough evaluation, considering both the patient's clinical presentation and laboratory results.

The main therapeutic goals for treating congenital HH include establishing regular menstrual cycles through HRT, inducing and maintaining secondary sex characteristics, ensuring normal sex hormone levels, preventing osteoporosis, and supporting psychological well-being. These measures are crucial for preparing the patient for later ovulation induction and achieving pregnancy.

For patients with acquired HH, the first priority is identifying and addressing the condition's underlying cause. In addition to this, HRT is essential to maintain menstruation and prevent the loss of secondary sex characteristics. Ovulation induction therapy is recommended for patients seeking fertility. In cases where fertility is not achieved with simpler treatments like intra-uterine insemination (IUI) or standard ovulation induction, IVF-ET may be considered, particularly in patients with combined fallopian tube issues, male factor infertility, or previous treatment failures.

Before initiating ovarian hyperstimulation, it is important to assess ovarian responsiveness. However, there are several challenges in evaluating ovarian reserve in patients with HH. Neither bFSH nor bFSH/bLH, which are typically used as markers for ovarian reserve, are effective in patients with HH. Additionally, the ovaries in HH patients often present with small, firm features on ultrasound, making it challenging to count antral follicles accurately. As a result, these patients are frequently misdiagnosed with POI or POF, leading to misleading ultrasound assessments of ovarian reserve (Fig. 4.8).

In contrast to these markers, AMH is a more reliable indicator of ovarian reserve in patients with HH. While a 2014 study questioned the validity of this assertion [26], AMH remains the most consistent approach to assessing ovarian reserve in these patients, as it is less influenced by the characteristics of HH.

When undergoing ovulation induction, HH patients typically require stepwise increases in medication dosages, including higher doses of GN and a longer duration of therapy. As the ovaries respond, they gradually enlarge, and antral follicles become visible on ultrasound and start to develop. It is critical to monitor the ovarian response throughout the treatment to minimize the risk of OHSS.

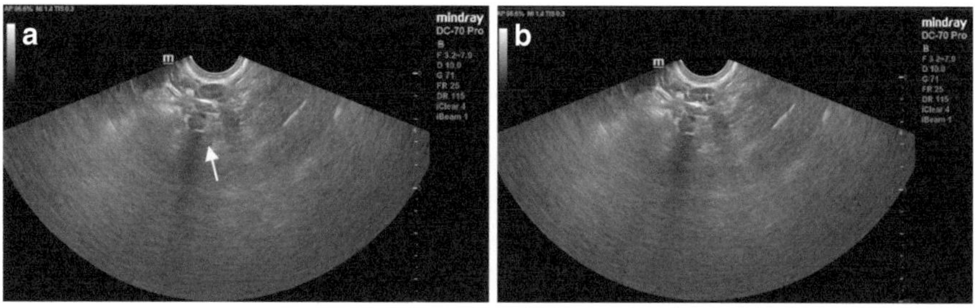

Fig. 4.8 (**a**) Ultrasound image of normal ovarian reserve in a patient with craniopharyngioma. (**b**) Measurement of ovarian size

4.2 Monitoring Ovulation in Natural Cycles and Follicular Development in Ovarian Hyperstimulation

Ovulation disorders are a common cause of female infertility. Transvaginal ultrasound is a valuable tool for assessing the location, size, morphology, development, and maturity of the developing follicles and monitoring the proliferation of the endometrium. When diagnosing infertility, it is essential to monitor ovulation in patients. Additionally, the presence of well-developed follicles, a receptive endometrium, and appropriate guidance on the timing of intercourse can enhance the chances of pregnancy. Ultrasound monitoring of ovulation is a key aspect of reproductive medicine that all clinical practitioners should be proficient in.

4.2.1 Ultrasound Monitoring of Ovulation in Natural Cycles

1. Prediction of ovulation and timing of follicle monitoring

In patients with regular menstrual cycles, antral follicles ranging from 2 mm to 7 mm in diameter can be observed in both ovaries between days 3 and 5 of the menstrual cycle. Among the recruited follicles, the one most sensitive to FSH (with the lowest threshold) becomes the dominant follicle, while the others undergo atresia. On day 6, the dominant follicle typically measures 7 mm to 8 mm in diameter. During the first half of the follicular phase, the dominant follicle grows at a rate of approximately 1 mm per day. After reaching a diameter of 10 mm, the growth rate accelerates to 2 mm per day. By day 12, the dominant follicle usually measures 16 mm to 18 mm in diameter.

A spontaneous LH peak occurs when the dominant follicle reaches 18 mm to 20 mm, followed by rapid follicular growth of 2 mm to 4 mm. The LH peak and the maximum follicular diameter typically occur almost simultaneously. By monitoring the size of the follicle and its growth rate from day 12 to day 14 of the menstrual cycle, we can predict the timing of the LH peak and ovulation. Ovulation generally occurs approximately 14 days before the onset of the next menstrual period. Thus, ovulation can be estimated by counting 14 days backward from the first day of the next menstrual period for patients with regular menstrual cycles.

Follicular monitoring in patients with regular menstrual cycles can begin daily, starting 3 to 5 days before the anticipated ovulation date, to track the size, tension, maturity of the follicles and the occurrence of ovulation. In patients with irregular menstrual cycles, monitoring may start on day 8 of menstruation. When the largest follicle reaches a diameter of 8 mm to 12 mm, a follow-up ultrasound should be scheduled two days later. If the follicle grows to 12 mm to 14 mm, the next ultrasound should be conducted the following day. Once the follicle reaches a diameter of ≥14 mm, daily monitoring is required until the follicle matures and ovulation occurs.

For patients with irregular menstrual cycles who cannot predict ovulation or frequently attend clinic visits for systematic monitoring, they may be advised to report to the clinic for ultrasound when they notice a clear, drawing-like vaginal discharge. This type of discharge is indicative of elevated estrogen levels and may signal an impending ovulation.

In irregular cycles, follicle monitoring can be done intermittently or continuously over an extended period, starting on day 5 of menstruation. Due to the unpredictable timing of ovulation and menstruation, extended monitoring may be necessary. Once an ovulation disorder is identified, ovulation induction therapy should be initiated in the subsequent menstrual cycle as part of the efforts to conceive.

Note: On day 4 of the menstrual cycle, antral follicles were observed in the ovaries, and the endometrium was thin. On day 8, the dominant follicle measured 8.8 mm in diameter, and the endometrium (triple line) was in the proliferative phase with a thickness of 7 mm. On day 12, the dominant follicle had grown to 12 mm in diameter, and the endometrium (triple line) was 9.2 mm thick. On day 15, the dominant follicle reached a diameter of 23 mm, the endometrium was 10.1 mm thick, and its morphological pattern was the transitional stage from triple line to homogeneous hyperechogenic. This change suggested the presence of an endogenous LH peak and a rising progesterone level, indicating that ovulation was likely to occur within the next 24 h. On day 16, the dominant follicle was no longer visible, and the endometrium had transitioned to a homogeneous hyperechogenic pattern, consistent with the secretory phase

2. Preovulatory Image of the Mature Follicle

The mature follicle typically measures 18 mm to 28 mm in diameter, is round or oval in shape, and moves toward the surface of the ovary. One side of the follicle is not covered by ovarian tissue and protrudes outward. Under ultrasound, if the follicle appears clear, smooth, and tense, with a dark, echo-less area and good translucency, it suggests that ovulation will occur within 24–48 h. The presence of the cumulus oophorus (a dot-like hyperechoic structure) on the inner wall of the follicle indicates that ovulation is imminent.

During the follicular phase, as the follicle grows, estrogen levels rise, causing the endometrium to thicken. At this stage, the endometrium is primarily influenced by estrogen, and its morphological pattern is a "triple line sign." As the follicle matures, the first estrogen peak triggers a positive feedback loop on the hypothalamic-pituitary-ovarian axis. This results in an LH peak and a small amount of progesterone begins to be produced, causing the endometrium to transition from triple line to homogeneous hyperechogenic (Fig. 4.9).

Ovulation is a sudden event and is difficult to capture with ultrasound. By combining ultrasound images of the follicle with peripheral blood hormone tests, we can estimate the timing of ovulation, helping guide the patient for intercourse aimed at conception. In some cases, observing the exact moment of ovulation during egg retrieval in an IVF procedure may be possible.

3. Postovulatory Ultrasound Imaging Features

   Postovulatory ultrasound imaging features (Fig. 4.10) include the following:

   (a) Sudden disappearance of the mature follicle: After ovulation, the mature follicle will suddenly disappear from the ultrasound image.
   (b) Significant shrinkage of the mature follicle: The mature follicle shrinks significantly, with blurred walls, irregular morphology, and uneven internal echogenicity.
   (c) Formation of corpus hemorrhagicum: Following ovulation, the follicular wall collapses, and small blood vessels covering the follicle rupture, causing blood to flow into the follicular cavity. This results in a cystic structure known as corpus hemorrhagicum, which typically lasts for about 72 h. It is generally filled with non-clotting blood and few blood clots. Ultrasound imaging shows fine, dotted echogenicity within the cyst. The corpus hemorrhagicum eventually develops into the corpus luteum. While the corpus hemorrhagicum is usually no larger than the original follicle, if bleeding occurs within the corpus luteum cavity, the diameter may exceed that of the normal corpus hemorrhagicum, forming a corpus luteum hematoma.
   (d) Presence of follicular fluid in the pelvic cavity: As the follicular fluid is discharged, a dark fluid area may appear around the ovary or in the recto-uterine pouch, indicating the completion of ovulation.

4. Ultrasonographic Features and Diagnosis of Undeveloped Follicles

   The absence of a dominant follicle in both ovaries, accompanied by multiple small follicles and a thin endometrium or proliferative endometrial changes (due to low estrogen levels), suggests a high likelihood of undeveloped follicles in the current menstrual cycle. However, it is important to differentiate this from ovarian images where ovulation has already occurred but without clear signs of ovulation. A more accurate diagnosis can be made through peripheral blood estrogen and progesterone tests:

   (a) Low levels of both estrogen and progesterone indicate that no follicles have developed in the current cycle (except in cases just before the menstrual period of the next cycle).

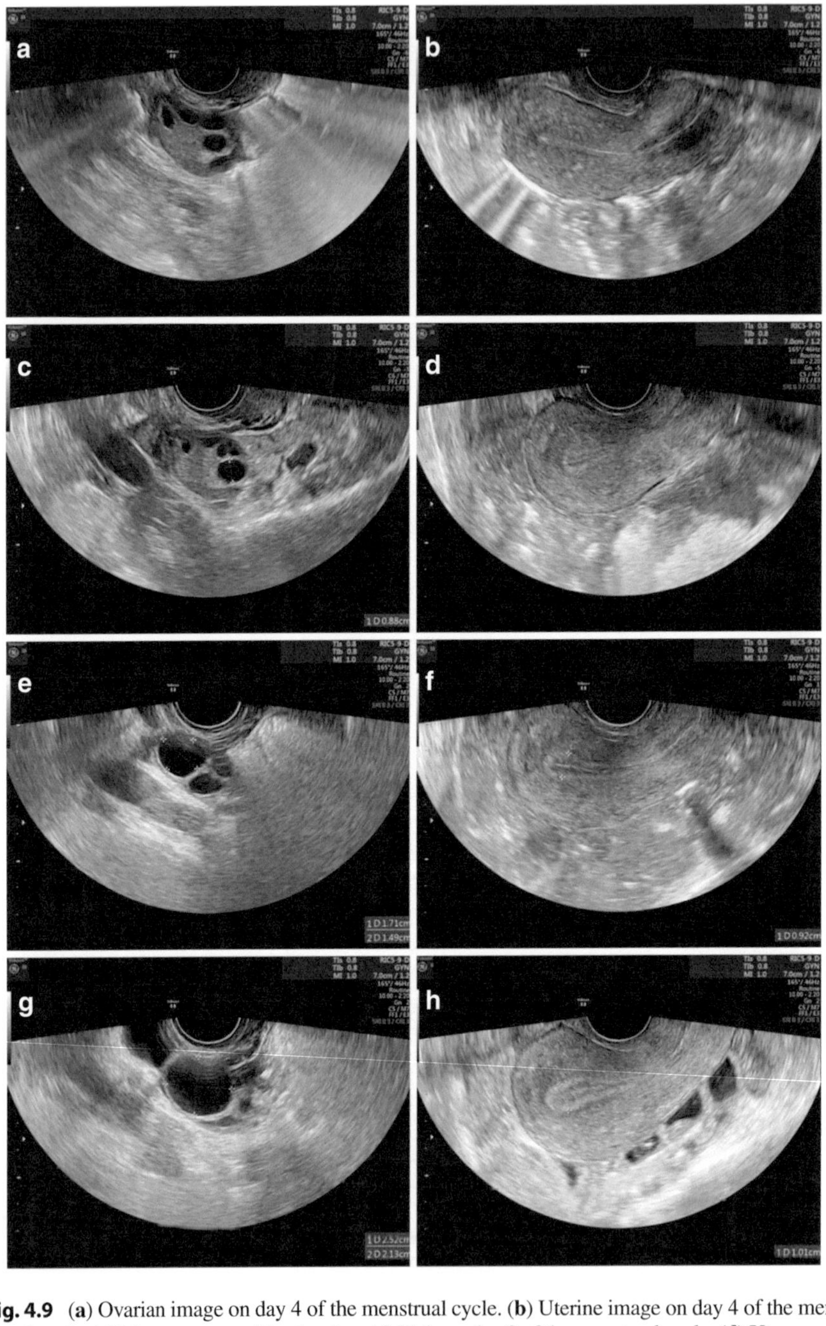

Fig. 4.9 (**a**) Ovarian image on day 4 of the menstrual cycle. (**b**) Uterine image on day 4 of the menstrual cycle. (**c**) Measurement of the dominant follicle on day 8 of the menstrual cycle. (**d**) Uterus and endometrium on day 8 of the menstrual cycle. (**e**) Measurement of the dominant follicle on day 12 of the menstrual cycle. (**f**) Measurement of endometrial thickness on day 12 of the menstrual cycle. (**g**) Measurement of the dominant follicle on day 15 of the menstrual cycle. (**h**) Measurement of endometrial thickness on day 15 of the menstrual cycle. (**i**) Ultrasound image after ovulation on day 16 of the menstrual cycle. (**j**) Uterus and endometrium on day 16 of the menstrual cycle

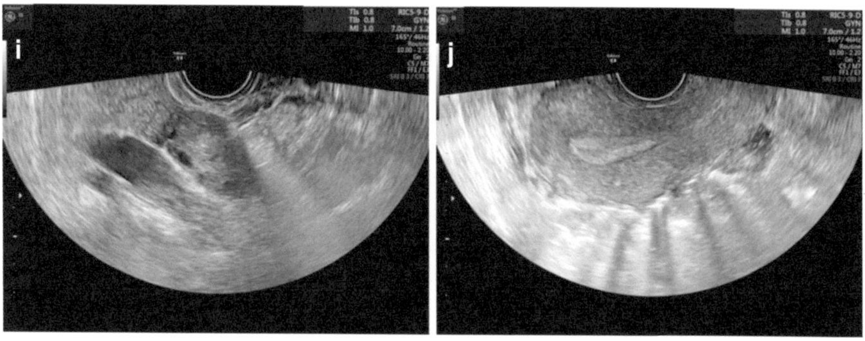

Fig. 4.9 (continued)

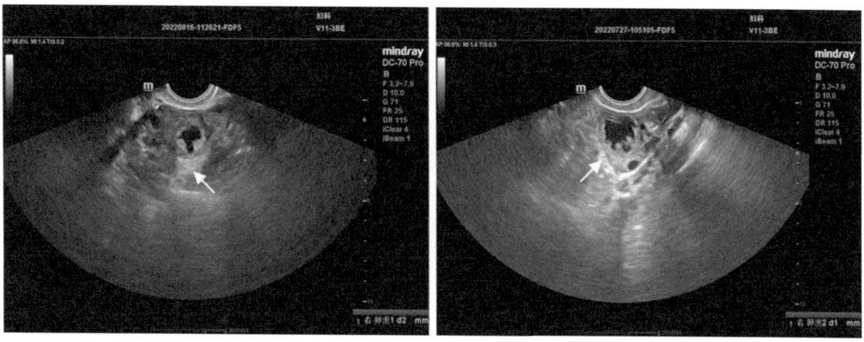

Fig. 4.10 Postovulatory imaging features of the ovary

(b) Progesterone >3 ng/mL suggests that ovulation has already occurred in the cycle.

(c) Progesterone >1.5 ng/mL, with a slight increase in estrogen, does not exclude recent ovulation. This suggests that progesterone is beginning to rise while estrogen decreases due to the expulsion of follicular fluid. To confirm the diagnosis, blood estrogen and progesterone levels should be rechecked after 3 to 5 days:

1. A continuous rise in progesterone indicates that the ovary has entered the luteal phase, confirming ovulation.
2. Little to no change in estrogen and progesterone suggests a high likelihood of follicular development failure in the current cycle.

If there is no dominant follicle in both ovaries but the endometrium is thickened with typical secretory changes (homogeneous hyperechogenic endometrium), it suggests that ovulation is more likely to have occurred in the current cycle, based on the patient's menstrual history. This can be further confirmed by blood estrogen and progesterone tests.

5. Luteinized Unruptured Follicle Syndrome (LUFS)

LUFS is defined as a mature follicle that does not rupture within 48 h after the LH peak. LH stimulates the granulosa cells in the follicle to luteinize and begin secreting progesterone. A range of clinical manifestations similar to those observed during a normal ovulatory cycle can occur due to the effects of progesterone. These include secretory changes in the endometrium, a biphasic basal body temperature, cervical mucus exhibiting normal ovulatory changes, and a regular menstrual cycle—leading to a false impression that ovulation has occurred. However, in LUFS, normal fertilization cannot occur despite the presence of an unruptured follicle.

The pathogenesis of LUFS is primarily attributed to a combination of endocrine and mechanical factors. Endocrine factors include dysfunction or deficiency of prostaglandin synthetase in the ovary, a diminished LH peak, insufficient progesterone secretion during peri-ovulation, hyperprolactinemia, or abnormal pituitary function [27]. Mechanical factors include pelvic adhesions, endometriosis, and thickening of the tunica albuginea, which can prevent follicular rupture [27]. Medically induced LUFS may also occur due to clomiphene-induced ovulation (as the anti-estrogenic effects of clomiphene lower LH peak levels) or incorrect timing of the hCG trigger.

The diagnosis of LUFS is primarily based on ultrasound monitoring. However, it must be differentiated from a corpus luteum or hemorrhagic corpus luteum. In terms of the course of events, LUFS lacks the obvious postovulatory signs seen in a corpus luteum or hemorrhagic corpus luteum. Therefore, daily ultrasonography should be performed a few days before ovulation for differential diagnosis. A normal corpus luteum is characterized by significant shrinkage or disappearance of the mature follicle, followed by enlargement during ovulation. In contrast, patients with LUFS experience no ovulation, with rapid and continuous enlargement of the follicle (without rupture). Hemorrhagic corpus luteum typically arises on the seventh to eighth day after ovulation, as luteal function peaks at this time, making luteal vessels prone to rupture and causing intracystic hemorrhage. Thus, hemorrhagic corpus luteum often occurs in the mid-luteal phase, secondary to trauma or strenuous physical activities (Fig. 4.11).

However, continuous daily monitoring can be challenging to implement in clinical practice. In some patients who develop a luteinizing cyst after ovulation, distinguishing between a corpus luteum formed after ovulation and LUFS can be challenging. There have also been occasional reports of spontaneous conception in patients newly diagnosed with LUFS. In such cases, observing whether a dark fluid area is present around the ovary or in the recto-uterine pouch can serve as a clue for determining whether ovulation has occurred.

The first step in treating LUFS is to address the underlying primary disease, either medically or surgically, such as hyperprolactinemia or endometriosis. Not all LUFS cases persist for several months in a row. If LUFS is detected during routine ovulation monitoring, intervention can be initiated in the subsequent menstrual cycle. For patients with LUFS, ovulation can be induced with medication once a mature follicle is present. The commonly used drug regimen includes high-dose hCG, low-dose progesterone injection, and oral dexamethasone.

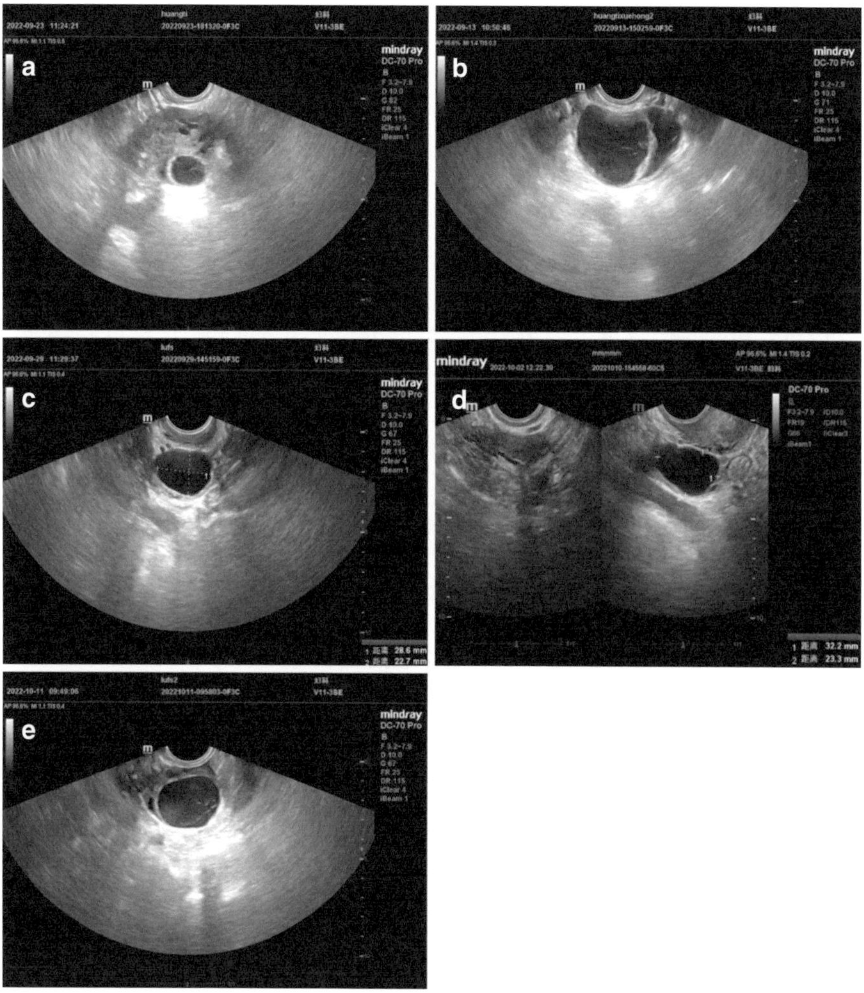

Fig. 4.11 (**a**) Corpus luteum after ovulation. (**b**) Hemorrhagic corpus luteum. (**c**) A patient with DOR and a 30-day menstrual cycle. The follicle diameter was monitored on day 15 of the menstrual cycle, measuring 18 mm. The patient was instructed to have intercourse on that day. Upon recheck on day 19 of the menstrual cycle, it was found that the follicle had not ovulated and had enlarged to 28 mm × 23 mm. (**d**) For the same patient upon recheck on day 22 of the menstrual cycle, it was found that the follicle had not ovulated and had enlarged to 32 mm × 23 mm. (**e**) For the same patient a repeat ultrasound on day 29 of the menstrual cycle revealed further increase in follicular diameter with decreased translucency and a few flocculent echoes, suggesting a suspected diagnosis of LUFS

The mechanism is as follows:

Intramuscular injection of 5000 IU to 10,000 IU hCG stimulates a natural-like LH peak. A small dose of progesterone is essential for follicular rupture, which is why 5 mg of progesterone is supplemented by intramuscular injection when the follicle reaches maturity. Dexamethasone reduces androgen secretion from the adrenal glands and improves the follicular microenvironment, increasing the follicle's responsiveness to gonadotropins. Therefore, patients with LUFS are given oral dexamethasone at a dose of 0.5 mg/day from the first day of menstruation until ovulation occurs [28].

It has been reported that transvaginal ultrasound-guided follicular puncture can mechanically rupture the follicle for ovulation while also decreasing blood androgen levels. This, in turn, alleviates the inhibition of follicular maturation by androgens [29]. Additionally, artificial insemination immediately following follicle puncture can increase the chances of conception in patients with LUFS. However, as an invasive procedure, follicular puncture may increase the risk of infection and bleeding and should be approached with caution in clinical practice.

Another proposed method is to localize the dominant follicle using transvaginal ultrasound, followed by external manipulation of the patient's abdomen to rupture the follicle using applied pressure. However, this approach may cause significant discomfort for the patient, and its safety and efficacy require further validation. In patients with recurrent LUFS, IVF-ET-assisted pregnancy (egg retrieval via direct puncture) may be considered. Some patients with LUFS may have functional defects in the follicular granulosa cells, leading to luteal insufficiency. In these cases, additional luteal support therapy is required after ovulation.

6. Small Follicle Ovulation and Atrophy

Small follicle ovulation, an abnormal type of ovulation, occurs due to insufficient secretion of pituitary gonadotropins or an early LH peak. This results in the follicle failing to develop and mature, leading to follicular atrophy or premature ovulation. In the small follicle ovulation cycle, the follicle diameter and growth rate are significantly smaller than in a normal cycle, with poor follicular development and cessation of growth at a certain point. Follicular maldevelopment leads to impaired fertilization capacity of the oocyte. Even if the oocyte is fertilized and implanted, the embryo's differentiation and development may be compromised, resulting in infertility or recurrent miscarriages [30]. The incidence of follicular maldevelopment in infertile patients has been reported to be between 16.5% and 29.6% [27].

There is no consensus on the diagnostic criteria for small follicle ovulation, although an average follicle diameter of ≥18 mm is commonly used as a marker of follicular maturity in clinical practice. If a small follicle is found to ovulate during follicular monitoring, subsequent pregnancy should be avoided.

Ovulation induction therapy can increase pregnancy chances, improve pregnancy outcomes, and reduce the risk of spontaneous abortion in patients with small follicle ovulation. The clomiphene + HMG + hCG regimen for ovulation induction has been shown to improve pregnancy outcomes: clomiphene (which has an anti-estrogenic effect and a long half-life) depletes a large number of estrogen receptors in the hypothalamus, reducing the sensitivity of hypothalamic gonadotropin-releasing hormone neurons to circulating estrogen. This results in a reduced or absent LH peak, thereby preventing premature ovulation. HMG enhances follicle growth, making the follicle grow faster. However, clomiphene is associated with the risk of LUFS, and high-dose hCG is required to induce ovulation after the follicle matures.

4.2.2 Precautions for Ultrasonography in Ovulation Induction Cycles

The ultrasound images of follicle monitoring in ovulation induction and natural menstrual cycles are similarly characterized, but some handling differences exist. Ovulation induction therapy is initiated on the third to fifth day of the menstrual cycle, provided that the following ultrasonic characteristics are observed before starting treatment:

(a) Endometrial thickness <6 mm: The endometrium typically reduces to <6 mm by days 3–5 of menstruation. If the endometrial thickness is ≥6 mm, it should be inspected to exclude space-occupying or endometrial pathologies.
(b) Count the number of antral follicles and check for ovarian cysts: Blood estrogen and progesterone levels should be measured in the presence of persistent clear cyst(s) >1 cm. Very low levels of both estrogen and progesterone suggest a high probability of simple cysts. In such cases, ovulation induction drugs should be initiated only after the patient has been fully informed of the risks of cyst enlargement associated with the drugs and informed consent has been obtained. After two days, a repeat ultrasound and progesterone test should be performed in patients with luteal cysts ≥1 cm and blood progesterone ≥1.0 ng/mL. In most patients, the progesterone level will decrease. If not, the patient's progesterone level and luteal cyst should be monitored until the luteal cyst is absorbed before initiating ovulation induction treatment. For patients with solid or mixed ovarian cyst(s), ovulation induction should be canceled. The cyst should be monitored, and additional examinations should be conducted to exclude possible pathologies if the cyst persists.
(c) Antral follicle count: If the number of antral follicles in each ovary exceeds 8–10, it indicates the risk of OHSS and multiple pregnancies, warranting a reduction in the dosage of ovulation induction medication.

In a natural cycle, ovulation follows the onset of the LH surge. However, the definition of the onset of the LH surge has not reached a consensus. Common criteria for its onset include an increase of 1.8 to 6 times the baseline LH level, an increase of at least two or three standard deviations (SD) above the mean of preceding measurements, and an LH level reaching 30% of the amplitude of the LH surge. In a natural cycle, the median duration between the onset of the LH surge and ovulation is 33.9 h, ranging from 22 to 56 h. The ovulation occurred at 17.6 h, with a range of 16–24 h following the LH peak [31].

Ultrasound combined with blood hormone testing provides a more accurate prediction of ovulation timing. In a study involving 20 women, the detected LH peaks ranged from 31 IU/L to 95 IU/L. Based on our clinic's experience, the highest LH peak observed during ovulation exceeded 200 IU/L. Changes in progesterone levels can be used as a reference to determine whether an elevated LH value occurs before or after the LH peak. For example, if the follicle diameter is 18 mm, with blood test results showing E2 200 pg/mL, LH 18 IU/L, and P 0.6 ng/mL, the very low progesterone level indicates that LH is in the early ascending phase, and ovulation is expected to occur within the next 24 to 48 h. However, if the progesterone level, in this case, is 1.7 ng/mL, this elevated progesterone level suggests that the granulosa cells of the dominant follicle have begun to luteinize and secrete progesterone in response to the LH peak. The elevated LH value at this point indicates that LH has peaked and is now falling, signaling ovulation within the next 24 h.

The timing of hCG administration in an ovulation induction cycle must be carefully determined based on follicular development. Premature administration of hCG can lead to follicular atresia, while delayed administration can cause follicular overaging and difficulties in ovulation. Ovulation can be induced by administering hCG when the dominant follicle is ≥18 mm in diameter and the blood estrogen level corresponds to the number of follicles. The serum estrogen level should be between 180 pg/mL and 250 pg/mL per mature follicle. After hCG administration, ovulation typically occurs 30 to 40 h later.

4.2.3 Precautions for Follicle Measurement in Controlled Ovarian Hyperstimulation Cycles

In patients undergoing IVF-ET, COH is used to maximize the number of oocytes retrieved, thereby increasing the chances of obtaining euploid embryos. However, follicle measurement in COH cycles is more challenging than in ovulation induction and natural cycles. The simultaneous growth of multiple follicles causes them to compress against each other, resulting in an irregular three-dimensional follicular pattern on ultrasonography. The most accurate approach is to measure follicular volume. However, the current measurement of follicular volume by 3D ultrasound has multiple limitations and is not widely available in clinical practice.

The standard method for measuring follicle size is to take the two mutually perpendicular diameters of the largest section of the follicle. The first challenge for irregularly shaped follicular sections is selecting the appropriate diameters for measurement. The commonly used area estimation method involves choosing two perpendicular diameters that best represent the area of the section (e.g., the length and width for a square-shaped section, the midline of both sides for a triangle- or trapezoid-shaped section). Caution should be exercised to avoid using diagonal lines for measurements, as this would inevitably increase the area results.

However, the question arises: Can the maximum sectional area of an irregular 3D object accurately represent its true size? The answer is no. When compressed, the maximum cross-sectional area of an elastic spherical object is always greater than in its natural state. When multiple follicles develop simultaneously and compress each other during ovulation hyperstimulation, the measured maximum section size of a squeezed follicle is inevitably larger than its true size. This represents the second challenge of follicle measurement during COH: selecting a representative cross-section.

Measurements of follicles with highly irregular spatial structures are bound to vary between operators. Some operators follow the principle of measuring the maximum sectional area, while others choose a representative section rather than the largest one for measurement. Unfortunately, no standardized norms or principles exist for measuring such irregular follicles. In clinical practice, measurement errors can be minimized when follicle monitoring is performed by the same operator, using the same ultrasound system, and adhering to consistent measurement standards.

The maturity of the follicle is not determined solely by the absolute value of the measured follicle size but also by daily fluctuations in blood hormone levels during the late follicular phase and the day-to-day changes in follicle size.

4.3 Ultrasound in Assisted Reproductive Procedures

ART includes IVF-ET and its derivatives, as well as IUI. Surgeries and procedures involved in ART include transvaginal ultrasound-guided oocyte retrieval, transabdominal ultrasound-guided embryo transfer, and artificial insemination with either the husband's sperm or donor sperm. Ultrasound monitoring plays a crucial role throughout assisted reproductive treatments. In this section, we will discuss the surgical procedures related to assisted reproductive technology.

4.3.1 Follicle Monitoring and Timing of Operation in IUI

IUI is an assisted reproductive technique in which semen is processed in vitro via density gradient centrifugation, followed by the injection of screened, highly viable sperm into the uterine cavity of the woman during her ovulation period using a catheter (Fig. 4.12). It is widely used for indications including oligozoospermia, asthenospermia, and sexual dysfunction in male partners, as well as unexplained infertility, cervical factor infertility, endometriosis, polycystic ovary syndrome, and ovarian dysfunction in women. Preoperative tubal patency testing (at least one fallopian tube must be patent) is required in all cases. However, the pregnancy success rate of IUI, influenced by various factors, remains relatively low (between 8% and 22%) [32]. Effective ovulation monitoring and the precise timing of insemination are critical to the success of IUI.

The follicle monitoring protocol in an IUI cycle can be the same as follicle monitoring in a natural cycle or an ovulation induction cycle. Several studies have evidenced that the ovulation induction cycle improves the pregnancy rate in IUI [33]. IUI with multiple developing follicles has a higher pregnancy success rate than with only one follicle but raises the risk of ovarian overstimulation and multiple pregnancies. For patients with ovulation disorders or failure to conceive after natural cycle

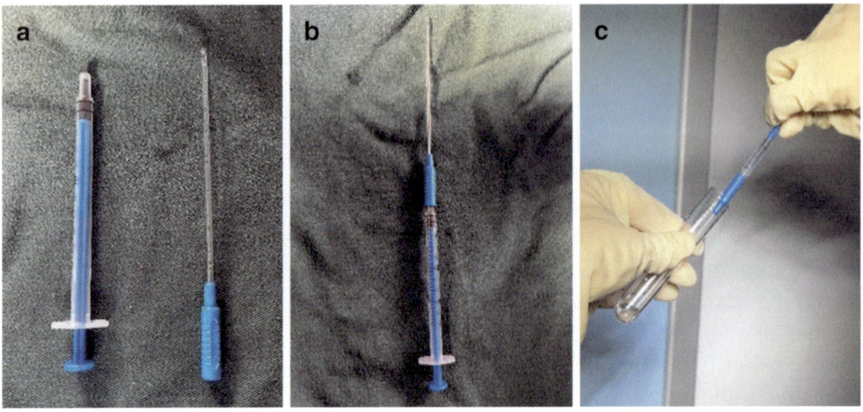

Fig. 4.12 Instruments used in IUI: (**a**) shows the artificial insemination catheter and syringe; (**b**) displays the connected catheter and syringe; and (**c**) demonstrates aspirating processed semen from a test tube through the artificial insemination catheter

IUI treatment, a mild ovulation induction regimen may be indicated, with the use of ovulation induction medications following the principle of stepwise increase in small dosages. The current treatment cycle should be aborted when more than three follicles have developed to prevent multiple pregnancies and ovarian hyperstimulation syndrome.

Concerning the choice of the number and timing of insemination, theoretically, dual IUIs (before and after ovulation) should have a higher pregnancy success rate than single IUI. This is because dual IUIs allow a certain number of motile sperm to be retained in the female uterine cavity during ovulation, increasing the chances of egg fertilization. However, most studies have shown that increasing the number of IUIs does not translate into an increase in successful pregnancy rates, with no statistically significant difference in pregnancy rates between dual insemination performed before and after ovulation and single insemination after ovulation [34]. In an ovulation induction cycle, IUI performed between 24 and 40 h after hCG administration yields the same pregnancy rate [35]. In natural cycles, the IUI procedure can be scheduled 24 h after the spontaneous LH rise [36].

In women with the uterus in an extremely anteverted or retroverted position, intrauterine intubation may be very challenging. In such cases, the patient should be instructed to relax and have a full bladder, which may reduce the cervical-uterine angle, or intubation may be attempted by pulling the cervix downward with cervical forceps. Alternatively, for patients struggling with IUI intubation, transabdominal ultrasound can be used to guide the direction of the intubation.

4.3.2 Transvaginal Ultrasound-Guided Egg Retrieval

Egg (oocyte) retrieval is a critical component of assisted reproductive procedures performed following COH. Historically, egg retrieval methods such as cesarean section, transabdominal laparoscopy, and transabdominal ultrasound-guided techniques were complex, posed significant challenges in egg collection, and caused considerable physical discomfort and pain for patients.

Transvaginal ultrasound, by positioning the transducer closer to the uterus, ovaries, and pelvic blood vessels, offers superior visualization of the pelvic organs and vasculature compared to transabdominal ultrasound. Consequently, transvaginal ultrasound-guided puncture and aspiration have become the standard method for egg retrieval.

In this procedure, a puncture needle connected to a negative-pressure suction device is secured to a transvaginal ultrasound transducer with a needle guide. The ultrasound accurately identifies the follicle's position, and follicular contents are aspirated through the puncture to retrieve the egg. This method achieves an egg acquisition rate of 80% to 90%.

This simple, convenient, safe, and minimally invasive technique enables continuous egg retrieval over multiple cycles, thereby improving the cumulative pregnancy rate for patients undergoing IVF.

1. Preparations before egg retrieval
   (a) Preoperative preparation of the patient

   The patient should undergo functional assessments of vital systems, including blood group typing, complete blood count, coagulation profile, liver and renal function tests, electrocardiogram (ECG), and chest X-ray. Screening for infectious and sexually transmitted diseases (STDs), such as acquired immunodeficiency syndrome (AIDS), vaginitis, chlamydia, and gonococcal infections, is also essential.

   Prior to the procedure, the patient should receive a thorough explanation of the process to foster positive cooperation and alleviate anxiety and nervousness. In order to minimize the risk of retrograde infections associated with egg retrieval, the patient's vagina should be disinfected using a sodium chloride solution or a 0.5% povidone-iodine solution on the day of hCG administration and the following day.

   Fasting protocols must be strictly followed for patients scheduled for general anesthesia. No food or fluids should be consumed after midnight on the night before the operation. On the day of the egg retrieval, the patient should remain fasting until the procedure is completed.

   (b) Instrument preparation

   The consumables required for the procedure include a 17 G or 18 G single- or double-lumen egg retrieval needle, test tubes, and a buffer or culture medium containing heparin and HEPES (4-(2-hydroxyethyl)-1-piperazineethanesulfonic acid). A thermostat container should be prepared in advance to hold test tubes during the procedure.

The connection of the negative pressure suction device must be verified to ensure it is secure and that the negative pressure is consistently maintained at 16 kPa (120 mmHg). A vaginal ultrasound transducer with a frequency of 5 kHz to 7.5 kHz should be disinfected by wiping it with saline.

After disinfection, a coupling agent is applied to the transducer, which is then enclosed in a sterile glove and a long plastic cover for the transducer's connecting cable. Subsequently, the puncture holder is mounted (Fig. 4.13).

2. Egg retrieval procedure
   (a) Egg retrieval is performed 34–36 h after hCG administration.
   (b) After verifying the patient's identity, the patient is placed in the lithotomy position, connected to a monitor, anesthetized, and intravenous access is established.
   (c) The surgeon washes and sterilizes their hands, dons a surgical gown and sterile gloves, and ensures that their hands do not come into contact with the puncture needle or any instruments that may come into contact with the follicular fluid.
   (d) After rinsing the vulva with saline, a sterile surgical hole towel is laid in place. The vagina is rinsed with saline until it is clean. For patients with vaginal infections, the vagina should first be disinfected with a 0.5% povidone-iodine solution, followed by multiple saline rinses to remove any iodine residue and prevent contamination of the aspirated follicular fluid.
   (e) The ultrasound transducer fitted with a needle guide is inserted into the vagina. The surgeon observes the position of the uterus and bilateral ovaries, evaluates the accessibility of the ovaries, counts the follicles to be punctured, plans the intended needle insertion route, and assesses its relationship to the pelvic organs and blood vessels.

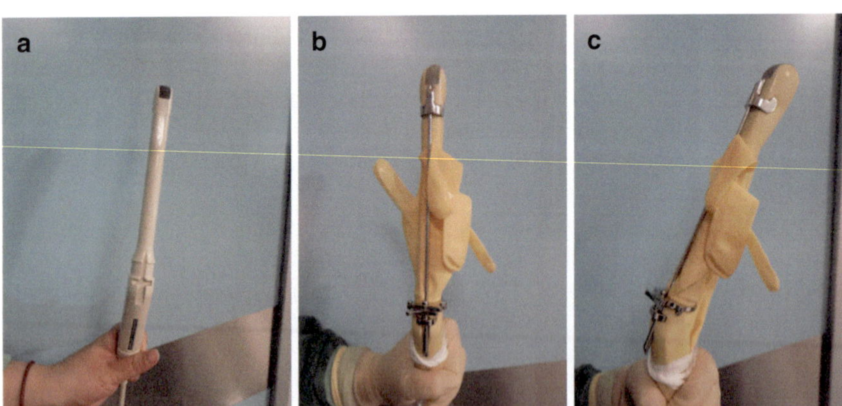

Fig. 4.13 Transvaginal ultrasound probe (transducer) prepared for egg retrieval. (**a**) The transvaginal ultrasound probe; (**b** and **c**) Mounted puncture holder, shown in front and side views, respectively

(f) Rinse the egg retrieval needle with a buffer or culture medium containing heparin and HEPES, ensuring the negative pressure system is functioning correctly, then discard the rinsing solution. Select the follicle closest to the vaginal wall for aspiration. Insert the puncture needle into the largest section of the follicle, ensuring the route avoids the vaginal blood vessels, cervix, bladder, pelvic blood vessels, and intestinal canal.

If the ovary is positioned high, an assistant may apply gentle pressure to the patient's abdomen to move the ovary closer to the ultrasound transducer. If the needle must pass through the uterus, avoid puncturing the endometrium as much as possible. Once the needle tip enters the follicle, initiate the negative pressure to aspirate the follicular fluid, fine-tuning the ultrasound transducer and slightly rotating the needle to keep its tip centered in the follicle during aspiration. Continue aspirating until the follicular fluid is completely drained and the follicular wall collapses. Rotate the needle again to gently scrape the follicular wall to ensure complete extraction of the follicular contents.

For patients with a small number of follicles, a double-lumen needle can be used to rinse the follicular cavity with culture medium after initial aspiration to increase egg retrieval yield. Test tubes containing the follicular fluid should always be stored in a thermostat container and immediately handed to the IVF laboratory technician to isolate the oocyte-corona-cumulus complexes, minimizing the risk of oocyte quality degradation due to prolonged in vitro storage.

(g) Follicles located along the same puncture route should be aspirated sequentially, from proximal to distal. Care must be taken to distinguish pelvic vascular cross-sections from follicles in the same plane. Vascular cross-sections, which may appear as ultrasound echoes similar to follicles, will transform into long tubular shapes when the ultrasound transducer is slightly rotated, preventing them from being mistaken for follicles.

After aspirating all follicles along one puncture route, retract the needle to the ovary's surface (without fully withdrawing it) while avoiding scratching the ovarian surface with the needle tip. Then, select a new puncture route to aspirate the remaining follicles sequentially. In most cases, all follicles in one ovary can be aspirated with a single puncture.

Once the puncture needle is removed from the body, it should be rinsed again with a heparin and HEPES-containing buffer or culture medium to clear any adherent oocyte-corona-cumulus complexes.

(h) Perform egg retrieval from the other ovary in the same manner. Once egg retrieval from both ovaries is complete, monitor for any signs of bleeding from the pelvic organs, including the uterus, ovaries, bladder, and retroperitoneum, as well as for active bleeding in the vagina.

In cases of active pelvic bleeding, hemostatic drugs may be administered intramuscularly to control the bleeding. For vaginal bleeding, the bleeding site can be clamped using cervical forceps, or gauze can be inserted into the vagina to apply pressure. The gauze should be removed after a few hours (Figs. 4.14 and 4.15).

(i) After egg retrieval, the patient should be monitored for 2 h. Her vital signs must be stable, and she should not experience any discomfort before being discharged from the clinic.

4.3.3 Transabdominal Ultrasound-Guided Embryo Transfer

Intrauterine embryo transfer is the process of placing in vitro-cultured embryos into the uterine cavity. It is the final and crucial step of the IVF procedure. Fresh embryo transfer is typically performed two to five days after egg retrieval. For frozen and resuscitated embryos from natural cycles, the transfer is usually performed three to five days after the LH peak, while the transfer of frozen and resuscitated embryos from artificial cycles typically occurs four to six days after hCG administration.

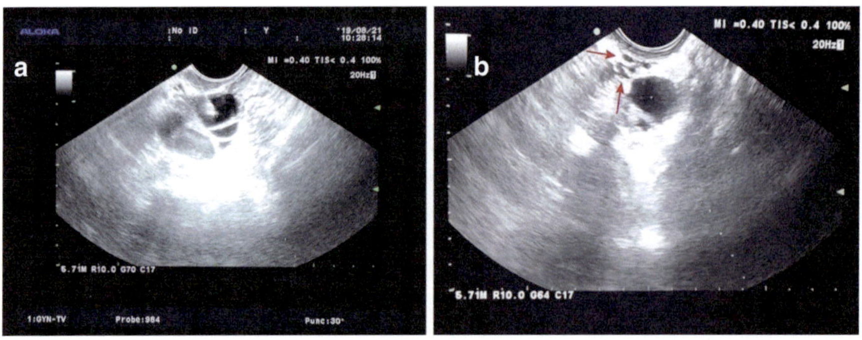

Fig. 4.14 (**a**) Selection of the puncture site. (**b**) Small anechoic areas in the vaginal wall and pelvis, which may represent blood vessels, should be avoided when inserting the puncture needle. The arrows indicate these small anechoic areas

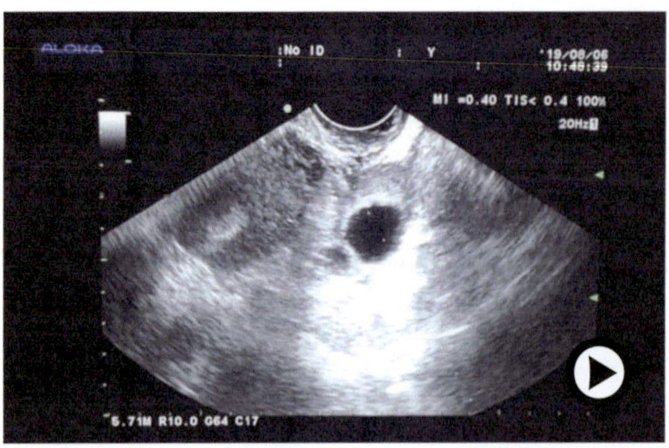

Fig. 4.15 Transvaginal ultrasound-guided egg retrieval (▶ https://doi.org/10.1007/000-hr3)

Transabdominal ultrasound-guided embryo transfer enables the operator to monitor the inclination of the uterus, facilitating the placement of the outer cannula of the transfer catheter along the cervical canal. This approach helps avoid bleeding caused by over-insertion of the outer cannula, which could damage the endometrium, while also ensuring the precise positioning of the tip of the inner transfer catheter.

1. Preoperative preparation for embryo transfer
   (a) For patients with a history of difficult embryo transfers or anticipated challenges (e.g., prior cervical conization, cervical adhesions, failed intrauterine catheterization during hysterosalpingography, overly inverted uterus, or reproductive tract malformations), a trial transfer may be performed a few days or up to one or two months before the actual procedure. The trial transfer allows the operator to assess the path of the outer cannula of the transfer catheter into the uterine cavity, which helps minimize the number of attempts during the actual embryo transfer, reduces the need for additional instruments (e.g., cervical forceps or probes), shortens the procedure time, and decreases the risk of uterine contractions and bleeding [37].
   (b) One week before the embryo transfer, the patient's vaginal discharge should be tested for potential infections.
   (c) The following equipment and instruments should be prepared: ultrasound machine, abdominal ultrasound probe, coupling agent, outer and inner cannulas of the transfer catheter, and 1 mL syringes.
   (d) The patient does not need to empty her bladder before the embryo transfer.
2. Embryo transfer procedure
   (a) The patient is placed in the lithotomy position, and a sterile drape is applied.
   (b) A speculum is inserted into the vagina to expose the cervix. The cervix is then wiped with cotton balls soaked in saline, and excess fluid is absorbed from the vagina with dry cotton balls. The mucus from the cervical canal is removed using cotton swabs dipped in a culture medium or saline to prevent it from obstructing the tip of the transfer catheter, which could cause the embryo to be retained in the catheter or expelled with the mucus during catheter withdrawal. Care should be taken to operate gently and avoid unnecessary pulling of the cervix to ensure the transfer process is as non-invasive and painless as possible.
   (c) Adjust the curvature of the transfer catheter's outer cannula according to the shape of the cervical canal and uterine cavity, as observed via transabdominal ultrasound. Gently insert the outer cannula into the cervical canal, positioning it just above the internal os to minimize irritation to the endometrium.
   (d) Insert the inner cannula, which contains the embryo and is connected to a 1 mL syringe, into the outer cannula of the transfer catheter. Slowly advance the inner cannula into the uterine cavity, positioning its tip at the target site in the mid-uterine cavity or at the best spot on the endometrium. Gently inject the embryo into the uterine cavity. According to the 2018 ASRM guidelines, the tip of the embryo transfer catheter should be placed in the

mid-uterine cavity, at least 1 cm from the uterine fundus. However, the placement should be individually assessed, and the fundus should be avoided during embryo transfer (Figs. 4.16 and 4.17).

(e) Slowly withdraw the transfer catheter while keeping the syringe in place to prevent the embryo from being aspirated back into the catheter, which could result in embryo retention. The practice of retaining the transfer catheter in the uterine cavity for a few seconds before withdrawal is controversial. However, studies have shown no statistically significant difference in pregnancy outcomes with or without this retention [37].

(f) Examine the transfer catheter under a microscope to check for retained embryos.

(g) Withdraw the speculum. The procedure is now complete. The patient can be moved from the operating room to the observation room, where she should rest for 15 to 30 min before being discharged from the clinic (Fig. 4.18).

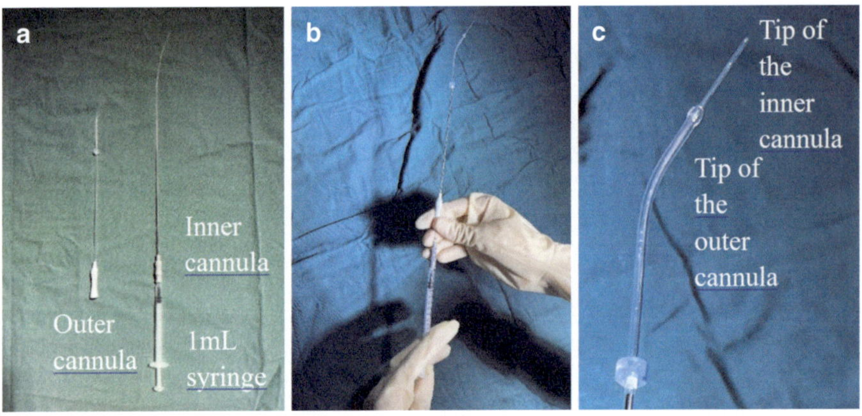

Fig. 4.16 Embryo transfer device. (**a**) The outer and inner cannula of the transfer catheter; (**b**) Insertion of the inner cannula into the outer cannula after the embryo has been aspirated into the inner cannula; (**c**) The tip of the inner cannula after it has been assembled with the outer cannula

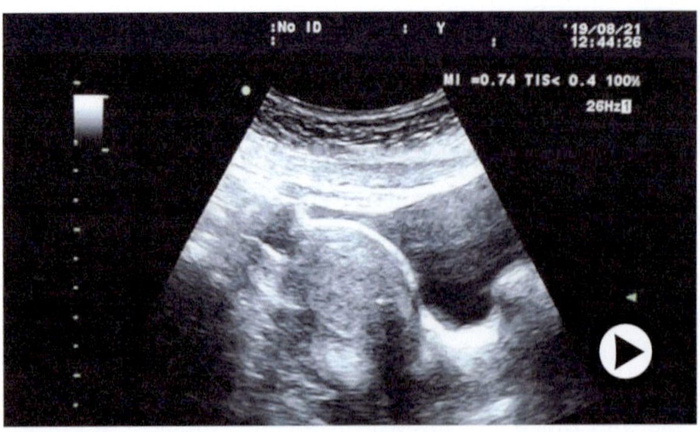

Fig. 4.17 Transabdominal ultrasound-guided embryo transfer (▶ https://doi.org/10.1007/000-hr2)

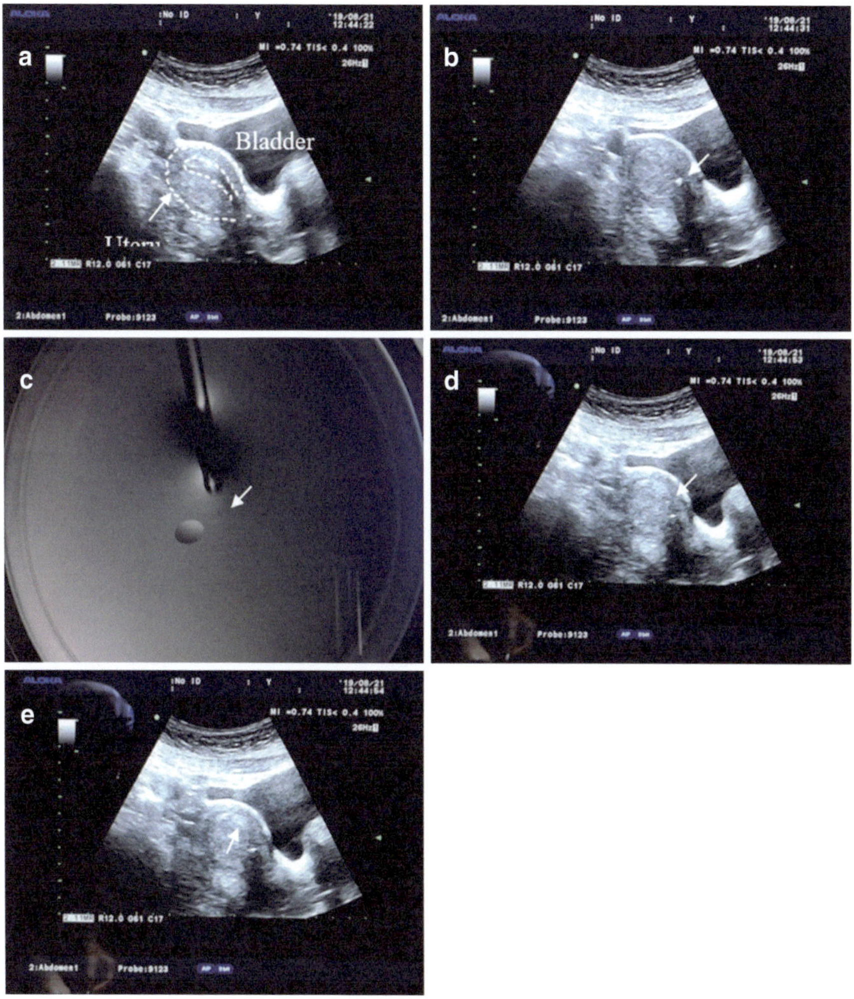

Fig. 4.18 (**a**) Transabdominal ultrasound visualization of the bladder, uterus, and endometrium. (**b**) Insertion of the outer cannula of the transfer catheter through the external os of the cervix, positioning the tip of the outer cannula just above the internal os. (**c**) Aspiration of the embryo into the inner cannula of the transfer catheter. (**d**) Insertion of the inner cannula into the outer cannula, advancing the tip of the inner cannula into the mid-upper endometrium of the uterine cavity. (**e**) Continued advancement of the inner cannula to the mid-upper uterine cavity, approximately 1 cm from the fundal endometrium, followed by gentle injection of the embryo into the cavity

4.4 Complications During Assisted Reproductive Treatment

4.4.1 Ovarian Hyperstimulation Syndrome (OHSS)

OHSS is the most common complication of ART, characterized by clinical manifestations such as abdominal distension, abdominal pain, ascites, oliguria (low urine output), anuria (absence of urine production), and hemoconcentration. Pathophysiological features include ovarian enlargement, increased vascular permeability, and, in severe cases, pleural effusion and ascites (Fig. 4.19). OHSS is categorized as mild, moderate, and severe based on the severity of symptoms [38] and as early-onset or late-onset based on the timing of onset.

(a) Early-onset OHSS occurs 3 to 7 days after hCG administration and is associated with the use of exogenous hCG. It typically lasts 7 to 10 days, is self-limiting, and, in most cases, resolves with symptomatic treatment.
(b) Late-onset OHSS occurs 12 to 17 days after hCG administration and is related to elevated endogenous hCG following pregnancy. It is often more severe, lasts longer (15–45 days), and can be more challenging to manage, especially when combined with pregnancy (Table 4.3).

Avoidance of OHSS is primarily focused on prevention. Predictors of OHSS include patient age, AFC, AMH level, BMI, the number of developed follicles, estrogen levels on the day of hCG injection, and the number of eggs retrieved. Monitoring bilateral ovarian AFC via ultrasound and measuring blood AMH levels are the most commonly used methods to assess ovarian reserve and responsiveness.

In patients at high risk for OHSS:

(a) For COH, the GnRH antagonist regimen with reduced GN dosage should be used instead of the GnRH agonist (GnRH-a) down-regulation regimen (long regimen).

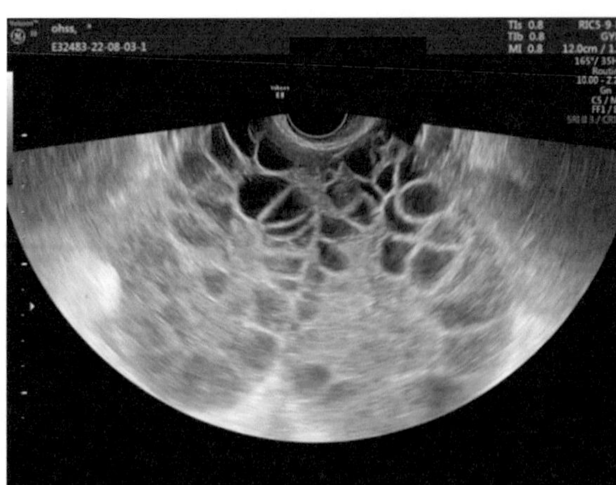

Fig. 4.19 Ovarian image of a patient with OHSS

Table 4.3 Golan classification of ovarian hyperstimulation

Severity	Grade	Clinical manifestations
Mild	Grade 1	Abdominal distension/abdominal discomfort
	Grade 2	Grade 1 manifestations + nausea, vomiting, and/or diarrhea, ovarian size 5–12 cm
Moderate	Grade 3	Features of mild OHSS + ascites on image
Severe	Grade 4	Features of moderate OHSS + clinical symptoms of ascites and/or pleural effusion and/or dyspnea
	Grade 5	Grade 4 manifestations + hemoconcentration, decreased blood volume, increased blood viscosity, coagulation abnormalities, renal hypoplasia

(b) When follicles reach maturity, GnRH-a should be used to trigger the endogenous LH peak rather than hCG, thereby reducing the risk of early-onset OHSS.
(c) After egg retrieval, a whole embryo freezing strategy should be adopted (i.e., cancel the fresh embryo transfer). While this does not entirely prevent early-onset OHSS, it helps prevent the patient's condition from worsening and the development of late-onset OHSS.
(d) Administration of an oral aromatase inhibitor (letrozole) after egg retrieval can help rapidly lower estrogen levels, eliminating the trigger for OHSS.
(e) Anticoagulant drugs may be prescribed to reduce the risk of thrombosis, provided active pelvic hemorrhage is ruled out.

Thrombosis, although rare in OHSS, is the leading cause of death in patients with severe OHSS. The major risk factors for thrombosis in ART include the following:

(a) Blood hypercoagulability due to elevated estrogen levels during COH and OHSS.
(b) Thrombophilia related to autoimmune disorders such as systemic lupus erythematosus and antiphospholipid syndrome.
(c) Decreased physical activity, a family history of thrombosis, and vascular malformations.

A detailed medical and family history is essential for patients undergoing ART, as prevention of OHSS is the key strategy for minimizing the risk of thrombosis.

4.4.2 Bleeding After Egg Retrieval

The most common emergency complication following egg retrieval is bleeding, which can occur in the vagina, ovaries, bladder, or abdominal cavity. This is often associated with coagulation disorders or injury from the puncture needle, which may scratch the surface of the ovaries or blood vessels in pelvic organs. Symptoms typically include abdominal pain, distension, nausea, and vomiting. Signs may include positive shifting dullness, abdominal tenderness, and rebound tenderness.

Retroperitoneal hemorrhage symptoms are often subtle and easily overlooked, potentially leading to shock in severe cases. Bleeding from the bladder may result in hematuria and dysuria. To minimize the risk of bleeding, patients should undergo coagulation function testing before egg retrieval and discontinue anticoagulant medications.

During the procedure, careful handling is crucial. Ultrasound imaging may reveal anechoic areas in the vaginal vault, which could indicate blood vessels in the vaginal wall. These areas should be avoided to prevent bleeding. Additionally, repeated puncturing of the vaginal wall should be avoided. The ovary should be positioned as close as possible to the vaginal wall, which can be achieved either by applying gentle downward pressure to the adnexal area with assistance or by pushing the cervix back to move the ovary downward. This technique helps guide the puncture needle into the follicle after passing through the vaginal vault and reduces the risk of injury to pelvic organs and tissues. Special care must also be taken to avoid torsion of the ovarian pedicle through gentle maneuvers.

After egg retrieval, the pelvis must be examined for active bleeding. If the bleeding is minor and slow, it can be observed for several minutes and may resolve with the body's natural clotting mechanisms. If bleeding is heavy and rapid, hemostatic drugs should be administered immediately during the procedure. The patient should remain bedridden, and her blood pressure and pulse should be closely monitored. If the patient shows signs of dizziness and pallor, intravenous access should be established immediately, and vital signs must be continuously monitored. In most cases, intra-pelvic bleeding after egg retrieval stops spontaneously and does not require surgery. However, significant and uncontrollable internal bleeding should be managed with immediate laparoscopic surgery or laparotomy, along with fluid and blood transfusions.

All patients must empty their bladder before egg retrieval to avoid bladder injury. However, the risk of bladder bleeding remains if transcystic puncture becomes necessary due to the anatomical position of the ovary or adhesions that place the ovary along the same puncture route as the bladder, with no possibility of circumvention. Immediately after the puncture needle is removed at the end of the transcystic egg retrieval, the bladder should be examined using ultrasound for active bleeding. The small puncture holes usually close quickly without causing bladder injury. If active bleeding in the bladder is detected, a urinary catheter must be inserted and kept flowing to prevent urine from filling the bladder. This will help the needle hole close and prevent persistent bleeding and blood clots. Hemostatic drugs should also be administered to stop the bleeding.

The urine bag should only be removed when the bloody urine in the bag gradually turns to clear, normal urine, and the patient should be observed for her ability to urinate independently. If the patient has blood clots in the bladder that prevent voluntary urination, a triple-lumen urethral catheter should be placed. The larger diameter of the catheter allows small clots to flow out of the bladder (Fig. 4.20). Large clots can also be flushed out by repeated bladder irrigation with sodium chloride injection. After the clots are removed by suction, the catheter should remain in place to observe changes in the urine. The nursing team at the clinic where the

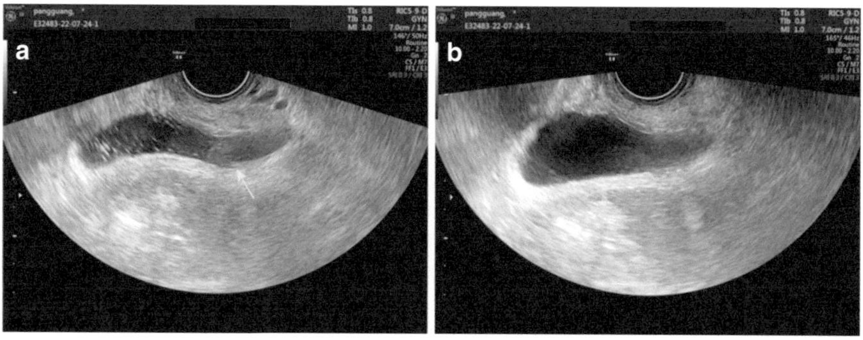

Fig. 4.20 (**a**) A small amount of bleeding and small blood clots in the bladder after egg retrieval. Although the patient urinated voluntarily several times, the clots could not be expelled (the arrow indicates the bladder). (**b**) Blood clots spontaneously flowed out of the bladder after insertion of the triple-lumen catheter, and the urine in the bladder became clear and free of clots

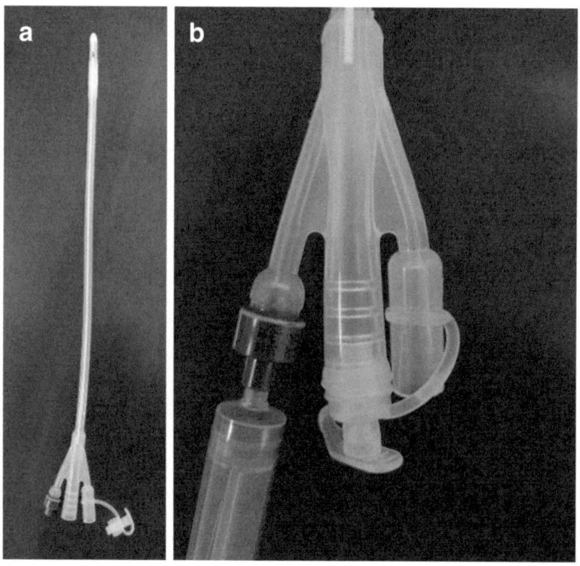

Fig. 4.21 Triple-lumen urethral catheter. (**a**) A standard triple-lumen urethral catheter: the three lumens are, from left to right, the injection port for bladder flushing, the outlet port for urine, and the balloon port. (**b**) A modified triple-lumen urethral catheter for bladder flushing: the outlet port for urine is sealed with the piston of the balloon port to prevent rapid outflow of the injected fluid. The injection port is connected to a syringe filled with saline for bladder irrigation. The tip of the urethral catheter is placed at the site of the blood clot under ultrasound guidance to aspirate it

author works has modified the triple-lumen urethral catheter, leading to more efficient aspiration of blood clots from the bladder (Fig. 4.21).

In managing bladder bleeding, care should be taken to prevent bladder filling due to patient retention of urine or catheter blockage, as this may reopen the closed needle hole and lead to continuous bleeding. Epinephrine may be added to the bladder irrigation solution to facilitate hemostasis by promoting vasoconstriction.

4.4.3 Torsion of the Ovarian Pedicle

The ovarian pedicle comprises the proper ovarian ligament, the suspensory ligament of the ovary, the fallopian tubes, and the mesosalpinx surrounding the ovary. Following COH, the increased size and uneven density of the ovary elevate the risk of ovarian pedicle torsion. This risk is further exacerbated in cases of combined OHSS. Patients with torsion of the ovarian pedicle typically present with pelvic pain and a palpable pelvic mass and may also experience nausea and vomiting.

When ovarian pedicle torsion occurs, venous reflux is initially compromised, leading to congestion and edema at the torsion site. Subsequently, arterial blood flow becomes impaired, resulting in local ischemia and necrosis, which can cause irreversible damage. Additionally, reversing adnexal torsion carries a risk of ischemia-reperfusion injury. These injuries may adversely affect ovarian reserve and future fertility [39], with prolonged torsion duration correlating with a greater decline in ovarian reserve [40]. Preventing ovarian pedicle torsion requires comprehensive patient education during COH treatment, particularly for those with OHSS. Patients should be advised to avoid strenuous physical activities or sudden changes in body position during ovulation induction and after egg retrieval to reduce the risk of adnexal torsion.

On ultrasonography, a "swirl sign" may indicate ovarian pedicle torsion. During torsion, the blood vessels, ligaments, or the fallopian tube at the pedicle twist clockwise or counterclockwise, forming an inhomogeneous mass. This mass appears as a round, oval, or tubular swirl on ultrasound, known as the "swirl sign", which is a key feature for the early diagnosis of ovarian torsion [41] (see Sect. 7.3 in Chap. 7 for additional details). The functionality of the torsioned ovary can be assessed by evaluating the blood flow signals in the torsioned pedicle and/or ovary. The presence of both arterial and venous blood flow indicates a low risk of ischemic necrosis and preserved ovarian function. If only arterial flow is detected, timely intervention can restore ovarian function in approximately 50% of cases. In contrast, the absence of blood flow signals significantly increases the risk of ischemic necrosis [41].

4.4.4 Infections

Transvaginal egg retrieval is an invasive procedure that carries a risk of retrograde infection, with the upward spread of vaginal pathogens being the primary source. The risk of pelvic infections is heightened in patients with pelvic inflammatory disorders, fallopian tube effusions, or ovarian endometriotic cysts. Additionally, repeated flushing of the follicular cavity with culture medium during egg retrieval using a double-lumen needle to enhance egg yield may increase the infection risk.

Pelvic infections typically manifest within a few days after egg retrieval but may also occur weeks or even months later [42].

Acute pelvic infections can lead to serious complications, including pelvic abscesses, sepsis, and, in severe cases, life-threatening infectious shock. Long-term effects of such infections, whether following acute recovery or chronic pelvic inflammatory conditions, can include chronic pelvic pain, infertility, or ectopic pregnancy, significantly impacting the patient's quality of life [43].

On ultrasound, a pelvic abscess is usually observed as a thick-walled cystic mass with weak dot-like echoes and stratified fluid level signs within the cystic lumen. Inflammatory cell infiltration can cause congestion and edema in the pelvic organs and tissues, often accompanied by oozing and the presence of fibro-membrane-like adhesion bands, which appear as strong band-like echoes. Diagnosis is generally straightforward when these imaging findings are correlated with the patient's clinical symptoms.

Preventing post-egg retrieval infections requires several precautionary measures, including preoperative screening of vaginal secretions for pathogens, thorough cleansing and rinsing of the vulva and vagina, minimizing the number of punctures during the procedure, and avoiding puncturing fluid-filled fallopian tubes or ovarian endometriotic cysts. Additionally, intestinal injury during the procedure should be avoided, and prophylactic antibiotics should be administered postoperatively.

If a patient develops symptoms such as abdominal pain or fever following egg retrieval, fresh embryo transfer must be canceled, and all embryos should be cryopreserved. The patient should receive prompt anti-infective and symptomatic treatment to contain and resolve the infection, thereby preventing the progression of pelvic abscesses or other complications.

In ART, estrogen and progesterone are commonly administered, with intravaginal routes being preferred in recent years, particularly for progesterone after embryo transfer. While this approach has largely replaced intramuscular administration, repeated intravaginal medication use can disrupt vaginal flora and compromise the natural vaginal barrier, increasing the risk of vaginitis during pregnancy. Patients are advised to maintain careful hygiene of the vulva and monitor changes in the appearance and odor of vaginal secretions. If abnormalities are noted, medical evaluation and testing for pathogens are recommended to prevent complications such as mid-pregnancy miscarriage or preterm labor resulting from ascending vaginal infections.

References

1. Moghadam ARE, Moghadam MT, Hemadi M, er al. Oocyte quality and aging. JBRA Assist Reprod. 2022;26(1):105–22.
2. Franasiak JM, Forman EJ, Hong KH, et al. The nature of aneuploidy with increasing age of the female partner: a review of 15,169 consecutive trophectoderm biopsies evaluated with comprehensive chromosomal screening. Fertil Steril. 2014;101(3):656–663.e1.
3. Female age-related fertility decline. Committee Opinion No. 589. Obstet Gynecol. 2014;123(3):719–21.

4. Steiner AZ, Pritchard D, Stanczyk FZ, et al. Association between biomarkers of ovarian reserve and infertility among older women of reproductive age. JAMA. 2017;318(14):1367–76.
5. Practice Committee of the American Society for Reproductive Medicine. Testing and interpreting measures of ovarian reserve: a committee opinion. Fertil Steril. 2020;114(6):1151–7.
6. Steiner AZ. Biomarkers of ovarian reserve as predictors of reproductive potential. Semin Reprod Med. 2013;31(6):437–42.
7. Arat Ö, Deveci D, Özkan ZS, et al. What is the effect of the early follicular phase FSH/LH ratio on the number of mature oocytes and embryo development? Turk J Med Sci. 2020;50(2):420–5.
8. Mukherjee T, Copperman AB, Lapinski R, et al. An elevated day three follicle-stimulating hormone: luteinizing hormone ratio (FSH:LH) in the presence of a normal day 3 FSH predicts a poor response to controlled ovarian hyperstimulation. Fertil Steril. 1996;65(3):588–93.
9. Broer SL, Broekmans FJ, Laven JS, et al. Anti-Müllerian hormone: ovarian reserve testing and its potential clinical implications. Hum Reprod Update. 2014;20(5):688–701.
10. Coelho Neto MA, Ludwin A, Borrell A, et al. Counting ovarian antral follicles by ultrasound: a practical guide. Ultrasound Obstet Gynecol. 2018;51(1):10–20.
11. Broekmans FJ, de Ziegler D, Howles CM, et al. The antral follicle count: practical recommendations for better standardization. Fertil Steril. 2010;94(3):1044–51.
12. Practice Committee of the American Society for Reproductive Medicine. Testing and interpreting measures of ovarian reserve: a committee opinion. Fertil Steril. 2015;103:e9–e17.
13. Pastore LM, Christianson MS, Stelling J, Kearns WG, Segars JH. Reproductive ovarian testing and the alphabet soup of diagnoses: DOR, POI, POF, POR, and FOR. J Assist Reprod Genet. 2018;35(1):17–23.
14. Steiner AZ, Herring AH, Kesner JS, et al. Anti-müllerian hormone as a predictor of natural fecundability in women aged 30–42 years. Obstet Gynecol. 2011;117(4):798–804.
15. Harris BS, Jukic AM, Truong T, et al. Markers of ovarian reserve as predictors of future fertility. Fertil Steril. 2023;119(1):99–106.
16. Amato P. "Ovarian reserve testing." Clinical reproductive medicine and surgery: a practical guide. Cham: Springer; 2022. p. 323–33.
17. European Society for Human Reproduction and Embryology (ESHRE) Guideline Group on POI, Webber L, Davies M, et al. ESHRE Guideline: management of women with premature ovarian insufficiency. Hum Reprod. 2016;31(5):926.
18. Chon SJ, Umair Z, Yoon MS. Premature ovarian insufficiency: past, present, and future. Front Cell Dev Biol. 2021;9:672890.
19. Katz S, Marshall J, Khorram O. An unusual case of ovarian resistance syndrome. Obstet Gynecol. 2003;101(5 Pt 2):1078–82.
20. Shulan LV, Cao Z. Insensitive ovary syndrome. Chin J Pract Gynecol Obstetr. 2006;22(5):336–8.
21. Shangold MM, Turksoy RN, Bashford RA, et al. Pregnancy following the 'insensitive ovary syndrome'. Fertil Steril. 1977;28(11):1179–81.
22. Conforti A, Esteves SC, Picarelli S, et al. Novel approaches for diagnosis and management of low prognosis patients in assisted reproductive technology: the POSEIDON concept. Panminerva Med. 2019;61:24–9.
23. Ferraretti AP, La Marca A, Fauser BC, et al. ESHRE consensus on the definition of 'poor response' to ovarian stimulation for in vitro fertilization: the Bologna criteria. Hum Reprod. 2011;26(7):1616–24.
24. Poseidon G, Alviggi C, Andersen CY, et al. A new more detailed stratification of low responders to ovarian stimulation: from a poor ovarian response to a low prognosis concept. Fertil Steril. 2016;105(6):1452–3.
25. Hayes F, Dwyer A, Pitteloud N, et al. Hypogonadotropic Hypogonadism (HH) and Gonadotropin Therapy.MDText.com, Inc. 2000.
26. Chan C, Liu K. Clinical pregnancy in a woman with idiopathic hypogonadotropic hypogonadism and low AMH: utility of ovarian reserve markers in IHH. J Assist Reprod Genet. 2014;31(10):1317–21.
27. Queenan JT, O'Brien GD, Bains LM, et al. Ultrasound scanning of ovaries at detect ovulation in women. Fertil Steril. 1980;34:99–105.

28. Lobo RA, Paul W, March CM, et al. Clomiphene and dexamethasone in women unresponsive to clomiphene alone. Obstet Gynecol. 1982;60(4):497–501.
29. Zhang J, Tang L, Kong L, et al. Ultrasound-guided transvaginal ovarian needle drilling for clomiphene-resistant polycystic ovarian syndrome in subfertile women. Cochrane Database Syst Rev. 2021;11(11):CD008583.
30. de Ziegler D, Frydman RF. Recurrent pregnancy losses, a lasting cause of infertility. Fertil Steril. 2021;115(3):531–2.
31. Erden M, Mumusoglu S, Polat M, et al. The LH surge and ovulation re-visited: a systematic review and meta-analysis and implications for true natural cycle frozen thawed embryo transfer. Hum Reprod Update. 2022;28(5):717–32.
32. Merviel P, Heraud MH, Grenier N, et al. Predictive factors for pregnancy after intrauterine insemination (IUI): an analysis of 1038 cycles and a review of the literature. Fertil Steril. 2010;93(1):79–88.
33. Khalil MR, Rasmussens PE, Erb K, et al. Homologous intrauterine insemination: an evaluation of prognostic factors based on a review of 2473 cycles. Acta Obstet Gynaecol Scand. 2001;80(1):74–81.
34. Alborzi S, Motazedian S, Parsanezhad ME, et al. Comparison of the effectiveness of single intrauterine insemination (IUI) versus double IUI per cycle in infertile patients. Fertil Steril. 2003;80(3):595–9.
35. Starosta A, Gordon CE, Hornstein MD. Predictive factors for intrauterine insemination outcomes: a review. Fertil Res Pract. 2020;6(1):23.
36. Blockeel C, Knez J, Polyzos NP, et al. Should an intrauterine insemination with donor semen be performed 1 or 2 days after the spontaneous LH rise? A prospective RCT. Hum Reprod. 2014;29:697–703.
37. Practice Committee of the American Society for Reproductive Medicine. Performing the embryo transfer: a guideline. Fertil Steril. 2017;107(4):882–96.
38. Golan A, Ron-el R, Herman A, et al. Ovarian hyperstimulation syndrome: an update review. Obstet Gynecol Surv. 1989;44:430–40.
39. Kaya C, Turgut H, Cengiz H, et al. Effect of detorsion alone and in combination with enoxaparin therapy on ovarian reserve and serum antimüllerian hormone levels in a rat ovarian torsion model. Fertil Steril. 2014;102(3):878–84.
40. Yasa C, Dural O, Bastu E, et al. Impact of laparoscopic ovarian detorsion on ovarian reserve. J Obstets Gynaecol Res. 2017;43(2):298–302.
41. Moro F, Bolomini G, Sibal M, et al. Imaging in gynecological disease (20): clinical and ultrasound characteristics of adnexal torsion. Ultrasound Obstet Gynecol. 2020;56(6):934–43.
42. El-Shawarby S, Margara R, Trew G, et al. A review of complications following transvaginal oocyte retrieval for in-vitro fertilization. Hum Fertil (Camb). 2004;7(2):127–33.
43. Brunham RC, Gottlieb SL, Paavonen J. Pelvic inflammatory disease. N Engl J Med. 2015;372(21):2039–48.

Assessment of Tubal Patency by Ultrasound

5

Da Li and Xinlu Wang

5.1 Overview

Tubal factors and ovulation disorders are among the leading causes of female infertility, alongside uterine factors, cervical factors, immune issues, and other less common causes. Tubal infertility is characterized by either a blockage of the fallopian tubes or the inability of the tubes to capture an oocyte from the ovary due to pelvic adhesions [1]. Tubal abnormalities are observed in 30–40% of women experiencing subfertility [2]. These abnormalities can affect the fallopian tubes' proximal, mid, or distal portions and often result from peritubal inflammation, abnormal tubal function, or congenital malformations [3, 4].

The severity of tubal abnormalities plays a crucial role in determining the most effective treatment approach. While laparoscopy (LSC) combined with chromopertubation and hysteroscopy is considered the gold standard for evaluating fallopian tube patency, hysterosalpingography (HSG) and hysterosalpingo-contrast sonography (HyCoSy) remain more commonly used in clinical practice [5].

The primary tests for assessing tubal patency include the following:

(a) Hydrotubation (HDT)
(b) X-ray hysterosalpingography (X-ray HSG)
(c) Hysterosalpingo-contrast sonography (HyCoSy)

Supplementary Information The online version contains supplementary material available at https://doi.org/10.1007/978-981-95-1373-4_5. The videos can be accessed individually by clicking the DOI link in the accompanying figure caption or by scanning this link with the SN More Media App.

D. Li (✉) · X. Wang
Shengjing Hospital of China Medical University, Shenyang, China
e-mail: wangxl1@sj-hospital.org

D. Li et al. (eds.), *Ultrasonography of the Female Reproductive System*,
https://doi.org/10.1007/978-981-95-1373-4_5

(d) Laparoscopy with chromopertubation ("lap and dye")
(e) Falloposcopy
(f) Computed tomography/magnetic resonance imaging hysterosalpingography (CT/MRI-HSG)

5.2 Comparison of Commonly Used Tubal Patency Tests

5.2.1 Hysterosalpingo-contrast Sonography

Nanini and colleagues first described the concept of intrauterine saline infusion during concurrent ultrasonography in 1981 [6]. Saline ultrasound has since emerged as a similarly accurate yet less invasive alternative to diagnostic hysteroscopy. Various contrast agents have gained popularity as these agents enhance the sonographic visualization of tubal patency [7].

HyCoSy is an ultrasound-guided procedure in which a contrast agent is injected into the uterine cavity and fallopian tubes through a catheter inserted into the uterus. The flow of the contrast agent is then monitored using an ultrasound transducer, allowing for the evaluation of both uterine cavity morphology and fallopian tube patency.

2D-HyCoSy enables clear visualization of the uterine cavity and the trajectory of the fallopian tubes. However, it has notable limitations, including difficulty in visualizing the entire tube within a single scanning plane and the need for significant skill and experience to perform effective follow-up scans [8].

In contrast, 3D-HyCoSy provides spatial stereoscopic images of the entire fallopian tube, enabling multiview observation of its spatial pattern. This improves the detection of significant abnormalities, reduces operator dependence [9], and shortens the time required to observe and assess tubal patency.

Real-time 3D techniques, referred to as 4D-HyCoSy, continuously display the entire process of hysterosalpingo-contrast sonography. These techniques visualize the sequential flow of the contrast agent, from its entry into the uterine cavity, then through the bilateral fallopian tubes, to its spillage from the fimbrial extremities and dispersion into the pelvic cavity. Assessment of tubal patency typically involves a comprehensive ultrasound examination based on 4D-HyCoSy, with static 3D and 2D-HyCoSy serving as supplementary techniques [10].

HyCoSy offers several advantages: it is noninvasive, safe, cost-effective, and reproducible. It does not involve radiation, nor does it carry risks of allergic reactions or embolic adverse events. The procedure demonstrates high accuracy, can potentially aid in unblocking fallopian tubes to a certain extent, and allows simultaneous visualization of the pelvis, ovaries, uterus, and other related structures or lesions.

Despite its benefits, HyCoSy results can be subject to a degree of uncertainty. The procedure requires performance by an experienced sonographer and is generally recommended as a secondary diagnostic method.

5.2.2 X-Ray Hysterosalpingography (X-Ray HSG)

X-ray HSG includes two primary techniques: hysterosalpingography (HSG) and selective salpingography (SSG).

1. HSG

   HSG remains the first-choice method for diagnosing tubal patency [11]. This diagnostic technique involves injecting a contrast agent into the uterus and fallopian tubes via a catheter, followed by obtaining X-rays or radiographs using a diagnostic X-ray device. The procedure assesses the following:
   - The patency of the fallopian tubes
   - The location of any obstruction
   - The morphology of the uterine cavity by the contrast agent's distribution in the uterus, fallopian tubes, and pelvic cavity

   HSG is also used to evaluate fallopian tube patency after surgical procedures, such as the following:
   - Re-anastomosis following tubal sterilization
   - Re-canalization of tubal blockage
   - Salpingostomy for hydrosalpinx

   Advantages of HSG

   HSG is relatively easy to perform, and both oil-based and water-based contrast agents used in this technique have been shown to offer beneficial effects in unblocking tubal obstructions [12].

   Disadvantages of HSG

   HSG has limitations, including the following:
   - Sensitivity of only 65% and specificity of 85% for diagnosing tubal patency compared to laparoscopy with chromopertubation [13]
   - Exposure to ionizing radiation
   - Risk of allergic reactions in patients sensitive to iodine
   - Inability to provide an accurate diagnosis of uterine or pelvic pathologies

2. HSG Contrast Agents

   HSG contrast agents are divided into two main categories: oil-based and water-based iodinated contrasts.

   (a) Oil-based iodinated contrasts

   These are further classified into normal iodized oils and super-liquefied iodized oils.

Advantages
- High viscosity and density
- Slow flow, producing clear images
- Ideal for assessing pelvic adhesions and cervical function [14]

Disadvantages
- Patients must return to the medical facility 24 h later for diffusion radiographs.
- If venous or lymphatic reflux occurs, the examination must be terminated to prevent oil embolism, which could potentially compromise the diagnosis.
- Slow absorption, posing a risk of granuloma formation [15, 16].
- High cost and risk of iodine allergy.

(b) Water-based iodinated contrasts

These are divided into ionic (e.g., meglucamine diatrizoate) and nonionic (e.g., Omnipaque/iohexol injection) agents.

Advantages
- Nonionic agents do not require an iodine allergy test.
- Delayed radiographs can be performed within 20 min, eliminating the need for a follow-up visit.
- The procedure can continue even in cases of venous or lymphatic reflux.
- Fast absorption and lower cost.

Disadvantages
- Lower viscosity and faster flow can complicate imaging.
- Higher diagnostic expertise is required to interpret results accurately.

3. SSG

SSG involves the insertion of a microcatheter into the opening of the fallopian tube, advancing it up to the interstitial part via the vaginal canal, cervix, uterine cavity, and uterine horn. Once in position, a contrast agent is injected. This technique helps distinguish between tubal spasm and true obstruction and is useful for clarifying conflicting results from other diagnostic tests [17].

Advantages of SSG
- High accuracy, with nearly 100% success in diagnosing tubal patency
- Effective in unblocking fallopian tube obstructions [18]

Disadvantages of SSG
- High cost
- Requires the use of disposable microcatheters
- Demands a skilled operator and involves exposure to a small amount of radiation

5.2.3 Hysteroscopy and Laparoscopy with Chromotubation

Hysteroscopy is regarded as the gold standard for intrauterine assessment and can also be used to evaluate fallopian tube patency. During hysteroscopy, the following methods are employed to assess and manage fallopian tube patency: (a) inspecting the fallopian tube opening to check for visible obstructions; (b) introducing a catheter into the fallopian tube opening and injecting a contrast agent or dye (e.g., methylene blue) to observe the flow and determine patency; (c) evaluating resistance or reflux during dye injection, where high pressure and reflux suggest possible blockage, while smooth flow without resistance or overflow indicates an unobstructed tube; and (d) treating mild blockages through therapeutic procedures such as tubal catheterization or balloon dilation to clear the obstruction.

In women with a history of pelvic infection, dysmenorrhea, or dyspareunia, laparoscopy with chromotubation is often preferred as it allows a comprehensive evaluation of pelvic organs [19]. This technique involves injecting a diluted methylene blue solution into the uterine cavity under laparoscopic visualization. Key aspects of the procedure include the following:

- Assess resistance to the injection and observe for abnormal swelling of the fallopian tubes.
- Identifying methylene blue solution flows from the fimbrial ends of the fallopian tubes into the pelvic cavity, indicating tubal patency.
- Evaluating the tubal morphology, alignment, distortion, atresia, and adhesions.
- Treating tubal obstruction, fimbrial adhesion, or other pelvic abnormalities simultaneously under laparoscopic guidance, if necessary [20].

Advantages
- Provides a definitive diagnosis with simultaneous therapeutic potential
- Allows detailed assessment of pelvic and ovarian structures and tubal morphology and adhesions

Disadvantages
- High cost of the procedure.
- Both methods are invasive and require general anesthesia.
- Associated with potential surgical complications.
- Limited in evaluating the internal structure of the fallopian tubes.
- Considered second-line diagnostic techniques.

5.2.4 Hydrotubation (HDT)

HDT is one of the earliest diagnostic methods for assessing tubal patency. This procedure involves injecting fluid into the uterine cavity via a catheter and determining tubal patency based on several factors:

- Resistance to the injection
- The volume of fluid required
- Presence or absence of reflux
- The patient's sensation during the procedure

Advantages
- Easy to perform and safe.
- Requires no specialized equipment.
- Cost-effective [21].
- It may offer therapeutic benefits for fallopian tubes with mild obstruction or insufficient patency.

Disadvantages
- Lacks objective diagnostic indicators and relies heavily on subjective judgment, leading to potential missed or false diagnoses
- A blind procedure that provides only a general assessment of tubal patency
- Cannot differentiate between unilateral and bilateral patency or identify the specific location of a blockage

5.2.5 Falloposcopy

Falloposcopy is a diagnostic technique that provides a direct view of the inner mucosa of the fallopian tubes. Depending on the access route, fluoroscopy can be performed via open surgery, laparoscopic surgery, or hysteroscopic surgery. However, due to its complexity and limitations, it is not commonly used as a routine screening method.

Advantages
- Offers detailed visualization of the inner mucosa of the fallopian tubes, which is not achievable with other diagnostic methods [22]

Disadvantages
- Expensive and resource-intensive
- Technically challenging to perform, requiring significant expertise
- Carries a risk of causing injuries to the tubal mucosa

5.2.6 CT/MRI Hysterosalpingography (CT/MRI-HSG)

1. CT-Hysterosalpingography (CT-HSG)

   CT-HSG is performed using a multidetector CT (MDCT) device. Modern MDCT devices with over 64 detectors can perform scans within 5 s, offering high temporal, spatial, and density resolution. Advanced 320-detector and 512-detector MDCT systems can complete scans in as little as 1 s. The technique operates on principles similar to X-HSG, utilizing a diluted nonionic iodinated water-based contrast agent. CT-HSG enables the acquisition of dynamic real-time data, tracking the diffusion of the contrast agent through the fallopian tubes into the pelvic cavity. However, it is not commonly used as a routine diagnostic test for tubal patency.

Advantages of CT-HSG

- Provides comprehensive and direct visualization of pathologies in the uterus, fallopian tubes, ovaries, and pelvic structures
- Offers superior image resolution compared to X-HSG
- Demonstrates higher diagnostic accuracy than X-HSG [23]

Disadvantages of CT-HSG

- High cost
- Risk of allergic reactions to iodinated contrast agents
- Involves modest exposure to ionizing radiation

2. MRI-Hysterosalpingography (MRI-HSG)

MRI-HSG involves an initial multisequence scan of the pelvis, followed by the intrauterine injection of a contrast agent to visualize the uterine cavity and fallopian tubes. Diagnosis is based on observing the morphology of the fallopian tubes, the smoothness of contrast agent passage, and its diffusion into the pelvic cavity during multitemporal scans.

Currently, the most widely used MRI-HSG techniques are

- Magnetic Resonance Hydrography (MRH): Utilizes fluid signals to assess tubal patency
- Contrast-Enhanced Magnetic Resonance Angiography (CE-MRA): Offers clearer visualization of tubal morphology by reducing interference from uterine and pelvic cavity fluid

The contrast media commonly used include saline or gadopentetate dextran solution diluted at a ratio of 1:20 in saline. Among these methods, CE-MRA is preferred due to its superior clarity and diagnostic accuracy. Despite its diagnostic potential, MRI-HSG has limited applications in routine clinical practice.

Advantages of MRI-HSG

- Noninvasive and free of radiation exposure
- Provides high-resolution imaging of soft tissues
- Simultaneously visualizes pelvic structures, including the ovaries, uterus, cervix, and vagina, with exceptional clarity [24]
- Demonstrates high diagnostic concordance with laparoscopy

Disadvantages of MRI-HSG
- Relatively high cost
- Long examination time [25]

5.3 4D HyCoSy

5.3.1 General Aspects of the Examination

1. Indications
   4D HyCoSy is indicated for
   (a) Assessment of female infertility: This should include evaluating tubal patency and identifying pathologies affecting the uterus, fallopian tubes, and ovaries, as well as detecting pelvic adhesions.
   (b) Posttreatment evaluation: Assess the efficacy of interventions such as tubal repair, re-canalization, plastic surgery, and treatments for tubal pregnancy.
2. Contraindications
   4D HyCoSy is contraindicated in the following conditions:
   (a) Infections: Acute or subacute infections of the reproductive tract or active tuberculosis
   (b) Menstruation or bleeding: Ongoing menstruation or vaginal bleeding
   (c) Unconfirmed pregnancy: If pregnancy has not been definitively ruled out
   (d) Postsurgical recovery: Within 8 weeks of pelvic surgery or 6 weeks of abortion or other intrauterine procedures
   (e) Malignancy: Known malignant tumors of the reproductive tract
   (f) Systemic conditions: Fever exceeding 37.5 °C or severe systemic illnesses, rendering the patient unable to tolerate the examination
   (g) Allergies: Known hypersensitivity to microbubble contrast agents
3. Timing of the Examination
   For optimal diagnostic results, 4D HyCoSy should be performed during the follicular phase, also known as the endometrial proliferation phase.
4. Preparations prior to contrast injection
   (a) Patient Preparation
   - Routine examinations: Conduct a blood cell count, coagulation function tests, infectious disease screening, vaginal secretion analysis, and an electrocardiogram (ECG) before the contrast imaging procedure.
   - Pregnancy exclusion: Confirm that the patient is not pregnant. Patients should avoid sexual intercourse from the end of their last menstruation until the time of the examination.
   - Bladder emptying: Instruct the patient to empty her bladder before the procedure.
   - Fasting: Fasting is not required for this procedure.

(b) Medical History and Consent
- Take a detailed medical history and ensure that the patient understands the procedure.
- Obtain informed consent signed by the patient.
- If necessary, consider administering antispasmodic or analgesic medications to improve patient's comfort during the procedure.

(c) Instrumentation and Adjustment
- Ultrasound equipment: Use a Color Doppler ultrasound system with contrast imaging capabilities, such as the GE Voluson E6, E8, or E10 models.
- Transducer specifications: Employ a transvaginal volume transducer (e.g., RIC5-9-D model) with a frequency range of 5–9 MHz and a mechanical index of 0.11–0.15.

5. Intrauterine catheterization

(a) Procedure

Step 1: Patient preparation:
- Position the patient in the lithotomy position.
- Perform routine sterilization of the vulva and thighs.
- Place a sterile surgical drape over the patient.

Step 2: Speculum placement and cervical preparation:
- Insert a speculum to expose the cervix.
- Sterilize the vagina and the external cervical orifice.

Step 3: Catheter preparation:
- Verify the balloon's sealing integrity on the angiographic catheter.
- Use a #12 double-lumen catheter for the procedure.
- Expel any air trapped in the catheter to ensure proper function.

Step 4: Catheter placement:
- Gently insert the catheter into the uterine cavity.
- Inflate the balloon by injecting 1–3 mL of saline, adjusting the volume based on the cervical laxity.
- Gently pull the catheter to seal the internal cervical orifice.

Step 5: Final step
- Carefully remove the speculum to avoid dislodging the catheter.

(b) Precautions
- Maintain strict aseptic conditions throughout the procedure to minimize infection risk.
- Perform all actions delicately, avoiding forceful manipulations that could lead to bleeding or vasovagal reactions.
- For patients with anomalies (e.g., double uterus or complete uterine septum), insert separate catheters into each uterine cavity as appropriate.

5.3.2 General Flow of HyCoSy

HyCoSy employs a classification method for tubal patency status, which typically includes categories such as patency, obstruction, or uncertain [26]. However, in

China, the classification system is more detailed and includes patency, partial patency, and complete obstruction. In cases of complete bilateral tubal obstruction, patients are advised to consider in vitro fertilization-embryo transfer (IVF-ET) as a treatment option [1].

Further differentiation of tubal obstruction is possible through laparoscopic chromopertubation, where the site of blockage is categorized as follows:

- Proximal Tubal Obstruction: Diagnosed when there is no passage of dye beyond the isthmus of the fallopian tube
- Distal Tubal Obstruction: Diagnosed when dye extends beyond the ampulla but fails to reach the infundibulum of the fallopian tube [27]

In China, two primary workflows are followed for HyCoSy, depending on the sequence of salpingo-contrast ultrasound and saline infusion sonohysterography (SIS) (Fig. 5.1):

Flow 1: Salpingo-contrast ultrasound before SIS

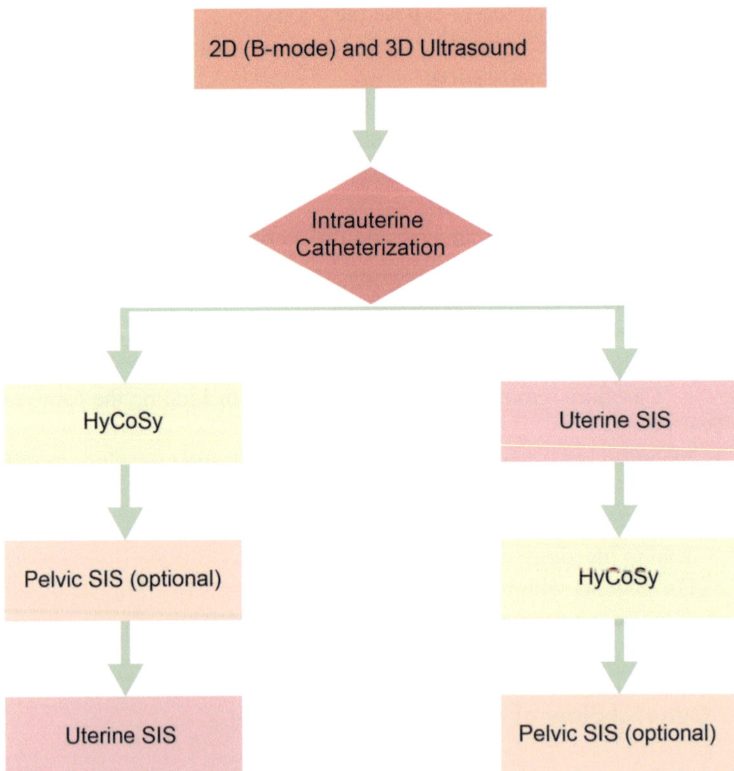

Fig. 5.1 The "one-stop solution" HyCoSy procedure

1. Sequence:
   - Perform salpingo-contrast ultrasound first.
   - Conduct SIS afterward.
2. Advantages:
   - Allows evaluation of the primordial status of the fallopian tubes without prior disturbance from SIS
3. Disadvantages:
   - Requires repeated rinsing of the uterine cavity to reduce the impact of residual microbubbles, which could hinder intrauterine visualization during the subsequent SIS session

Flow 2: Salpingo-Contrast Ultrasound After SIS

1. Sequence:
   - Perform SIS first.
   - Follow with salpingo-contrast ultrasound.
2. Advantages:
   - Eliminates interference from microbubbles during SIS, ensuring high-quality imaging of the uterine cavity
   - Facilitates better 3D visualization of the relative spatial position of the contrast catheter within the uterine cavity, reducing the likelihood of false-positive results caused by improper catheter placement

When the primary purpose is evaluating tubal patency, Flow 1 is recommended, with the following step-by-step procedure for HyCoSy:

1. Routine 2D and 3D ultrasonography
   (a) Observe the uterus, bilateral adnexa, and pelvis

   Put the transvaginal probe into a sterilized cover and insert it into the vagina to
   - Observe the thickness of the endometrium.
   - Look for any intrauterine lesions or malformations.
   - Assess for lesions of the uterus, ovaries, and fallopian tubes.
   - Examine the echogenicity of the uterine serosa (noting whether calcification is present).
   - Check for fluid accumulation or any strip-like echoes in the pelvic cavity.

   (b) Adjust the size and position of the water balloon

   The position of the contrast catheter and the size of the water balloon significantly affect both the procedure and results.

   Oversized water balloon:
   - May cause discomfort and pain due to excessive pressure on the uterine cavity
   - Increases the likelihood of contrast reflux or tubal spasms

Undersized water balloon:

- Prone to catheter dislodgement, which may compromise the procedure

Optimal size and position of the water balloon:

- The water balloon should match the uterine cavity's dimensions and the cervix's elasticity.
- Ideal Proportions: The balloon's upper and lower diameters should account for 1/3 to 1/2 of the uterine cavity length.
- The lower edge of the balloon should align with the internal cervical os.
- The balloon should be either spherical or ellipsoidal.
- The catheter should be gently pulled to ensure that the balloon is not dislodged, and the catheter tip should avoid positioning in the uterine horns (as shown in Figs. 5.2, 5.3, and 5.4).

(c) Position of the uterus and ovaries and the sliding sign

Observe the position of the ovaries in relation to the uterus and predetermine the area of tubal alignment. Gently manipulate the uterus and ovaries with the probe or apply gentle pressure on the patient's lower abdomen with a hand to observe any sliding of the uterus or ovaries relative to the surrounding tissues. During this process, the patient should be questioned about any tenderness (as shown in Figs. 5.5 and 5.6).

- Sliding sign (+): The presence of relative movement between the uterus, ovaries, and surrounding tissues indicates a positive sliding sign, suggesting no adhesions.
- Sliding sign (−): Poor mobility or the absence of sliding may indicate the presence of adhesions. This requires further investigation for conditions such as pelvic infection or endometriosis.

2. Real-time 3D contrast ultrasonography

(a) Initial preparation and positioning

The procedure begins with a 3D trial scan to identify the contrast plane and determine the best position for visualizing the uterine horns and fallopian tubes. The goal is to include the uterine cavity and both ovaries within

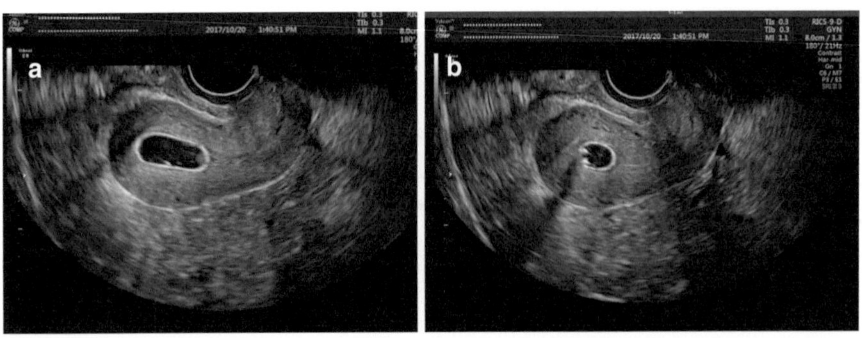

Fig. 5.2 (**a**) Adjusting balloon size. Before adjustment, the balloon occupied the entire uterine cavity. (**b**) After adjustment, the balloon occupied 1/3 of the uterine cavity

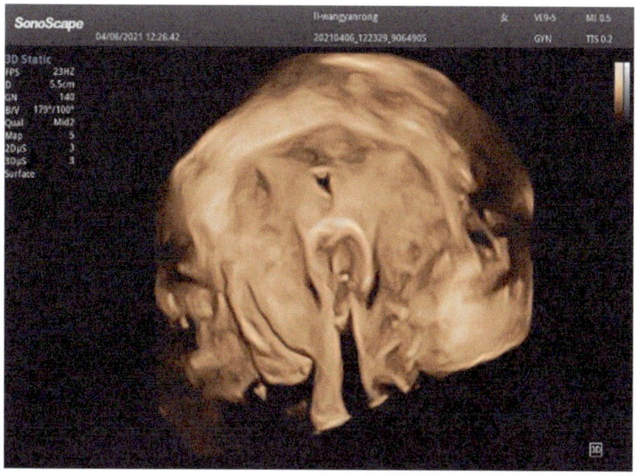

Fig. 5.3 3D imaging demonstrates a balloon with a proper position and size. The lower edge of the balloon was at the level of the internal cervical os

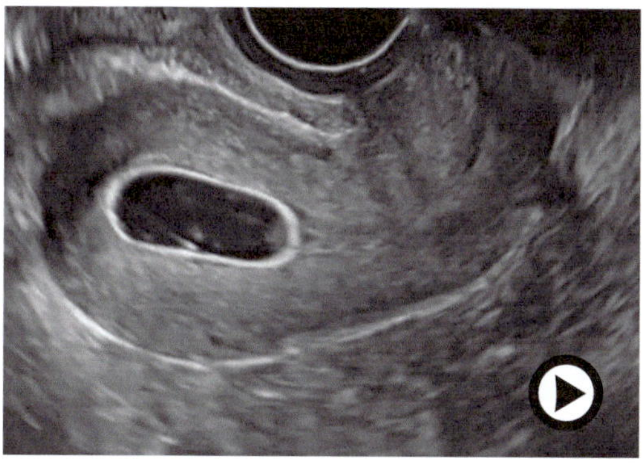

Fig. 5.4 Adjusting the balloon size (▶ https://doi.org/10.1007/000-hrs)

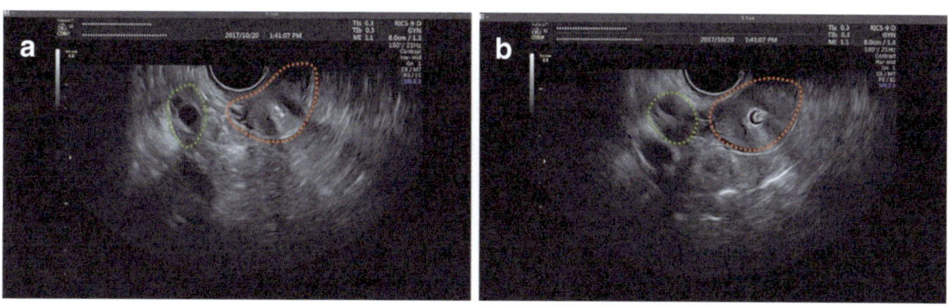

Fig. 5.5 (**a**) Ovarian and uterine mobility before pressure application (ovary circled in green, uterus circled in orange). (**b**) Ovarian and uterine mobility after pressure application (ovary circled in green, uterus circled in orange)

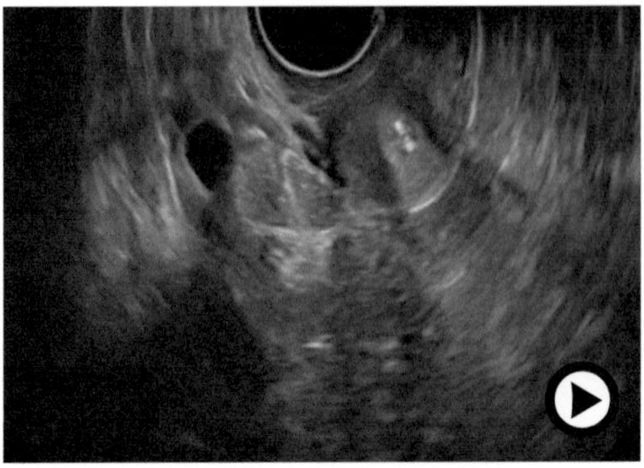

Fig. 5.6 Sliding sign (+) (▶ https://doi.org/10.1007/000-hr5)

the volume scan. If it is not possible to capture both uterine horns and ovaries simultaneously, the contrast procedure can be performed separately on each side.

Transvaginal ultrasonography is typically used, with the uterus positioned in either an anteverted or retroverted orientation to improve tubal visualization. If the uterus is positioned too horizontally, causing the uterine horns to appear in the far field and making tubal imaging difficult, transabdominal ultrasonography may be considered as an alternative. To ensure optimal imaging, adjust the contrast settings, maximize the image frame, and minimize background noise.

(b) Performing the contrast procedure

Activate the 4D contrast mode and have an assistant slowly administer the contrast agent or operate the delivery device. Carefully observe the process, starting with the injection of the contrast agent into the uterus and continuing until the agent diffuses into the pelvis.

The timing of image acquisition is influenced by the level of fallopian tube patency and the patient's tolerance. Typically, imaging begins when the contrast catheter is visible and continues until a stable diffusion image of the pelvis is achieved. In cases of partial or complete fallopian tube obstruction, imaging may need to stop if the patient experiences significant discomfort or if uterine cavity pressure exceeds safety limits.

After obtaining satisfactory images, save the video recordings for review (refer to Figs. 5.7 and 5.8).

(c) (Optional) high-resolution imaging

For additional details, high-resolution static 3D ultrasonograms of the fallopian tubes can be captured. To ensure precise visualization, acquire volume images of the left and right fallopian tubes separately.

3. Real-time 2D contrast ultrasonography

Real-time 2D contrast ultrasonography utilizes multimodal imaging, often performed in dual-frame mode, for enhanced visualization and comparison.

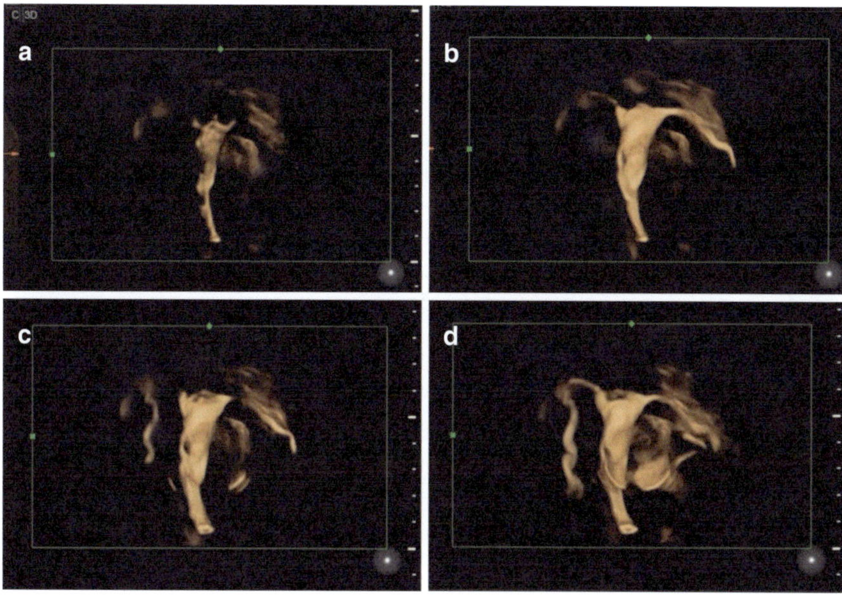

Fig. 5.7 (**a**) Visualization of the uterine cavity in real-time 3D contrast image of multiple time phases. (**b**) Visualization of the proximal fallopian tube. (**c**) Visualization of the distal fallopian tube. (**d**) Pelvic diffusion

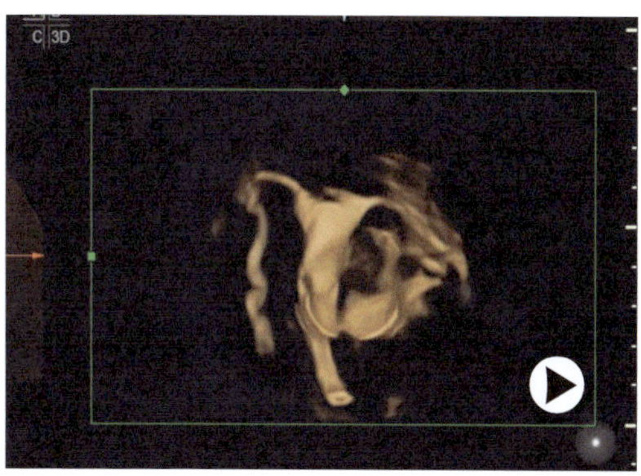

Fig. 5.8 Real-time 3D contrast ultrasonography procedure (▶ https://doi.org/10.1007/000-hr6)

(a) 2D observation in contrast mode

Begin by tracing the trajectory of the fallopian tubes in contrast mode (refer to Figs. 5.9, 5.10, and 5.11). Focus on evaluating the fluidity of the contrast agent, paying close attention to how it flows around the periovarian region and disperses throughout the pelvis (refer to Fig. 5.12).

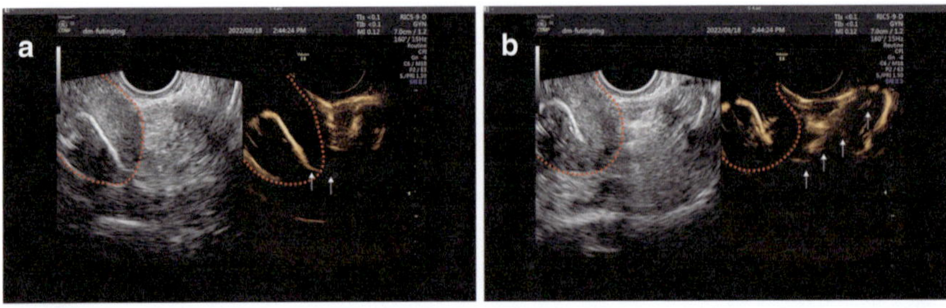

Fig. 5.9 (**a**) Visualization of the left fallopian tube trajectory. The proximal segment of the left fallopian tube was shown (uterus outlined in orange; arrows indicate the tubal trajectory). (**b**) Visualization of the left fallopian tube trajectory. The distal segment of the left fallopian tube was shown (uterus outlined in orange; arrows indicate the tubal trajectory)

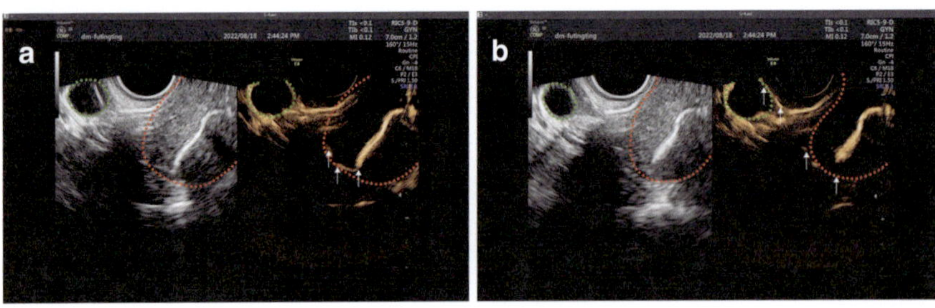

Fig. 5.10 (**a**) Visualization of the right fallopian tube trajectory. The proximal segment of the right fallopian tube is shown (uterus outlined in orange; right ovary outlined in green; arrows indicate the tubal trajectory). (**b**) Visualization of the right fallopian tube trajectory. The distal segment of the right fallopian tube is shown (uterus outlined in orange; right ovary outlined in green; arrows indicate the tubal trajectory)

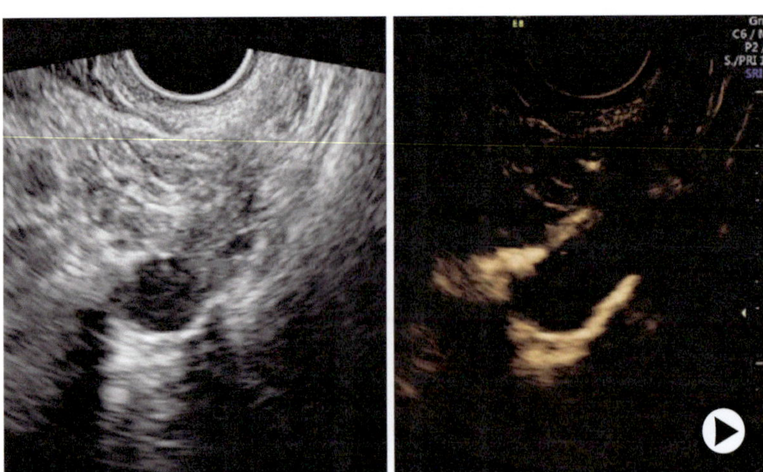

Fig. 5.11 Visualization of the tubal trajectory (▶ https://doi.org/10.1007/000-hr7)

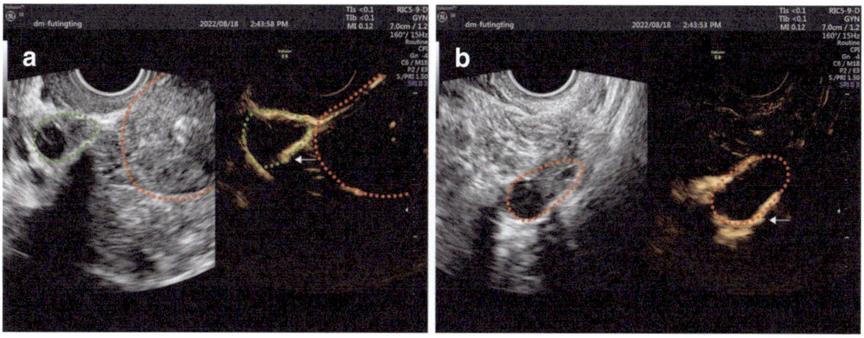

Fig. 5.12 (**a**) The right ovary enveloped by contrast agent. The uterus is outlined in orange, and the right ovary is outlined in green. Strong echoes (indicated by the arrow) represent the contrast agent surrounding the ovary. (**b**) The left ovary enveloped by contrast agent. The left ovary is outlined in orange. Strong echoes (indicated by the arrow) represent the contrast agent surrounding the ovary

(b) B-mode or color doppler mode

Switch to B-mode or color Doppler mode to observe the contrast agent in relation to surrounding anatomical structures. Track the agent's trajectory within the fallopian tubes, ensuring detailed evaluation of the following:

- The presence of dilatation in the fallopian tubes
- The morphology of the fimbrial part
- The echogenicity of the tubal wall

This step provides critical complementary information to the previously assessed contrast patterns (refer to Figs. 5.13, 5.14, 5.15, and 5.16).

4. Pelvic SIS

Pelvic SIS is performed by continuing the injection of 50–200 mL of 0.9% saline through the original contrast catheter. The anechoic fluid can be visualized by ultrasound as it enters the pelvis through the fallopian tubes and accumulates in the pelvic cavity. SIS effectively demonstrates the movement of the tubal fimbriae, revealing whether they are swinging freely or are restricted (refer to Figs. 5.17 and 5.18).

Additionally, SIS allows for the identification of strip-like or abnormal mass echoes within the pelvis. However, this examination may only be successfully performed in some patients due to varying degrees of tubal patency.

5. Uterine SIS

(a) Reduction of the balloon:

The fluid in the balloon should be reduced to 0.5–1.0 mL to obtain a clear view of the uterine cavity while preventing the catheter from dislodging. The upper and lower diameters of the balloon should account for approximately 1/5 to 1/4 of the length of the uterine cavity.

(b) 2D negative contrast

The uterine cavity is repeatedly rinsed by injecting saline through the catheter. This procedure minimizes residual microbubbles' impact on the

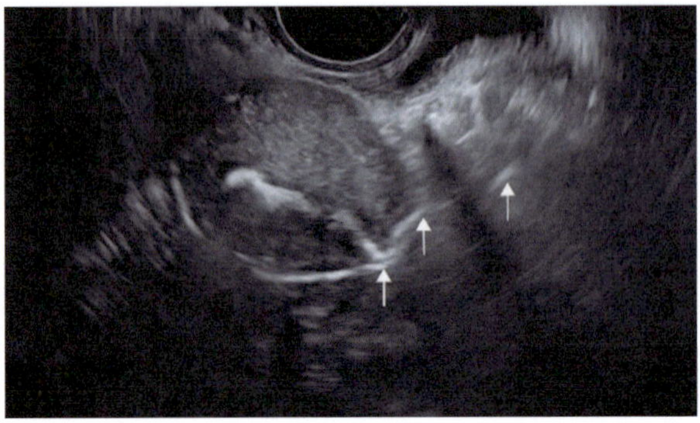

Fig. 5.13 B-mode visualization of the fallopian tube. Arrows indicate the tubal trajectory

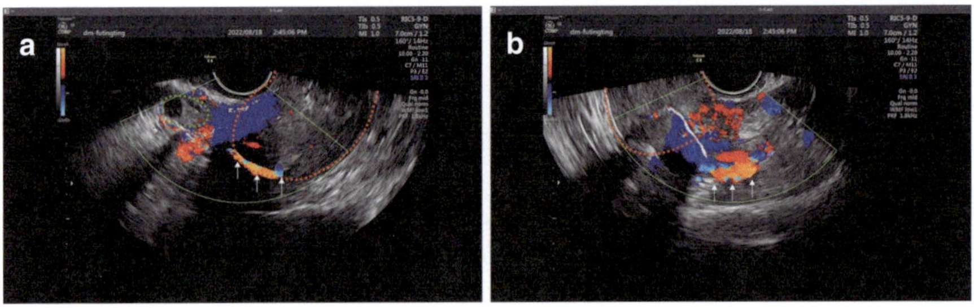

Fig. 5.14 (**a**) Contrast agent flow in the right fallopian tube shown in color Doppler mode. The uterus is outlined in orange, the right ovary is outlined in green, and arrows indicate the tubal trajectory. (**b**) Contrast agent flow in the left fallopian tube shown in color Doppler mode. The uterus is outlined in orange, and arrows indicate the tubal trajectory

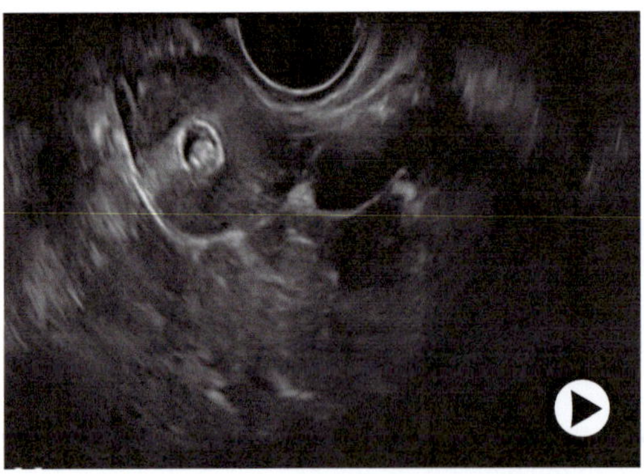

Fig. 5.15 Visualization of fallopian tube trajectory in B-mode (▶ https://doi.org/10.1007/000-hr8)

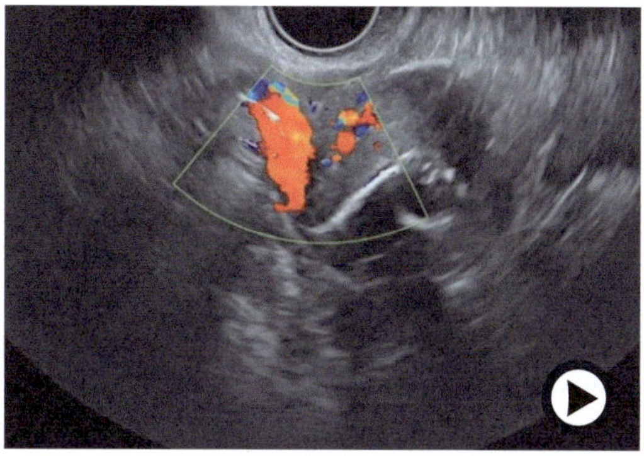

Fig. 5.16 Observation of tubal trajectory and contrast agent flow in color Doppler mode (▶ https://doi.org/10.1007/000-hr9)

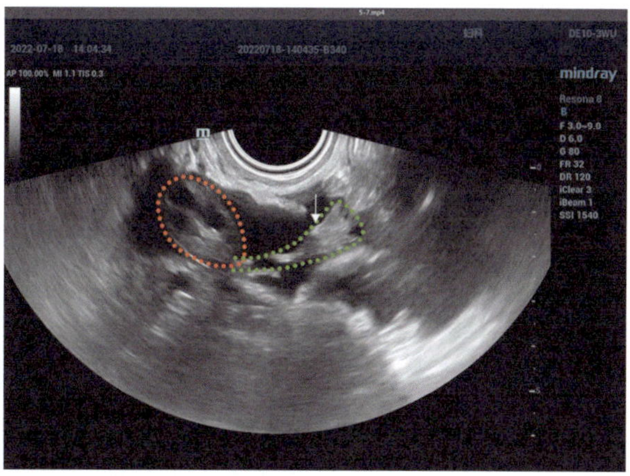

Fig. 5.17 Visualization of the tubal fimbriae using SIS. The ovary is outlined in orange, the fimbriae are marked by the arrow, and the fallopian tube is outlined in green

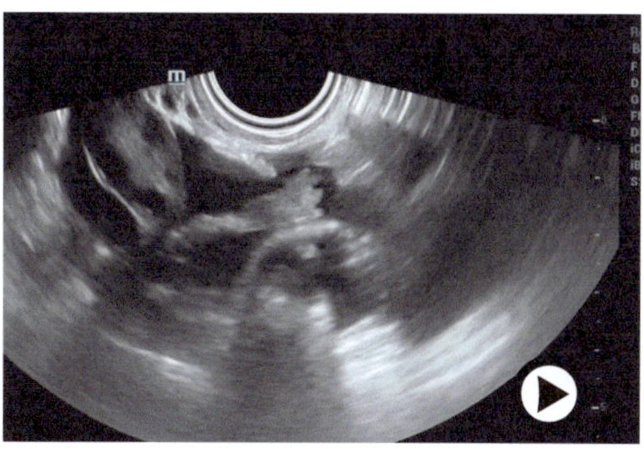

Fig. 5.18 Natural swinging motion of the tubal fimbriae observed using SIS (▶ https://doi.org/10.1007/000-hra)

uterine cavity display and helps expand it. Uterine SIS is particularly effective for assessing abnormalities that are difficult to distinguish on conventional 2D and 3D ultrasound, such as endometrial polyps, intrauterine adhesions, submucosal leiomyomas, and cesarean scar defects (refer to Figs. 5.19 and 5.20).

6. Image analysis and reporting

Replay the captured images and perform postprocessing to refine the quality. Select the necessary images based on the specific times and directions of the contrast agent's flow and compile these into a comprehensive report.

The report should include four key sections:

(a) Routine ultrasound findings: A description of the uterus, ovaries, and pelvis as observed during the standard ultrasound scan

(b) Uterine morphology and diseases: A detailed assessment of the uterine structure and any abnormalities or diseases detected

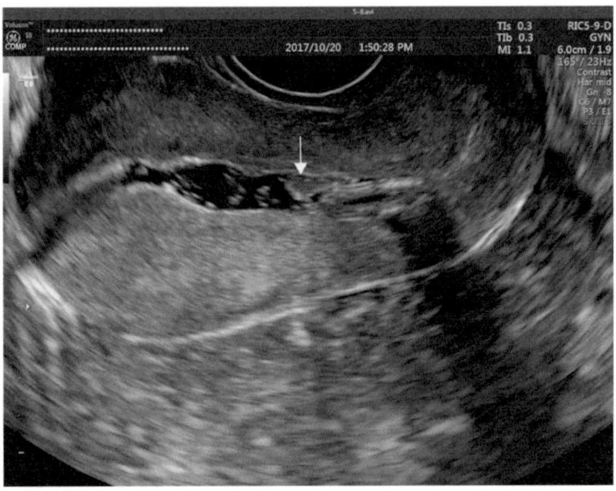

Fig. 5.19 Uterine SIS showing a polyp in the lower segment of the intrauterine cavity (indicated by the arrow)

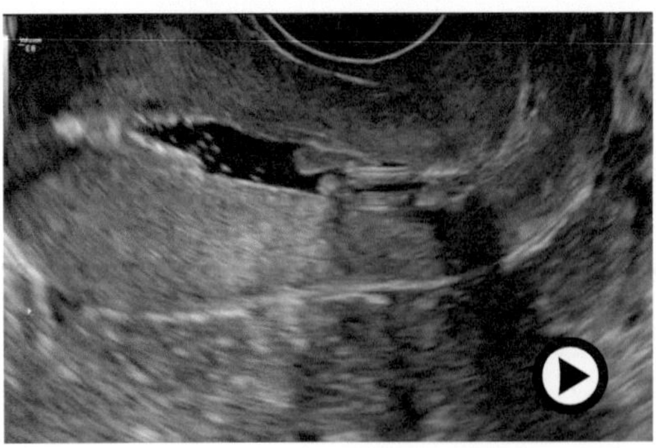

Fig. 5.20 Uterine SIS showing a polyp in the lower segment of the intrauterine cavity (▶ https://doi.org/10.1007/000-hrb)

(c) Tubal patency: An evaluation and diagnosis of the fallopian tubes' patency based on contrast imaging
(d) Contrast dispersion in the pelvis: A description of how the contrast agent disperses within the pelvic cavity, providing insights into the anatomy and potential issues

5.3.3 Normal Images and Analysis of Ultrasound Images

1. Normal manifestations of the uterus

   In a normal uterus, the myometrium shows no contrast echoes. The contrast medium fills the uterine cavity without any filling defects. The uterine cavity typically has a triangular shape (refer to Fig. 5.21), with a flat fundus and a well-defined cavity surface. Its volume ranges from 3 to 5 mL, and it can usually be filled with 5–7 mL of fluid.

   A balloon placed in the lower part of the uterine cavity may appear as a filling defect. The uterus's tension can affect the visualization of the cavity, where local contractions may cause partial defects that seem to disrupt the flow of contrast. The uterine horns may appear pointed, strangulated, or obtuse, but in most cases, they are symmetrically shaped on both sides.

2. Normal manifestations of the fallopian tubes

   When assessing the patency of the fallopian tubes, they are typically divided into three segments for detailed observation: the proximal segment, the mid-distal segment, and the distal fimbriae. Each fallopian tube (six segments in total) is visualized and described separately, as shown in Figs. 5.22 and 5.23.

   - *Proximal segment*: Focus on the connection between the fallopian tube and the uterine horn.
   - *Mid-distal segment*: Pay attention to the direction of the fallopian tube's course, its diameter, and whether the tubal wall appears smooth.
   - *Fimbriae*: Observe the overflow of the contrast agent, checking for any aggregation of the contrast.

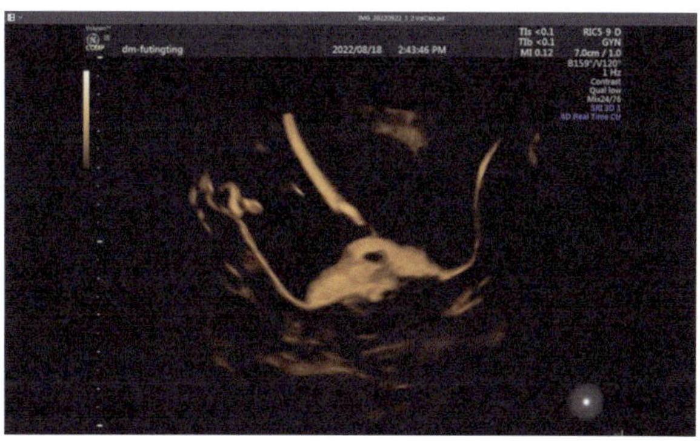

Fig. 5.21 Contrast-enhanced ultrasonography showing the morphology of the uterine cavity

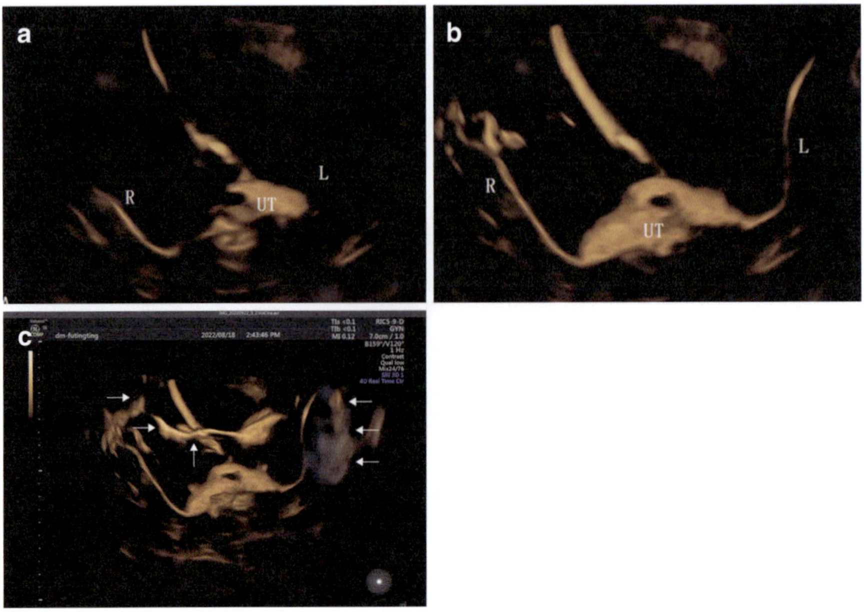

Fig. 5.22 (**a**) View of the proximal segments of both fallopian tubes. R indicates the right fallopian tube, L indicates the left fallopian tube, and UT indicates the uterus. (**b**) View of the mid-distal segments of both fallopian tubes. R indicates the right fallopian tube, L indicates the left fallopian tube, and UT indicates the uterus. (**c**) View of the bilateral tubal fimbriae and contrast diffusion. Arrows indicate contrast diffusion

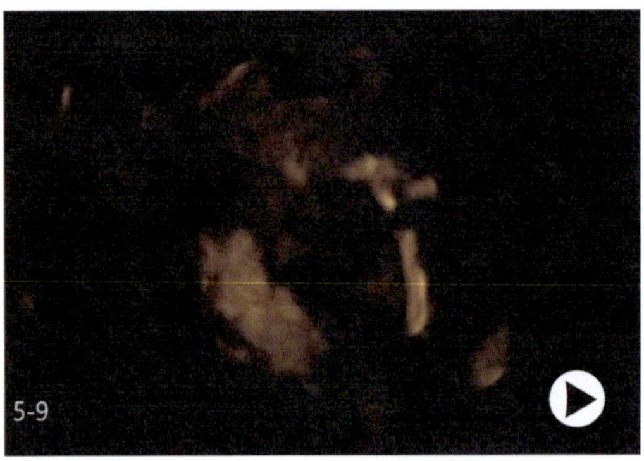

Fig. 5.23 Real-time 3D continuous dynamic visualization of both fallopian tube segments (▶ https://doi.org/10.1007/000-hrc)

(a) Normal tubal trajectory (Fig. 5.24):

The normal trajectory of the fallopian tubes can be classified into four types based on their position relative to the uterine cavity:

- Ascending type: The tubes curve upward on both sides of the uterine fundus.
- Descending type: The tubes curve downward on both sides of the uterus.
- Reversed type: One tube ascends, while the other descends.
- Horizontal type: The tubes extend from the level of the uterine body to both sides.

(b) Patent fallopian tubes (Figs. 5.25 and 5.26):

In cases of patent fallopian tubes, both tubes are visualized throughout the entire process. The contrast agent enters the fallopian tubes from the uterine cavity and quickly reaches the distal part. The fallopian tubes appear clear, with smooth walls, a natural trajectory, and no swelling. Key observations include the following:

- A large amount of contrast agent is expelled from the fimbriae of both tubes.
- The contrast agent disperses uniformly throughout the pelvis.
- The uterine cavity does not exhibit significant swelling.
- When injecting the contrast agent, no resistance is encountered, or the resistance disappears suddenly when additional pressure is applied.
- The patient experiences little to no pain during the procedure or only mild discomfort.

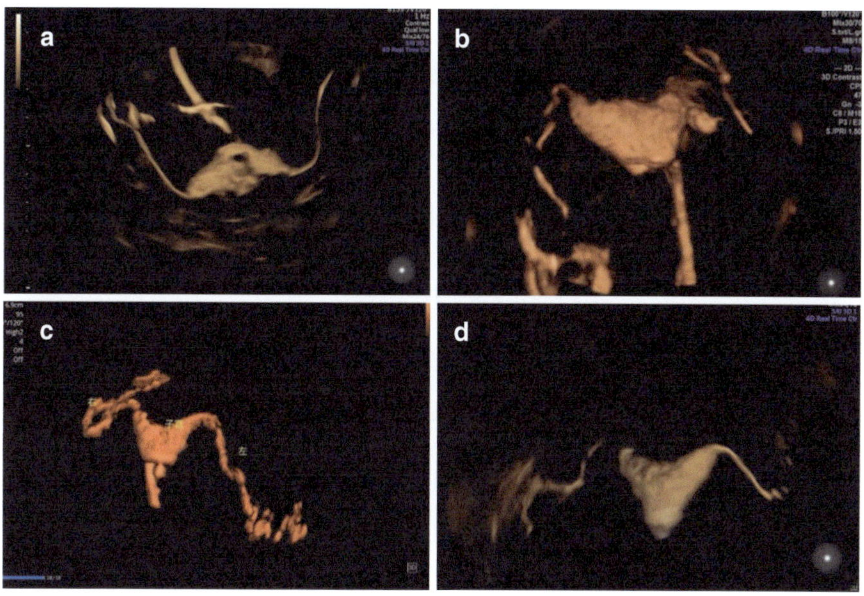

Fig. 5.24 (**a**) Bilateral fallopian tubes traveling in an ascending direction. (**b**) Bilateral fallopian tubes traveling in a descending direction. (**c**) Bilateral fallopian tubes traveling in opposite directions. (**d**) Bilateral fallopian tubes in traveling in a horizontal direction

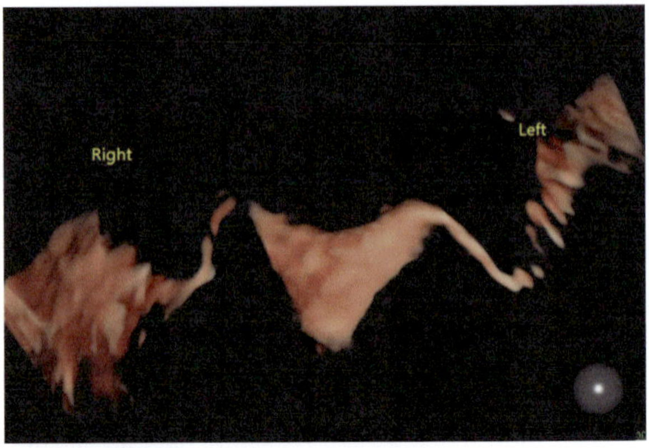

Fig. 5.25 Visualization of patent bilateral fallopian tubes

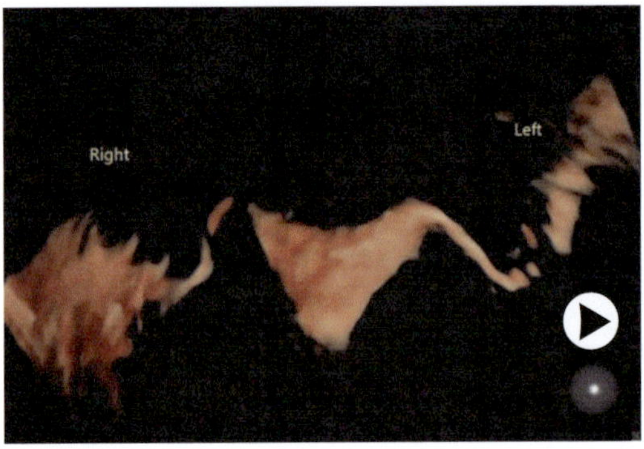

Fig. 5.26 Real-time visualization of patent bilateral fallopian tubes (▶ https://doi.org/10.1007/000-hrd)

5.3.4 Abnormal Images and Analysis of Ultrasound Images

1. Abnormal manifestations of the uterine cavity
   (a) Congenital uterine anomalies:

   Abnormalities in the morphology of the uterine cavity, such as a unicornuate uterus, septate uterus, or double uterus, are typically visible on contrast imaging. The diagnostic accuracy for identifying uterine anomalies is approximately 97.6% when assessed in the coronal plane with 3D ultrasound and about 96.5% with SIS [28]. Therefore, it is crucial to incorporate regular 3D imaging to assess potential uterine malformations during contrast imaging.

   Additionally, the depth of the depression in cases of a septate uterus should not be measured during contrast imaging but should be evaluated in the 3D coronal plane (Fig. 5.27).

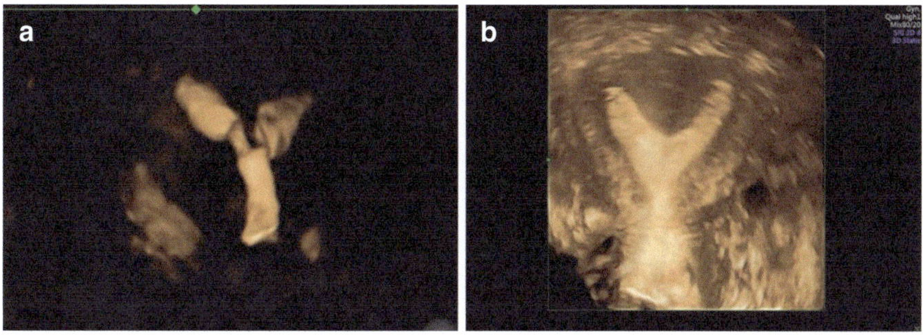

Fig. 5.27 (**a**) Incomplete septate uterus displayed in contrast mode. (**b**) Incomplete septate uterus shown in the 3D ultrasound coronal plane

(b) Intrauterine adhesion:

Intrauterine adhesions present as irregular filling defects across the uterine cavity (Figs. 5.28 and 5.29). These adhesions lead to a reduction in the volume of the uterine cavity. As the volume of the contrast agent increases, the position of the filling defect remains unchanged, and there is an increase in peripheral tension.

(c) Intrauterine space-occupying pathologies:

Space-occupying lesions such as endometrial polyps or submucosal fibroids may appear as single or multiple round filling defects with well-defined borders within the uterine cavity when using contrast imaging. Uterine SIS provides clearer visualization of the lesion's location, size, number, and extent, as well as the relationship of its base to the endometrium or myometrium (Fig. 5.30), aiding in a definitive diagnosis.

(d) Cesarean scar defects:

Cesarean scar defects are observed as contrast filling at the scar on the anterior uterine wall. Discontinuity of the myometrium at the cesarean scar in the lower part of the anterior wall of the uterus can be visualized on uterine SIS as a triangular, wedge-shaped, or irregular indentation (Figs. 5.31 and 5.32).

2. Reflux of contrast agent

Contrast agent reflux refers to the unintended movement of the contrast agent from the uterus into the myometrium, the muscular layer of the fallopian tubes, para-uterine veins, and pelvic lymphatic vessels through abnormal pathways. This leads to its eventual re-entry into the circulatory system [29]. Reflux typically manifests as abnormal imaging patterns, including cloudy, earthworm-like, or grid-like formations within the uterus and/or surrounding the fallopian tubes. These patterns can closely resemble the fallopian tubes, presenting a significant challenge in analyzing tubal contrast images.

There are three distinct types of contrast agent reflux, as shown in Figs. 5.33 and 5.34:

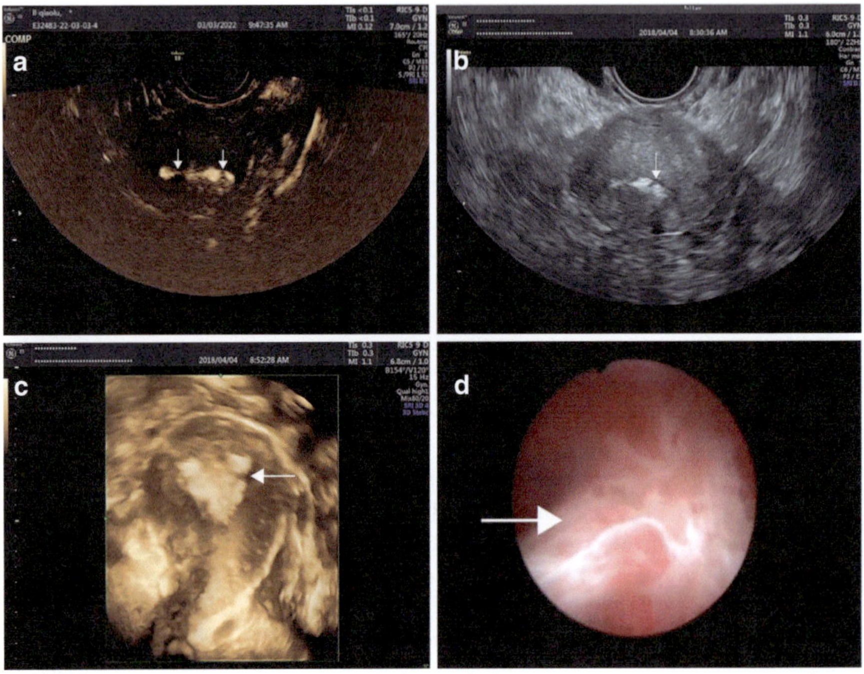

Fig. 5.28 (**a**) Intrauterine adhesion visualized in contrast mode (arrows indicate the adhesion bands). (**b**) Intrauterine adhesion visualized on uterine SIS (the arrow indicates the adhesion band). (**c**) Intrauterine adhesion displayed in the coronal plane on 3D ultrasound (the arrow indicates the adhesion band). (**d**) Intrauterine adhesion observed under hysteroscopy (the arrow indicates the adhesion band)

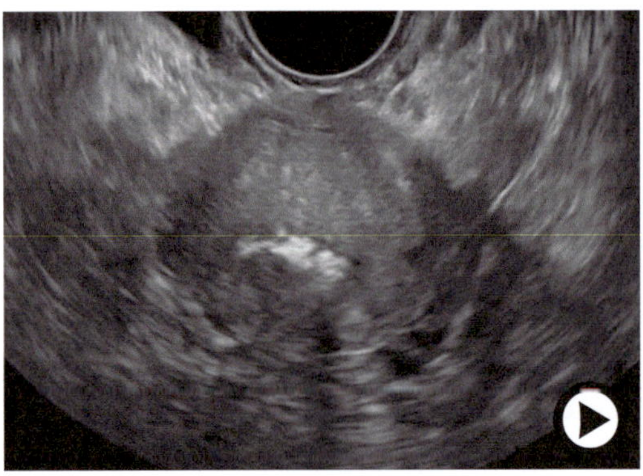

Fig. 5.29 Visualization of intrauterine adhesion bands using uterine SIS (▶ https://doi.org/10.1007/000-hre)

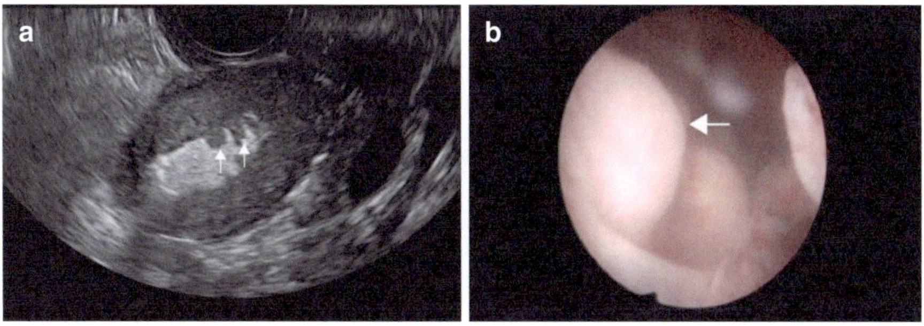

Fig. 5.30 (**a**) Multiple endometrial polyps visualized in uterine SIS (arrows indicate the polyps). (**b**) Endometrial polyps observed under hysteroscopy (the arrow indicates the polyps)

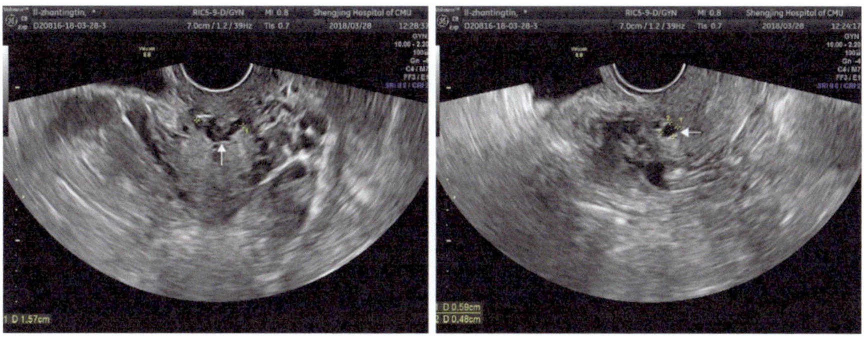

Fig. 5.31 Uterine SIS showing cesarean scar defects (indicated by the arrow)

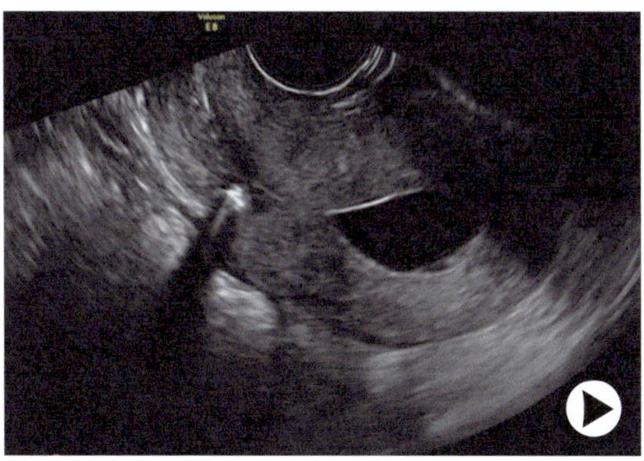

Fig. 5.32 Uterine SIS demonstrating cesarean scar defects (▶ https://doi.org/10.1007/000-hrf)

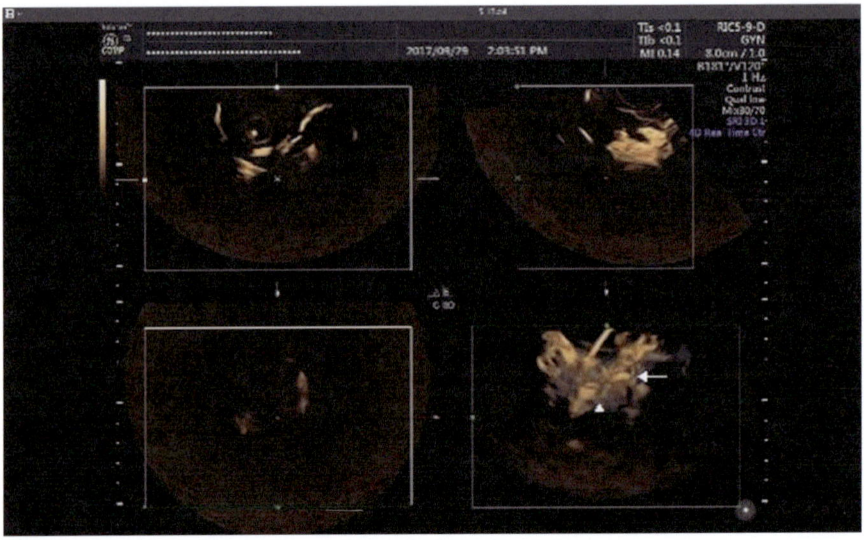

Fig. 5.33 Contrast agent reflux (arrows indicate reflux into the myometrium)

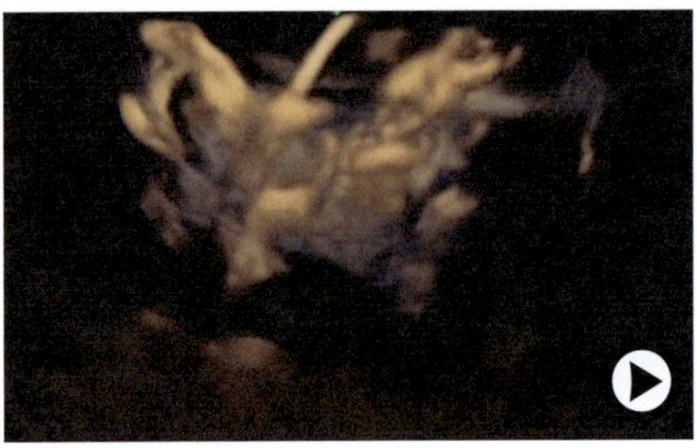

Fig. 5.34 Contrast agent reflux (▶ https://doi.org/10.1007/000-hrg)

- Interstitial-lymphatic reflux
- Venous reflux
- Mixed reflux: The most common type, characterized by ductal venous reflux and fine mesh-like or cloudy lymphatic reflux on contrast imaging.

The primary causes of contrast agent reflux include the following:

- High intrauterine pressure: Often caused by a complete or partial obstruction of the fallopian tubes
- Endometrial and tubal wall injuries: Typically resulting from organic pathologies of the uterus or fallopian tubes
- Spasms of the uterus or fallopian tubes

When contrast agent reflux is observed during an examination, the procedure should be paused to evaluate the images carefully. Dynamic frame-by-frame playback can help analyze the reflux, focusing on the following:

- Tubal images
- Pelvic contrast dispersion
- The specific patterns of contrast agent reflux

Adjusting the gain and rotating the image for different perspectives is often useful. Additionally, switching to 2D contrast mode or B-mode allows better visualization of the reflux site and its relationship to surrounding structures.

A second contrast examination may be considered after the patient rests for approximately 15 min in severe reflux that remains unclearly visualized. During the second attempt, the contrast agent should be injected more slowly. This method often reduces reflux, facilitating improved visualization of the fallopian tubes.

3. Abnormal tubal patency

Tubal patency is commonly categorized using a dichotomous approach: patent or obstructed [30]. In contrast, the classification system in China divides tubal patency into three grades: patent, partially obstructed, and obstructed.

(a) Partially obstructed fallopian tubes (Figs. 5.35 and 5.36)

Partially obstructed fallopian tubes exhibit the following characteristics:

- The tubes may appear thin, rigid, or tortuously coiled, with a discontinuous bead-like appearance.
- Alternatively, they may be swollen and dilated, with a small amount of contrast agent spilling from the fimbriae.
- The contrast agent disperses unevenly in the pelvis.
- The uterine cavity may show distension.
- Resistance may be felt during contrast injection; the patient typically reports mild to moderate pain.

(b) Obstructed fallopian tubes (Figs. 5.37, 5.38, and 5.39)

Tubal obstruction is divided into two categories based on the location of the blockage:

- Proximal obstruction: Affects the interstitial part and isthmus
- Distal obstruction: Affects the ampulla and infundibulum

Key imaging characteristics include the following:

- The obstructed fallopian tube may appear absent, partially or fully visualized, often with irregular, thin, stiff, or nodular walls.
- A "cut-off sign" is often seen in the distal section, and no contrast agent spills from the fimbriae.
- The uterine cavity may appear enlarged, with rounded uterine horns, and contrast reflux into the myometrium may be observed.
- During the procedure, the operator perceives high resistance when injecting the contrast agent.
- The patient typically experiences significant pain.

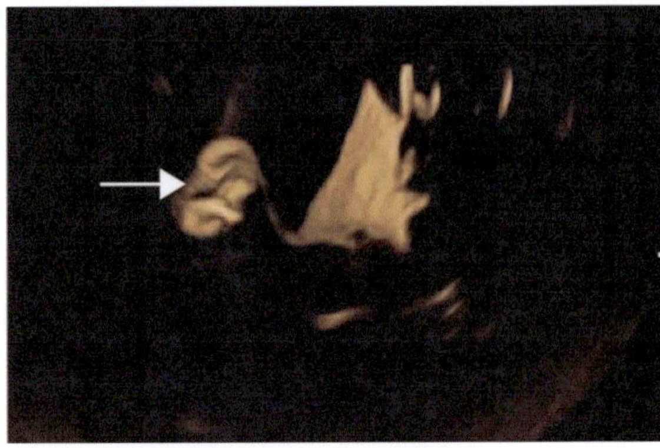

Fig. 5.35 Tortuous and slightly enlarged mid-distal segments of the right fallopian tube (arrow indicates tubal tortuosity)

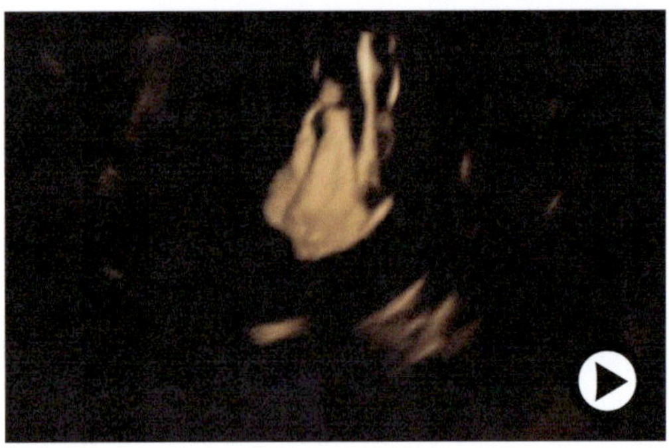

Fig. 5.36 Tortuous right fallopian tube with a small amount of contrast spilled from the fimbriae (▶ https://doi.org/10.1007/000-hrh)

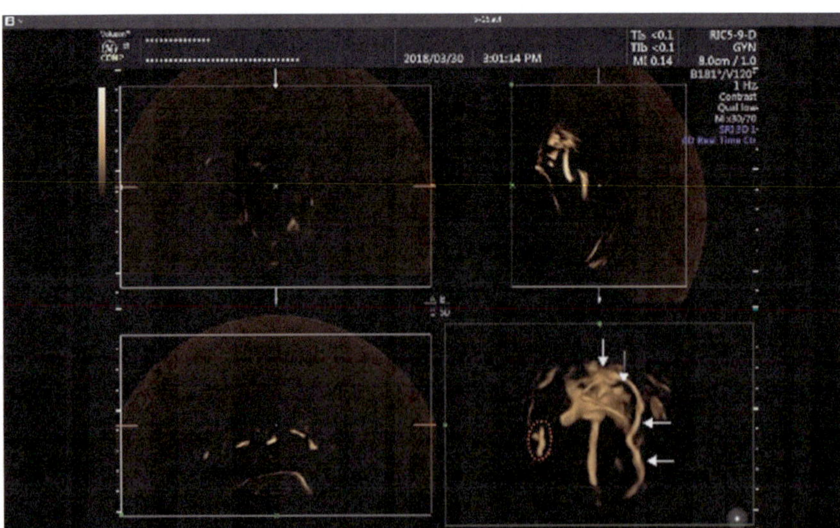

Fig. 5.37 Proximal obstruction of the left fallopian tube; distal obstruction of the right fallopian tube (circled), with contrast reflux into the myometrium (arrows indicate reflux)

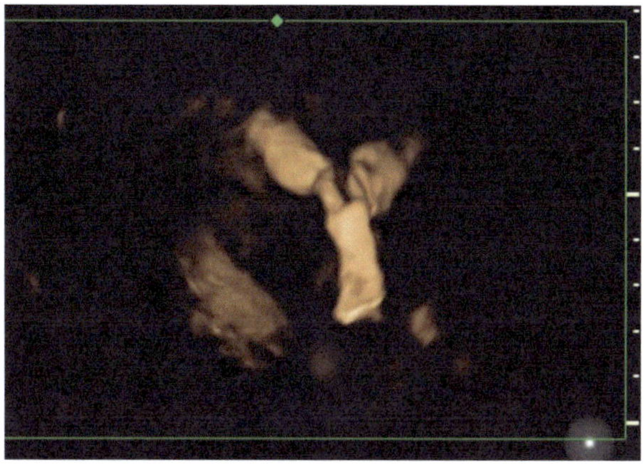

Fig. 5.38 Bilateral proximal tubal obstruction

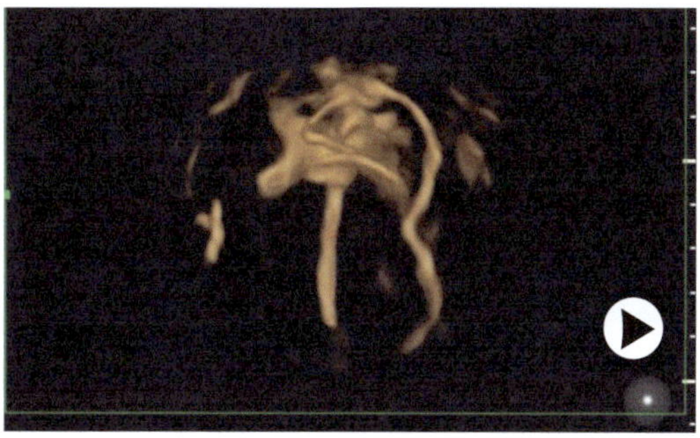

Fig. 5.39 Proximal obstruction of the left fallopian tube; distal obstruction of the right fallopian tube with contrast reflux into the myometrium (▶ https://doi.org/10.1007/000-hrj)

(c) Hydrosalpinx (Figs. 5.40, 5.41, 5.42, and 5.43)

Hydrosalpinx, a condition resulting from distal tubal obstruction, is categorized based on the patency of the proximal segment of the fallopian tube to the uterine cavity:

- The proximal segment is patent to the uterine cavity.
- The proximal segment is not patent to the uterine cavity.

These two conditions have different implications for clinical management:

- When the proximal segment is patent, effusion may reflux into the uterine cavity, often requiring surgical intervention such as resection, ligation, or plugging of the affected fallopian tube to improve the success of embryo transfer [31].
- When the proximal segment is not patent, the contrast agent cannot enter the fallopian tube and does not appear on contrast imaging.

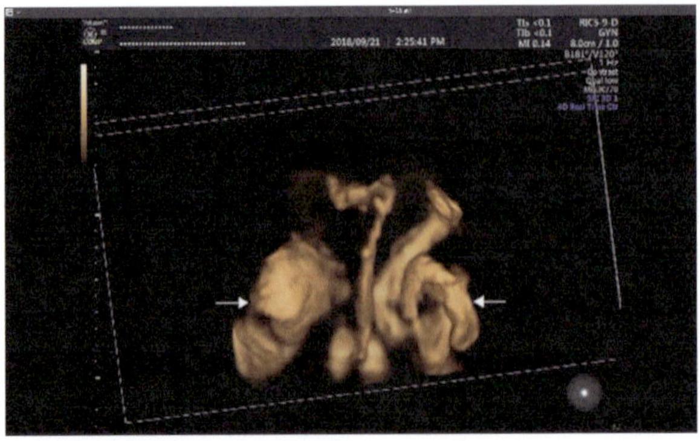

Fig. 5.40 3D contrast image showing fluid accumulation in both fallopian tubes (arrows indicate contrast filling in the enlarged fallopian tubes)

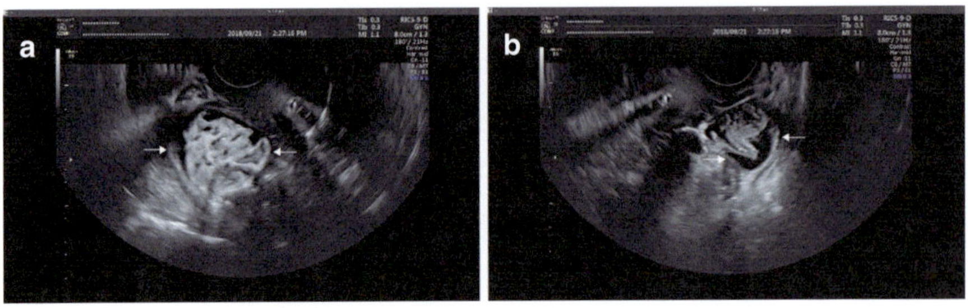

Fig. 5.41 (**a**) 2D B-mode ultrasound showing contrast agent aggregates in the enlarged right fallopian tube (arrows indicate the aggregates). (**b**) 2D B-mode ultrasound showing contrast agent aggregates in the enlarged left fallopian tube (arrow indicates the aggregate)

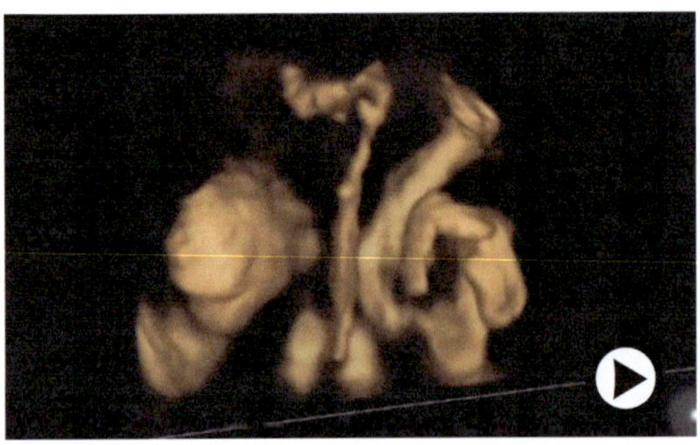

Fig. 5.42 Real-time 3D contrast imaging showing bilateral tubal dilatation and tortuosity (▶ https://doi.org/10.1007/000-hrk)

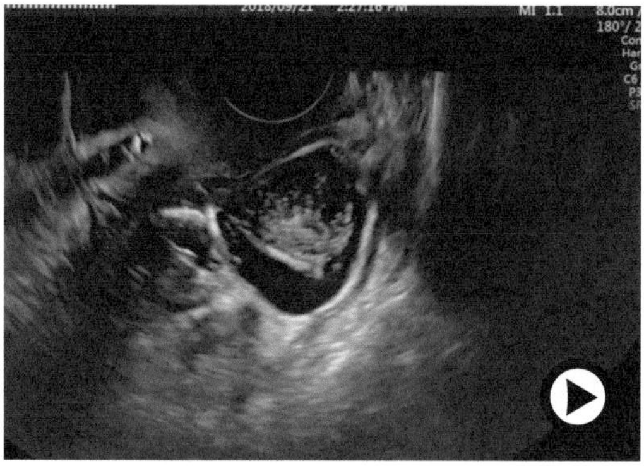

Fig. 5.43 2D B-mode ultrasound showing contrast agent accumulation in the dilated bilateral fallopian tubes (▶ https://doi.org/10.1007/000-hrm)

Key imaging characteristics include the following:

- For proximal patency, contrast imaging shows the contrast agent filling a tortuous, dilated fallopian tube with distal tubal atresia, but no contrast agent exits the fimbriae.
- The operator may perceive resistance during injection, and it often persists.

4. Pelvic adhesions (Figs. 5.44, 5.45, and 5.46)

   Pelvic adhesions are characterized by uneven diffusion or zonal confinement of the contrast agent within the pelvis, resulting in strip-like echogenic patterns visible on ultrasound imaging (Figs. 5.44, 5.45, and 5.46). These patterns reflect the restriction of normal pelvic anatomy caused by adhesion bands.

5.3.5 Clinical Applications and Diagnostic Tips

While HyCoSy is highly accurate in detecting tubal factor infertility, false diagnoses or missed cases can occur due to factors such as abnormal ciliary movement, tubal stenosis, and improper contrast agent usage. In clinical practice, it is essential to combine multiple ultrasound modalities with the patient's clinical history to arrive at a comprehensive diagnosis of uterine, tubal, and pelvic pathologies. The following clinical cases will provide a more intuitive and concrete understanding of the diagnostic process. The following section will present several patient cases to provide a more intuitive and concrete understanding of the diagnostic process.

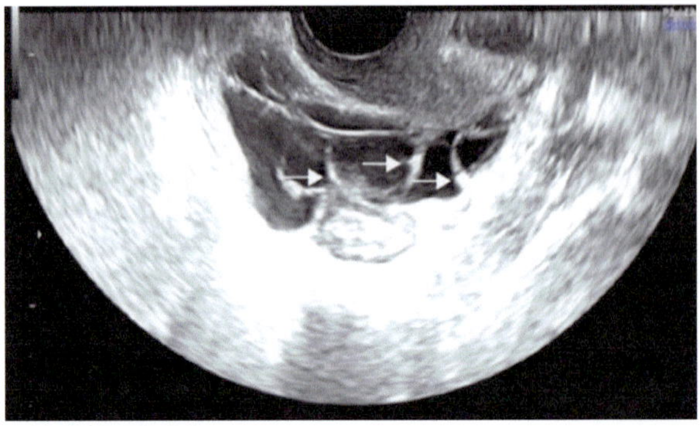

Fig. 5.44 Stripe-like patterns in the pelvis caused by intrapelvic adhesions (arrows indicate adhesions)

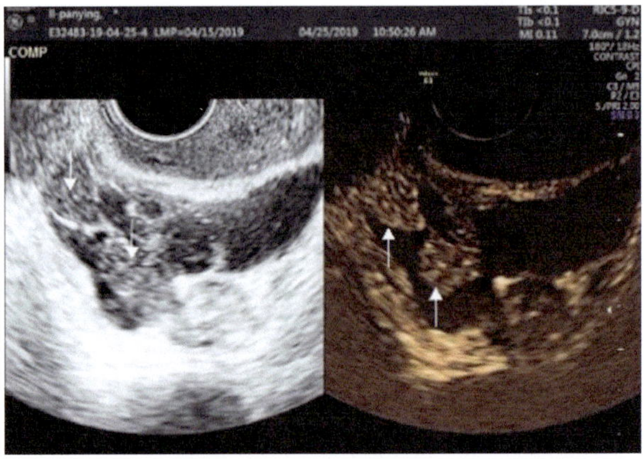

Fig. 5.45 Contrast agent segregated by strip-like echogenic shadows in the pelvis, indicating restricted diffusion (as indicated by the arrows)

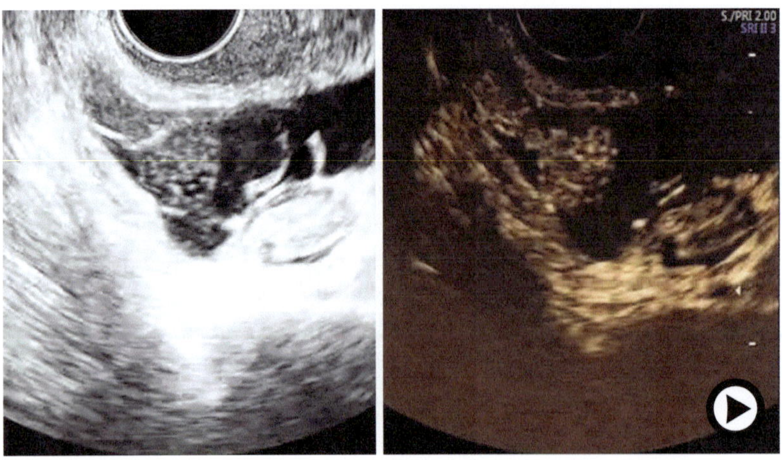

Fig. 5.46 Real-time imaging showing restricted diffusion of the contrast agent, with strip-like echogenic shadows in the pelvis (▶ https://doi.org/10.1007/000-hrn)

Case 1

1. Patient history:
   A 24-year-old female with irregular menstruation (cycle length: 32–90 days, menstrual period length: 4 days), normal menstrual volume, and no dysmenorrhea. She had been diagnosed with polycystic ovary syndrome (PCOS) several years ago, had not been pregnant, and had been struggling with infertility for 2 years.
2. HyCoSy imaging (Figs. 5.47 and 5.48)
3. Analysis and diagnosis
   (a) B-mode ultrasound:
   The uterus was anteverted with smooth, intact contours and homogeneous echogenicity. A water balloon was clearly visualized in the uterine cavity. No apparent lesions were observed in the myometrium. The left ovary was located away from the uterus and had good mobility, while the right ovary was positioned closer to the uterus and had good mobility. Bilateral ovarian polycystic changes were noted (Fig. 5.48). No significant lesions were observed in the bilateral adnexal areas.
   (b) Contrast-enhanced ultrasound:
   The bilateral fallopian tubes were fully visualized, with well-defined walls and normal alignment. The morphology appeared smooth, with the contrast agent being discharged from the fimbriae of both fallopian tubes. The contrast medium dispersed evenly around the ovaries on both sides, and no contrast reflux was seen in the myometrium.
   (c) Intrapelvic findings:
   Contrast enhancement revealed the even encapsulation of the contrast medium around both ovaries, with a homogeneous distribution in the pelvis (Fig. 5.48). No abnormal findings were noted, indicating the absence of intrapelvic adhesions. No resistance was felt during the injection, and the patient reported no pain during the procedure. These findings suggest bilateral patent fallopian tubes.
   (d) SIS imaging:

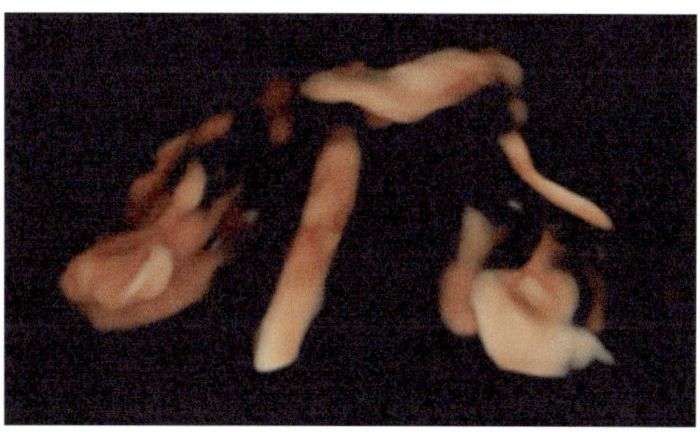

Fig. 5.47 Bilateral fallopian tubes were patent

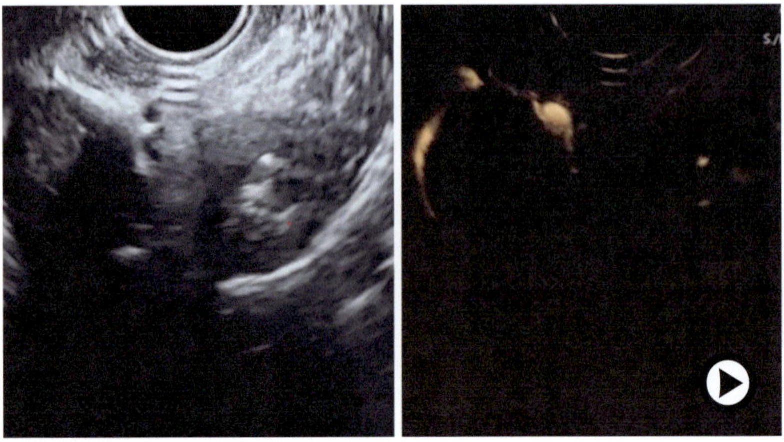

Fig. 5.48 Case 1 (▶ https://doi.org/10.1007/000-hrp)

SIS showed normal uterine cavity morphology with no obvious abnormalities.

4. Medical advice:

   Given the presence of patent fallopian tubes and the patient's age (under 35 years), it was advised that she attempt to conceive naturally. Due to her PCOS, assisted ovulation or artificial insemination may be considered if natural conception does not occur.

Case 2

1. Patient history:

   A 37-year-old female with regular menstruation (cycle length: 26–30 days, menstrual period length: 3–5 days), low menstrual volume, and no dysmenorrhea. She had two pregnancies with no live births and had been struggling with infertility for 1 year. The patient experienced two embryo arrests and two IVF failures. The male partner's test results were normal.
2. HyCoSy imaging (Figs. 5.49, 5.50, and 5.51)
3. Analysis and diagnosis
   (a) B-mode ultrasound:

   The uterus was anteverted with smooth, intact contours and homogeneous echogenicity. A water balloon was clearly visualized in the uterine cavity. No obvious lesions were observed in the myometrium. The left ovary was situated posteriorly and close to the uterine body with good mobility, while the right ovary was located distant from the uterine body, also with good mobility. No lesions were noted in the bilateral adnexal areas.

   (b) Contrast-enhanced ultrasound (Fig. 5.51):

   The uterine cavity was well-defined, with regular morphology. Bilateral fallopian tubes were fully visualized, with a slight delay in the left tube. The tubal walls were well-defined, with normal alignment and smooth morphol-

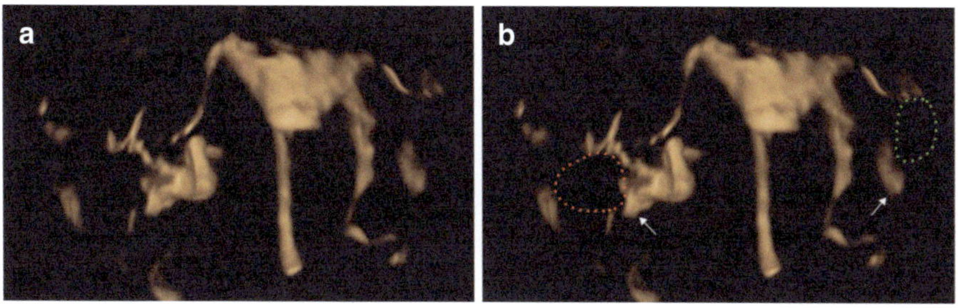

Fig. 5.49 (**a**) Bilateral fallopian tubes were patent; contrast reflux was observed in the myometrium. (**b**) The right ovary is circled in orange; the left ovary is circled in green; the arrow indicates the contrast agent surrounding the ovary

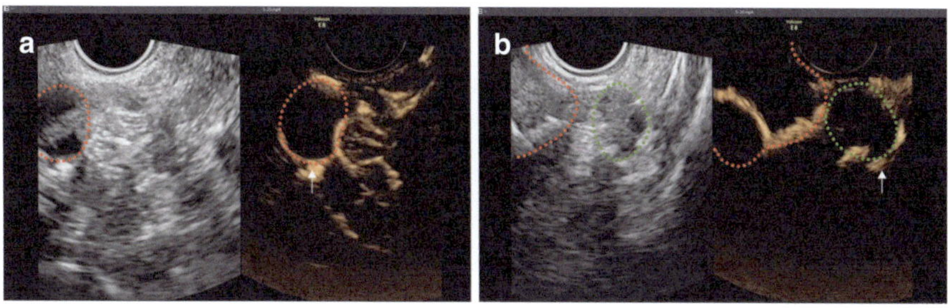

Fig. 5.50 (**a**) Contrast medium surrounding the right ovary (the right ovary is circled in orange, and the strong echo indicated by the arrow is the contrast medium encircling the ovary). (**b**) Contrast medium surrounding the left ovary (the uterus is circled in orange; the left ovary is circled in green; the strong echo indicated by the arrow is the contrast medium encircling the ovary)

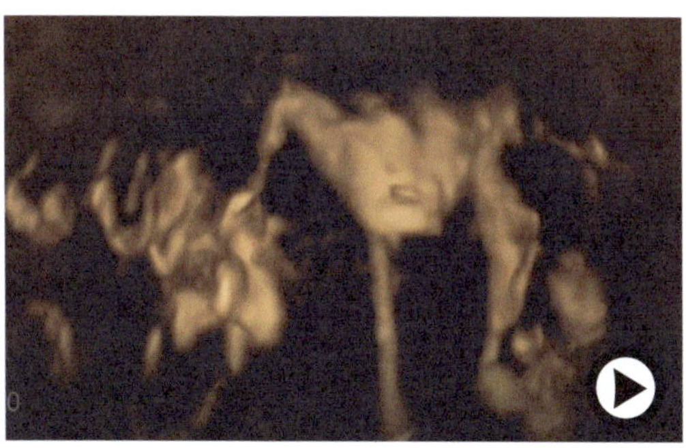

Fig. 5.51 Case 2 (▶ https://doi.org/10.1007/000-hrq)

ogy. Discharge of the contrast agent from fimbriae was observed. The contrast medium was dispersed evenly around the ovaries. No contrast reflux was seen in the myometrium, and little resistance was felt during injection, with no pain reported by the patient.

(c) Intrapelvic findings:

Contrast enhancement revealed even encapsulation of the contrast medium around both ovaries, with a homogeneous distribution in the pelvis (Figs. 5.50 and 5.51). No abnormal findings were noted, indicating the absence of intrapelvic adhesions.

(d) SIS imaging:

SIS showed normal uterine cavity morphology with no obvious abnormalities.

4. Medical advice:

Given the patient's age (over 35 years) and history of failed IVF attempts, she was advised to try to conceive for a short period. In light of the patient's repeated fetal arrests, she was also advised to undergo an endometrial tolerance examination and treatment in preparation for another IVF cycle.

Case 3

1. Patient history:

A 32-year-old female with regular menstruation (cycle length: 30 days, menstrual period length: 4–5 days), low menstrual volume, and no dysmenorrhea. She had one pregnancy with no delivery and had been struggling with infertility for 3 years. Six months ago, the patient's HSG examination showed smooth contrast agent injection, normal shape and size of the uterine cavity with no definite filling defects. Bilateral tubal alignment was stiff, with no dilatation or fluid accumulation, and bilateral distal contrast agent diffusion was slightly restricted.

2. HyCoSy imaging (Figs. 5.52, 5.53, and 5.54)
3. Analysis and diagnosis

(a) B-mode ultrasound:

The uterus was anteverted, with smooth and intact contours and homogeneous echogenicity. The water balloon was visualized in the uterine cavity. No lesions were observed in the myometrium. The left ovary was positioned posteriorly and distantly from the uterine body with good mobility, while the right ovary was situated closer to the uterine body, also with good mobility. No lesions were seen in the bilateral adnexal areas.

(b) Contrast-enhanced ultrasound:

The uterine cavity was well-defined with regular morphology. The bilateral fallopian tubes were fully visualized, with smooth walls and rigid alignment. A very small amount of contrast agent overflowed from the fimbriae of both fallopian tubes. Contrast agent diffusion was seen around the left ovary during the late phase of contrast enhancement. A small amount of contrast agent was discharged slowly from the fimbriae of the right fallopian tube, exhibiting a bunch-like pattern. A homogeneous diffusion of contrast medium was seen around the right ovary, along with a small amount of con-

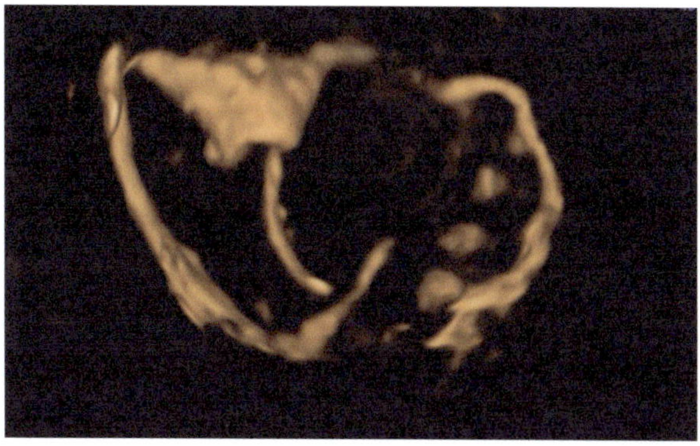

Fig. 5.52 Bilateral fallopian tubes with partial obstruction and rigid morphology

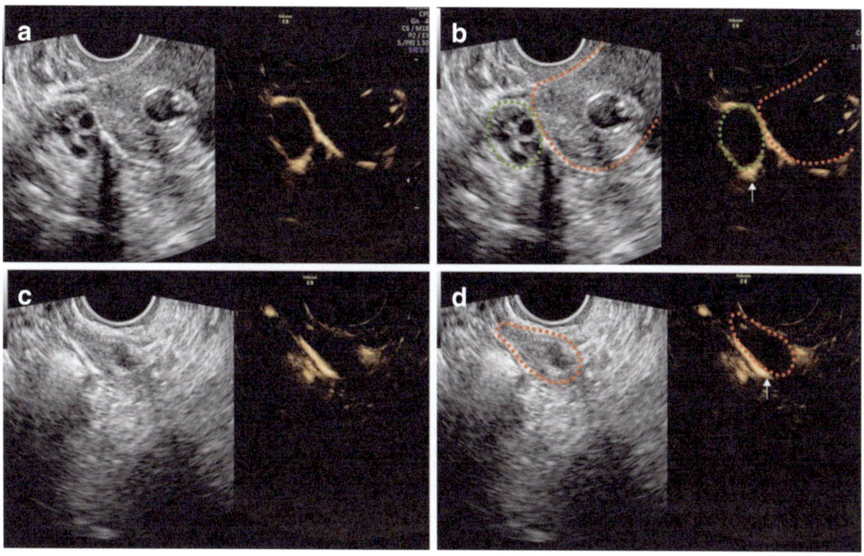

Fig. 5.53 (**a**) Contrast agent surrounding the right ovary. (**b**) The right ovary is circled in green; the arrow represents the contrast agent surrounding the ovary; the uterus is circled in orange. (**c**) Contrast agent surrounding the left ovary. (**d**) The left ovary is circled in orange; the arrow represents the contrast agent surrounding the ovary

trast agent reflux in the myometrium. Based on these findings, the diagnosis was partial obstruction of both fallopian tubes, with the left fallopian tube being more severely affected.

(c) Intrapelvic findings:

During intrapelvic scanning, ultrasound revealed good mobility of both ovaries with no tenderness. Contrast enhancement showed homogeneous diffusion of the contrast medium in the pelvic cavity (Fig. 5.54), indicating no significant adhesions.

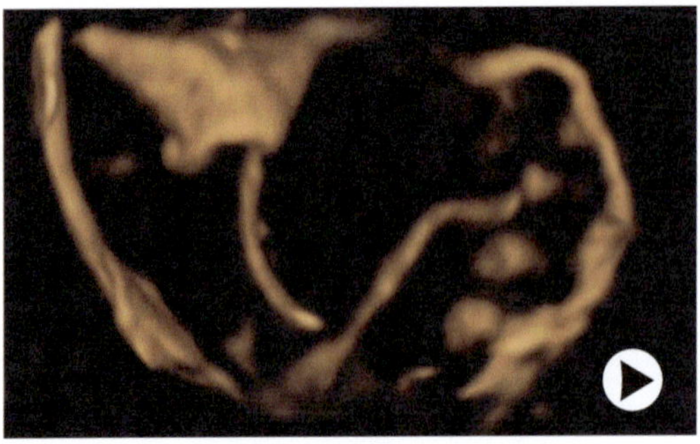

Fig. 5.54 Case 3 (▶ https://doi.org/10.1007/000-hrr)

(d) SIS imaging:

SIS showed normal uterine cavity morphology with no significant abnormalities.

4. Medical advice:

Given the patient's age, medical history, and the marked stiffness of both fallopian tubes with slow and minimal discharge of contrast medium, it was recommended that the patient undergo IVF treatment at the earliest opportunity.

Case 4

1. Patient history:

The patient was a 34-year-old female with irregular menstrual cycles. She had one pregnancy with no delivery and one embryonic arrest and reported infertility for one and a half years. An HSG performed 2 years ago showed a smooth injection of contrast medium with a normal uterine cavity size and shape. However, the left fallopian tube was not visualized, and the right fallopian tube showed partial visualization without distal end visualization.

2. HyCoSy imaging (Figs. 5.55, 5.56, 5.57, 5.58, and 5.59)
3. Analysis and diagnosis

(a) B-mode ultrasound findings:

The uterus was anteverted, with smooth, intact contours and homogeneous echogenicity. A well-defined water balloon was visible in the uterine cavity. No lesions were observed in the myometrium. With good mobility, the left ovary was positioned posteriorly and away from the left uterine body. Similarly, the right ovary was located posteriorly and away from the uterus and had good mobility. No lesions or tenderness were noted in the bilateral adnexal areas.

(b) 3D ultrasound measurement of uterine depression:

A depression in the endometrium at the fundus of the uterus was visible in both B-mode and contrast mode (Figs. 5.55 and 5.56). It is important to note that the depth of this depression should be measured in the coronal plane in 3D mode, not in contrast mode. The depression depth was measured at 1.0 cm (Fig. 5.55). This finding did not support the diagnosis of an incom-

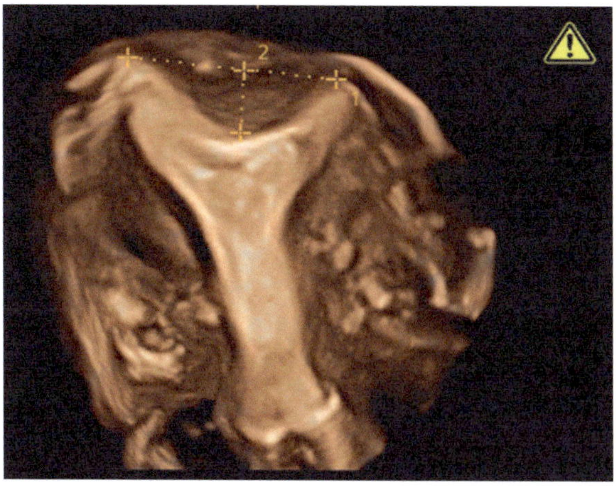

Fig. 5.55 The uterus appears Y-shaped in coronal view on 3D mode ultrasound

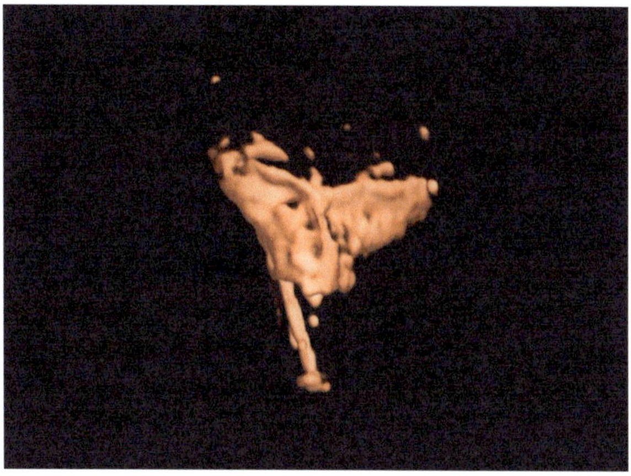

Fig. 5.56 The bilateral fallopian tubes were obstructed at their proximal ends and were not visualized during the first contrast injection

plete septate uterus. Therefore, an arcuate uterus was considered a more likely diagnosis.

(c) Contrast-enhanced ultrasound—fallopian tubes and pelvic findings:

The uterine cavity was distended at the initiation of contrast medium injection, but the bilateral fallopian tubes were not visualized (Fig. 5.56). Significant resistive pressure against the injection was observed, and the patient experienced severe, intolerable pain. A diagnosis of bilateral proximal tubal obstruction was suggested.

Proximal tubal pathology is typically characterized by obstruction, which can be classified as follows:

- Nodal obstruction (due to nodulitis, endometriosis)
- Nonnodal obstruction (due to fibrosis)
- Pseudo-obstruction (caused by debris, mucus plugs, polyps, or spasms) [4].

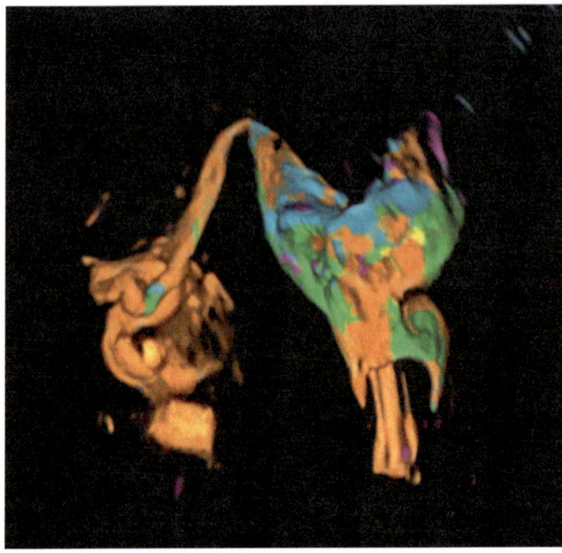

Fig. 5.57 Second contrast injection: uterus was clearly visible; the left fallopian tube was obstructed; the right fallopian tube was partially obstructed and distorted

To rule out pseudo-obstruction (e.g., caused by spasms), a second contrast-enhanced imaging was recommended.

This time, the contrast medium was injected slowly at a low rate. The patient experienced mild pain but was cooperative. After gradually increasing the injection pressure, the right fallopian tube was visualized (Figs. 5.57 and 5.59), showing a distorted alignment of the distal segment, with contrast overflow seen at the fimbrial end. Based on these findings, a diagnosis of partial obstruction of the right fallopian tube was made. The left fallopian tube was never visualized, with no contrast overflow at the fimbrial end and no diffusion of contrast around the left ovary, leading to the diagnosis of proximal obstruction of the left fallopian tube.

No significant adhesions or abnormal imaging findings were present in the pelvic cavity.

(d) SIS findings (Figs. 5.58 and 5.59):

Although a significant amount of contrast medium remained in the uterine cavity, the pressurized injection of saline diluted the contrast agent, which did not affect the diagnosis of uterine pathology. A diagnosis of an endometrial polyp was considered, as a moderately echogenic mass measuring approximately 1.0 × 0.5 cm with clear borders was seen in the anterior wall of the uterus.

4. Medical advice:

The patient was advised to attempt conception naturally for a short period. If this approach is unsuccessful, hysteroscopy may be considered to further evaluate and treat the endometrial polyp and proximal tubal obstruction.

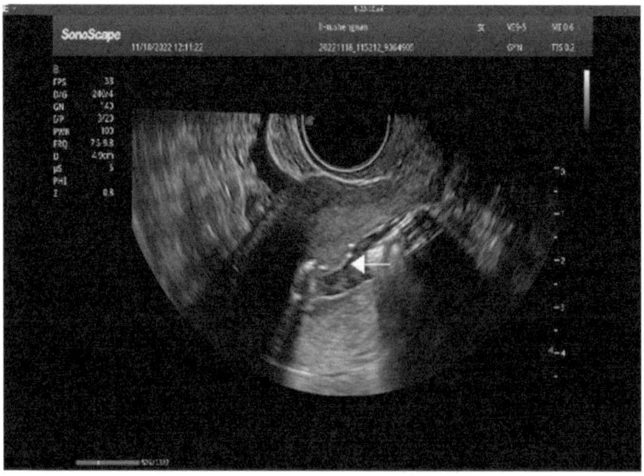

Fig. 5.58 SIS showing endometrial polyps (as indicated by the arrow)

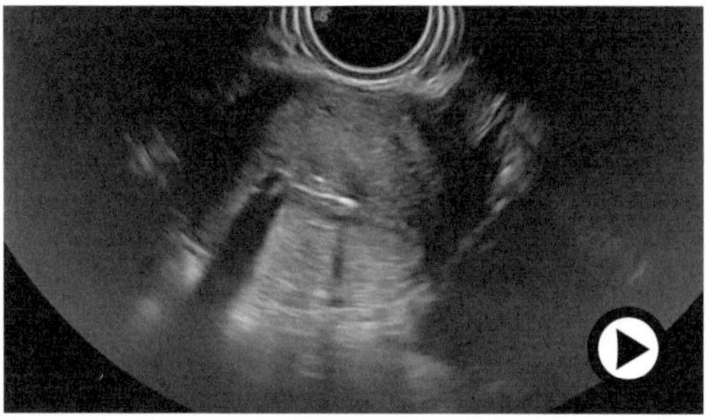

Fig. 5.59 Case 4 (▶ https://doi.org/10.1007/000-hr4)

Case 5

1. Patient history:

   The patient was a 39-year-old woman with regular menstrual cycles and no dysmenorrhea. She had one pregnancy (with no delivery) and had been experiencing infertility for 10 years.
2. HyCoSy imaging (Figs. 5.60 and 5.61)
3. Analysis and diagnosis
   (a) B-mode ultrasound:

   The uterus was retroverted, with smooth and intact contours and homogeneous echogenicity. A water balloon was clearly visualized in the uterine cavity. Multiple fibroids were observed, the largest of which was located in the posterior wall of the uterus. The left ovary was positioned close to the uterine body, with limited mobility. The right ovary was located away from the cervix on the right side of the uterus and showed good mobility. No lesions were observed in the bilateral adnexal regions.

   (b) Contrast-enhanced ultrasound:

   The uterine cavity appeared smooth and regular in shape. Regarding tubal patency, contrast-enhanced ultrasound (Fig. 5.61) showed the entire

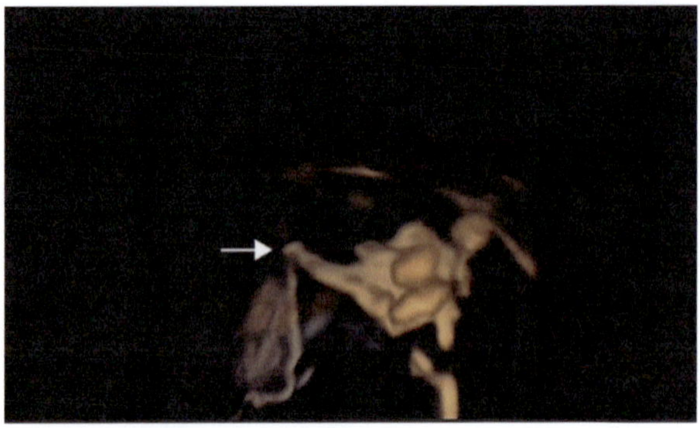

Fig. 5.60 The right fallopian tube was partially obstructed and reflexed (the arrow shows the reflexed angle); the distal part of the left fallopian tube was blocked; there was contrast reflux in the myometrium

right fallopian tube visualized with a stiff alignment and obvious localized reflection. Contrast overflow was seen at the fimbrial end, and the contrast medium dispersed evenly around the right ovary. The left fallopian tube was intermittently visualized, showing truncation at the mid-section, a slightly tortuous course, and a rather rigid morphology, with no contrast overflow at the fimbrial end. The contrast agent was unevenly distributed around the left ovary.

Echoes of contrast reflux within the myometrium were observed, and the contrast agent was unevenly distributed in the pelvis, with significantly less contrast on the left side compared to the right side. Based on these findings, a diagnosis of partial obstruction of the right fallopian tube and complete obstruction of the distal section of the left fallopian tube was made.

(c) Intrapelvic findings:

B-mode ultrasound showed limited mobility of the left ovary. Contrast-enhanced ultrasound revealed minimal contrast agent encircling the left ovary, with uneven contrast diffusion and band-like echoes in the pelvis (Fig. 5.61), indicating adhesions.

(d) SIS imaging:

SIS showed a mid-echogenic mass in the uterine cavity with clear borders, consistent with an endometrial polyp.

4. Medical advice:

Given the patient's advanced age, the partial obstruction of the right fallopian tube, and the complete obstruction of the distal section of the left fallopian tube, the patient was advised to proceed with IVF treatment as soon as possible.

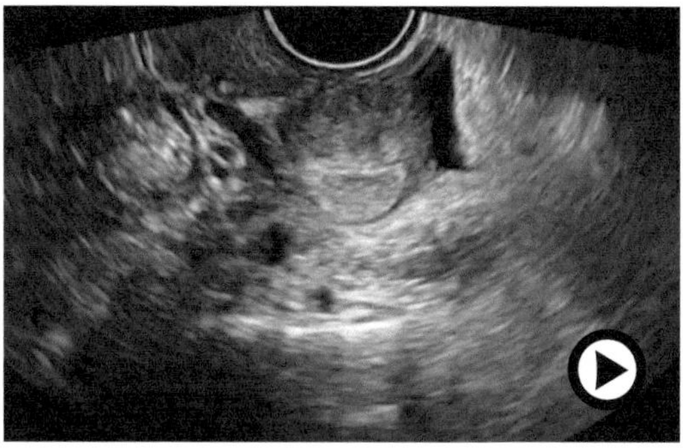

Fig. 5.61 Case 5 (▶ https://doi.org/10.1007/000-hrt)

5.4 Management of Intracontrast and Postcontrast Adverse Events and Postcontrast Cautions

5.4.1 Management of Intracontrast and Postcontrast Adverse Events

Common adverse reactions following contrast injection include lower abdominal pain, vaginal bleeding, abortion syndrome, and contrast agent allergies. Most of these events can be managed with symptomatic treatment, and hospitalization for observation may be necessary in some cases.

1. Abdominal Pain

   Mild-to-moderate abdominal and pelvic pain can occur during or after the contrast injection, often due to the dilatation of the uterus and fallopian tubes following contrast medium administration [32].

   Pain during the procedure should significantly subside within 30 min. If abdominal pain persists or worsens after the examination, further evaluation and consultation are recommended.
2. Vaginal Bleeding

   Vaginal bleeding is a common complication during the peri-HyCoSy period and is most often caused by trauma to the cervix or endometrium during procedures like intrauterine catheterization. In some cases, postoperative vaginal bleeding may also occur due to the presence of cervical polyps, endometrial polyps, submucosal fibroids, or other underlying conditions.

   It is important to perform the intrauterine catheterization gently to minimize trauma. Generally, vaginal bleeding less than the volume of a typical menstrual period does not require special treatment and usually resolves within 1 week. However, if bleeding exceeds the menstrual volume, the cause should be investigated, and appropriate treatment should be initiated.

3. Vasovagal Reactions

   Mechanical stimulation of the cervix and uterine wall, or excessive pressure in the uterine cavity, may trigger vagus nerve excitation. This can lead to a range of effects on the cardiovascular system, including insufficient cerebrovascular blood supply [33, 34].

   Vasovagal reactions may present as nausea, vomiting, dizziness, shortness of breath, pallor, profuse sweating, a drop in blood pressure, cardiac arrhythmias, chest tightness, and, in severe cases, shock. These symptoms may occur during and/or after contrast injection and are often associated with emotional stress, difficulty in dilating the cervical canal, rough handling by the operator, excessive negative pressure, or strong uterine contractions in the patient.

   Vasovagal reactions can be categorized according to the severity of the patient's symptoms:

   - Mild: A feeling of lower abdominal cramping or vague pain, often accompanied by nausea
   - Moderate: Significant pain that is tolerable, possibly accompanied by nausea and vomiting
   - Severe: Severe pain, often accompanied by nausea, vomiting, cold sweats, pallor, a drop in blood pressure, and a slowed pulse rate

   Preventive measures:

   - Create a comfortable surgical environment.
   - Use gentle techniques to minimize trauma, including limiting the use of cervical forceps.
   - Minimize irritation to the cervical os and uterus.
   - Use minimal balloon filling (typically 1.0–1.5 mL) to prevent catheter slippage.
   - Consider administering atropine 0.5 mg intramuscularly 30 min before the procedure to help prevent vasovagal reactions.

   Treatment measures:

   - For mild symptoms, instruct the patient to lie down and rest. Most symptoms resolve spontaneously with symptomatic treatment (e.g., oxygenation).
   - For severe cases, administer intravenous atropine 0.5 mg and prepare for resuscitation if necessary.

4. Allergy to the Contrast Agent

   Using sulfur hexafluoride microbubble contrast agent as an example, the main manifestations of an allergic reaction may include skin rash, flushing, and, in more severe cases, shortness of breath and a drop in blood pressure [35].

   Treatment measures:

   - If an allergic reaction occurs, the examination should be stopped immediately, and treatment should be tailored to the patient's clinical symptoms. Anti-allergy medications such as promethazine hydrochloride and dexamethasone may be administered. In addition, the patient should receive oxygen and, if necessary, support for respiratory and circulatory functions. Patients with a known history of allergies to medications or foods should be closely monitored and observed during the procedure.

5.4.2 Postcontrast Cautions

1. Staying for observation

   After completing the contrast-enhanced ultrasound examination, the patient should be instructed to rest in a comfortable position, either lying down or sitting quietly for 15–30 min. Warm compresses may be applied to the lower abdomen, and the patient can consume warm water. The patient should be informed that most discomforts will resolve with rest. However, if any serious adverse symptoms occur, the patient should contact medical staff immediately for appropriate treatment.
2. Prevention of infections

   As the uterine cavity and fallopian tubes communicate with the external environment via the vagina, there is a risk of infection, particularly due to potential cervical or endometrial injury during intrauterine manipulation. To mitigate this risk, a 3-day course of preventative antibiotics is recommended. While rare, some patients may develop acute vaginitis, endometritis, or pelvic inflammation postprocedure, which should be treated promptly with appropriate anti-infective therapy.
3. Other periperiodic management

   After the contrast-enhanced ultrasound, the patient should rest adequately and avoid strenuous exercise for at least 1 week. Alcohol and spicy foods should also be avoided during this period. Sexual intercourse, tub baths, and swimming should be avoided for 2 weeks post procedure.

References

1. Carson SA, Kallen AN. Diagnosis and management of infertility: a review. JAMA. 2021;326(1):65–76.
2. Exalto N, Emanuel MH. Clinical aspects of HyFoSy as tubal patency test in subfertility workup. Biomed Res Int. 2019;2019:4827376.
3. Honoré GM, Holden AE, Schenken RS. Pathophysiology and management of proximal tubal blockage. Fertil Steril. 1999;71(5):785–95.
4. Zafarani F, Ghaffari F, Ahmadi F, et al. Hysterosalpingography in the assessment of proximal tubal pathology: a review of congenital and acquired abnormalities. Br J Radiol. 2021;94(1122):20201386.
5. Canday M, Yurtkal A, Kirat S. Evaluation and perspectives on hysterosalpingography (HSG) procedure in infertility: a comprehensive study. Eur Rev Med Pharmacol Sci. 2023;27(15):7107–17.
6. Saunders RD, Shwayder JM, Nakajima ST. Current methods of tubal patency assessment. Fertil Steril. 2011;95(7):2171–9.

7. Dishuck CF, Perchik JD, Porter KK, et al. Advanced imaging in female infertility. Curr Urol Rep. 2019;20(11):77.
8. Sladkevicius P, Ojha K, Campbell S, et al. Three-dimensional power Doppler imaging in the assessment of fallopian tube patency. Ultrasound Obstet Gynecol. 2000;16(7):644–7.
9. Qu E, Zhang M, Ju J, et al. Is hysterosalpingo-contrast sonography (HyCoSy) using sulfur hexafluoride microbubbles (SonoVue) sufficient for the assessment of fallopian tube patency? A systematic review and meta-analysis. J Ultrasound Med. 2023;42(1):7–15.
10. Grigovich M, Kacharia VS, Bharwani N, et al. Evaluating fallopian tube patency: what the radiologist needs to know. Radiographics. 2021;41(6):1876–18961.
11. Devine K, Dolitsky S, Ludwin I, et al. Modern assessment of the uterine cavity and fallopian tubes in the era of high-efficacy assisted reproductive technology. Fertil Steril. 2022;118(1):19–28.
12. Zhang J, Lan W, Wang Y, et al. Ethiodized poppyseed oil-based contrast medium is superior to water-based contrast medium during hysterosalpingography regarding image quality improvement and fertility enhancement: a multicentric, randomized and controlled trial. EClinicalMedicine. 2022;46:101363.
13. Swart P, Mol BW, van der Veen F, et al. The accuracy of hysterosalpingography in the diagnosis of tubal pathology: a meta-analysis. Fertil Steril. 1995;64:486–91.
14. Chen J, Liu S, Lu J. Comparison of fertility outcomes between oil-based and water-based contrast media during hysterosalpingography: a meta-analysis. Exp Ther Med. 2023;26(3):449.
15. Fang F, Bai Y, Zhang Y, et al. Oil-based versus water-based contrast for hysterosalpingography in infertile women: a systematic review and meta-analysis of randomized controlled trials. Fertil Steril. 2018;110(1):153–160.e3.
16. Yang JJ, Chapman M. What are the risks associated with lipiodol hysterosalpingography? A literature review. Radiography (Lond). 2023;29(6):1041–5.
17. Cobellis L, Argano F, Castaldi MA, et al. Selective salpingography: preliminary experience of an office operative option for proximal tubal recanalization. Eur J Obstet Gynecol Reprod Biol. 2012;163(1):62–6.
18. Thurmond AS, Machan LS, Maubon AJ, et al. A review of selective salpingography and fallopian tube catheterization. Radiographics. 2000;20(6):1759–68.
19. Younas K, Majoko F, Sheard K, et al. Select and treat at laparoscopy and dye test improves the spontaneous pregnancy. Hum Fertil (Camb). 2014;17(1):56–9.
20. Kamath MS, Rikken JFW, Bosteels J. Does laparoscopy and hysteroscopy have a place in the diagnosis of unexplained infertility? Semin Reprod Med. 2020;38(1):29–35.
21. Adesiyun AG, Cole B, Ogwuche P. Hydrotubation in the management of female infertility: outcome in low resource settings. East Afr Med J. 2009;86(1):31–6.
22. Lundberg S, Rasmussen C, Berg AA, et al. Falloposcopy in conjunction with laparoscopy: possibilities and limitations. Hum Reprod. 1998;13(6):1490–2.
23. Carrascosa P, Capuñay C, Baronio M, et al. 64-Row multidetector CT virtual hysterosalpingography. Abdom Imaging. 2009;34(1):121–33.
24. Duan N, Chen X, Yin Y, et al. Comparison between magnetic resonance hysterosalpingography and conventional hysterosalpingography: direct visualization of the fallopian tubes using a novel MRI contrast agent mixture. Acta Radiol. 2020;61(7):1001–7.
25. Chen LS, Zhu ZQ, Li J, et al. Hysterosalpingo-contrast-sonography vs. magnetic resonance-hysterosalpingography for diagnosing fallopian tubal patency: a systematic review and meta-analysis. Eur J Radiol. 2020;125:108891.
26. Lindborg L, Thorburn J, Bergh C, et al. Influence of HyCoSy on spontaneous pregnancy: a randomized controlled trial. Hum Reprod. 2009;24(5):1075–9.
27. Ott J, Hager M, Nouri K, et al. Assessment of tubal patency: a prospective comparison of diagnostic hysteroscopy and laparoscopic chromopertubation. J Minim Invasive Gynecol. 2020;27(1):135–40.
28. Grimbizis GF, Di Spiezio Sardo A, Saravelos SH, et al. The Thessaloniki ESHRE/ESGE consensus on diagnosis of female genital anomalies. Hum Reprod. 2016;31:2–7.

29. Yang P, Zhong Y, Zhang C, et al. Contrast agent reflux in transvaginal 4-D hysterosalpingo-contrast sonography: influencing factors and coping strategies. Ultrasound Q. 2024;40(1):61–5.
30. Reis MM, Soares SR, Cancado ML, et al. Hysterosalpingo contrast sonography (HyCoSy) with SH U 454 (Echovist) for the assessment of tubal patency. Hum Reprod. 1998;13:3049–52.
31. Ng KYB, Cheong Y. Hydrosalpinx – salpingostomy, salpingectomy or tubal occlusion. Best Pract Res Clin Obstet Gynaecol. 2019;59:41–7.
32. Guney M, Oral B, Bayhan G, et al. Intrauterine lidocaine infusion for pain relief during saline solution infusion sonohysterography: a randomized, controlled trial. J Minim Invasive Gynecol. 2007;14(3):304–10.
33. Dessole S, Farina M, Capobianco G, et al. Determining the best catheter for sonohysterography. Fertil Steril. 2001;76:605–9.
34. Xie H, Zhang X, Tian D, et al. Effect of acupoint application of Chinese medicine combined with a hot compress on pain of uterine and fallopian tube contrast agent in infertile women. Altern Ther Health Med. 2024;30(9):65–71.
35. Longhino D, Buonomo A, Zocco MA, et al. Anaphylaxis after SonoVue: a case report and a literature review. J Clin Med. 2024;13(17):5018.

6 Ultrasound Assessment of Endometrial Receptivity

Da Li, Na Zuo, and Zhijing Na

6.1 Overview

Endometrial receptivity (ER) refers to the endometrium's capacity to allow the embryo to settle, adhere, and invade. Favorable ER triggers changes in the endometrial stroma at specific stages, facilitating embryo implantation. The receptive period of the endometrium, also known as the implantation window, typically lasts between 30 and 36 h. For women with a 28-day menstrual cycle, this window usually occurs on the 19th or 20th day of the cycle [1]. For women undergoing artificial cycles induced by hormone replacement therapy, the implantation window typically occurs between 4 and 7 days after progesterone administration.

A successful pregnancy through in vitro fertilization and embryo transfer (IVF-ET) depends on several factors, including embryo quality, ER, and the synchronization between endometrial and embryonic development [2, 3]. With the advancement of diagnostic and laboratory techniques, as well as genetic testing before embryo transfer, embryo quality is no longer the most critical factor influencing pregnancy outcomes. In fact, studies suggest that two-thirds of embryo implantation failures are attributed to poor ER and altered embryo-endometrial dialogue [4].

Endometrial biopsy is commonly used to evaluate ER [5, 6]. However, endometrial receptivity analysis (ERA), a more recent development, can detect the implantation window with precise hourly accuracy. Despite its precision, ERA is not the preferred method for assessing ER due to its invasive nature and limited

Supplementary Information The online version contains supplementary material available at https://doi.org/10.1007/978-981-95-1373-4_6. The videos can be accessed individually by clicking the DOI link in the accompanying figure caption or by scanning this link with the SN More Media App.

D. Li (✉) · N. Zuo · Z. Na
Shengjing Hospital of China Medical University, Shenyang, China

D. Li et al. (eds.), *Ultrasonography of the Female Reproductive System*,
https://doi.org/10.1007/978-981-95-1373-4_6

repeatability. In contrast, ultrasonography is a noninvasive and repeatable tool used extensively in assisted reproduction. It allows for dynamic, real-time observation of the endometrium [7]. The ultrasonographic evaluation of ER, including the measurement of endometrial thickness, morphology, and hemodynamic profile, plays a crucial role in guiding treatment regimens and determining the appropriate therapeutic approach [8].

6.2 Markers of Endometrial Morphology for Evaluating Endometrial Receptivity by Ultrasound

6.2.1 Thickness of the Endometrium

The functional layer of the endometrium undergoes cyclic changes in response to estrogen and progesterone secreted by the ovaries. Endometrial thickness is the most commonly used ultrasound marker for evaluating ER and significantly impacts pregnancy outcomes [4]. It is generally recommended that the endometrium be measured in the sagittal plane by transvaginal ultrasound [9].

1. Timing of endometrial thickness measurement and ER evaluation

   Although the implantation window falls during the secretory phase of the endometrium, in clinical practice, the timing of ultrasound evaluation of ER is typically set at the end of the proliferative phase of the endometrium. This corresponds to the day before ovulation in a natural cycle, the day of hCG injection in an ovarian stimulation cycle, and the day of progesterone administration in a hormone replacement cycle. This timing is used to guide subsequent consultation and treatment. A meta-analysis comparing endometrial thickness at different stages of the menstrual cycle between pregnant and nonpregnant groups showed a statistically significant difference in endometrial thickness at the end of the proliferative phase (hCG day and progesterone supplementation day) between the two groups. However, no significant difference was observed in endometrial thickness measured on the egg retrieval day, the day of embryo transfer in a frozen-thaw cycle, or during the midluteal phase in the cycle before implantation [8].

   It has been shown that the optimal endometrial thickness for embryo implantation on the progesterone supplementation day in medical frozen-thawed embryo replacement cycles is between 9 and 14 mm [10]. The thin endometrium is widely recognized as detrimental to pregnancy [11] and serves as a negative predictor of pregnancy outcomes. That is, patients diagnosed with thin endometrium are more likely to experience pregnancy failure. However, different studies define "thin endometrium" in varying ways. A study involving 24,000 fresh embryo transfer and 20,000 frozen-thawed embryo transfer cycles across 33 centers found that clinical pregnancy and live birth rates decreased for each millimeter of endometrial thickness below 8 mm in fresh IVF cycles and below 7 mm in frozen-thaw IVF cycles [12]. Other studies have shown that an endometrial thickness of <7 mm is associated with a significant decline in live birth rates, and endometrial thickness <6 mm is linked to a dramatic decline in live birth rates [13]. Some studies also suggest that endometrial thickness greater than 14 mm may be associated with decreased pregnancy rates. However, others have concluded that an upper limit for endometrial thickness does not exist, and a "too-thick" endometrium should not automatically lead to the cancellation of an embryo transfer cycle, provided that no pathological condition is present [13].

The significance of assessing endometrial thickness on the day of embryo transfer in an IVF cycle remains controversial. Some studies have shown that an endometrial thickness of ≥ 9 mm on the day of transfer is associated with a higher rate of sustained pregnancy. In contrast, other studies have indicated that endometrial thickness on the day of transfer is a poor predictor of pregnancy outcomes, offering limited clinical guidance. These studies suggest that there may be no need to intervene in cases of thin endometrium on the day of embryo transfer and propose eliminating the requirement for a specific endometrial thickness range on the day of implantation (e.g., 3–22 mm) [14].

The endometrium undergoes a series of changes during the secretory phase under the influence of progesterone. Recently, researchers have proposed that the dynamic changes in endometrial thickness throughout the secretory phase may be more informative than evaluating the absolute thickness at any single time point.

2. Changes in endometrial thickness and ER during the secretory phase

   Although textbooks and gynecologic ultrasound guidelines suggest that the endometrium thickens during the secretory phase compared to the proliferative phase [15], a decrease in endometrial thickness during the secretory phase is not uncommon in clinical practice. The presence of this phenomenon on the day of embryo transfer has raised concern among patients, but at this stage, such concerns appear to be unwarranted. Some studies have shown that endometrial thickness decreased in 1/3 of patients during the secretory phase compared to the proliferative phase, while it increased or remained unchanged in 2/3 of patients [16].

   It has been reported that the sustained pregnancy rate in patients with a 10% decrease in endometrial thickness after progesterone administration was significantly higher than that of patients with increased or unchanged endometrial thickness (52% vs. 24%). Moreover, the greater the decrease in endometrial thickness, the higher the pregnancy rate [16, 17].

   Researchers have suggested that, as progesterone receptors are activated during the secretory phase, ultrasound imaging may show enhanced and denser endometrial echogenicity, along with varying degrees of thickness, all of which are considered normal (Fig. 6.1). In contrast, a persistent increase in endometrial thickness during this phase could indicate a poor endometrial response to progesterone, a lack of progesterone receptors, or progesterone resistance due to conditions like chronic inflammation or endometriosis. These factors may negatively impact pregnancy outcomes [16, 17]. However, this hypothesis requires further investigation.

   A recent study demonstrated that endometrial thickness did not correlate with pregnancy outcomes in patients undergoing IVF, regardless of whether it increased, decreased, or remained unchanged on the day of embryo transfer [18].

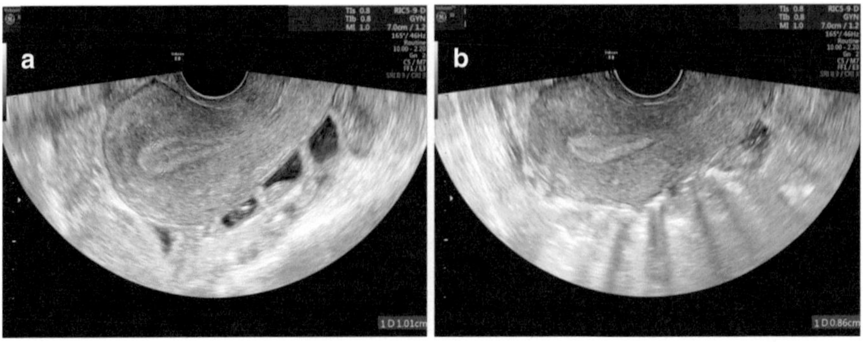

Fig. 6.1 (**a**) Endometrial thickness before ovulation. (**b**) Endometrial thickness after ovulation

6.2.2 Endometrial Morphology

In clinical practice, the morphology of the endometrium is typically categorized into three types (see details in Sect. 3.2 of Chap. 3). The physiological basis for these cyclic changes in morphology lies in the fluctuations of estrogen and progesterone levels throughout the menstrual cycle. Before ovulation, the endometrium is primarily influenced by estrogen, and it appears as a "triple-line" endometrium on ultrasound, representing the proliferative phase. Following ovulation, as progesterone levels rise, the endometrium gradually transforms from an "isoechogenic" to a "homogeneous hyperechogenic" appearance.

A meta-analysis involving patients treated with intrauterine insemination (IUI) found that those with a "triple-line" endometrium on the day of hCG injection or IUI day had a higher clinical pregnancy rate. In contrast, among patients undergoing in vitro fertilization (IVF), pregnancy outcomes were similar regardless of whether the endometrium displayed the "triple line" on the day of hCG injection, 1 day after hCG injection, on the day of egg retrieval, the day of progesterone administration, or the day of embryo implantation [8].

Although many clinicians believe that a "triple-line" endometrium on the day of hCG injection in fresh embryo transfer cycles or on the day of progesterone administration in frozen-thawed cycles leads to better pregnancy outcomes, the recent meta-analysis does not provide sufficient evidence to support this view.

6.2.3 Endometrial Volume

Endometrial volume is a 3D ultrasound index used to evaluate ER. It is obtained by manually outlining the entire endometrial border on 3D ultrasound, with measurements taken using virtual organ computer-assisted analysis (VOCAL) software (Fig. 6.2). There is a significant correlation between endometrial thickness and endometrial volume.

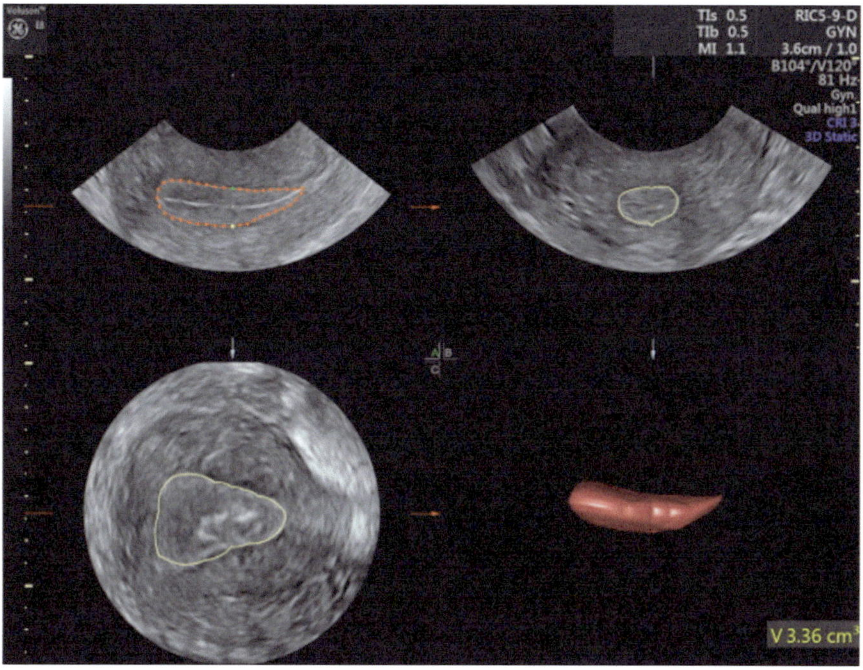

Fig. 6.2 Measurement of endometrial volume

A study of 550 intrauterine insemination (IUI) cycles found that the pregnant group had a higher endometrial volume on the day of IUI compared to the nonpregnant group. However, results from eight clinical trials on in vitro fertilization (IVF) showed no significant difference in endometrial volume between pregnant and non-pregnant groups, whether measured on the day of hCG injection or the day of embryo transfer [8].

Despite the lack of conclusive evidence supporting the predictive value of endometrial volume for pregnancy outcomes, many studies have used a threshold of 2.5 mL [19]. One study analyzing patients with pregnancy failure found that an endometrial volume threshold of 3.2 mL predicted pregnancy failure with 96% accuracy in frozen-thawed cycles [20]. However, the value of endometrial volume as a predictor of negative pregnancy outcomes remains to be confirmed through further studies.

6.2.4 Endometrial Peristalsis (EP)

Unlike the out-layer uterine muscle contractions that cause dysmenorrhea and labor pain, EP results from the contraction of the sub-endometrial myometrial layer. This contraction generates endometrial wave motion, similar to intestinal peristalsis (Fig. 6.3). The sub-endometrial myometrial layer, also known as the junctional

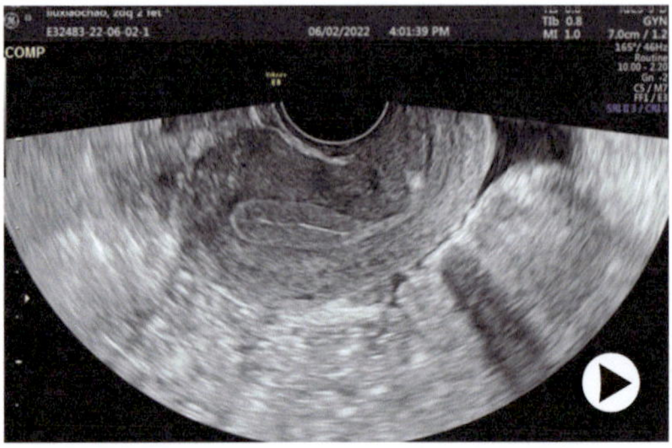

Fig. 6.3 Endometrial peristalsis (▶ https://doi.org/10.1007/000-hrx)

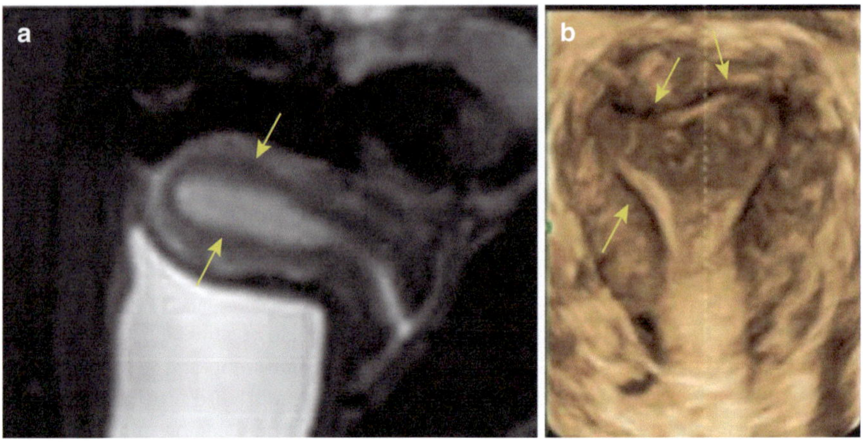

Fig. 6.4 The uterine junctional zone: panel (**a**) is an MRI image of the uterine junctional zone, and panel (**b**) is an ultrasound image of the uterine junctional zone

zone, consists of the basal layer of the endometrium and the inner third of the myometrium. Due to this region's relatively low water content, magnetic resonance imaging (MRI) shows a low-signal band distinct from the high-signal endometrium and the homogeneous-signal outer myometrium on T2-weighted images.

Transvaginal ultrasonography can detect the junctional zone (Fig. 6.4). Contractions of this zone and their frequency are regulated by cyclic hormonal fluctuations produced by the ovaries. They can be influenced by lesions near the junctional zone, such as uterine fibroids, endometrial polyps, and adenomyosis. Abnormal contractions of the junctional zone may lead to poor pregnancy outcomes. However, the assessment of junctional zone contractions is currently not part of routine gynecologic ultrasound practices due to its time-consuming and labor-intensive nature, and it is not addressed in clinical guidelines.

EP begins with the contraction of the junctional zone. Studies have categorized EP waves into five types based on their directionality: (a) peristalsis waves moving from the cervix to the fundus; (b) peristalsis waves moving from the fundus to the cervix; (c) waves emanating simultaneously from both the uterine fundus and cervix in opposite directions; (d) random peristalsis waves of variable directions; and (e) no motion [21, 22].

EP plays a crucial role in normal reproductive function and embryo implantation. In the early follicular phase, EP is characterized by waves moving from the uterine fundus to the cervix, primarily promoting the discharge of secretions and preventing microbial infections. As follicles develop and estrogen levels increase, EP intensifies, reaching its peak in the periovulatory period, with waves predominantly directed from the cervix to the fundus, which aids in the sperm transport. Following ovulation, EP frequency decreases, and random waves in opposite directions dominate until the midluteal phase, providing time and opportunity for the embryo to fully engage with the endometrium. During the late luteal phase, the endometrium becomes relatively quiescent, which is favorable for embryo implantation [23].

Dysregulation of EP, including excessive frequency and amplitude of peristalsis, can adversely affect embryo implantation and increase the likelihood of ectopic pregnancy. Research indicates that the highest clinical pregnancy rates are found in women with an EP frequency of less than two waves per minute prior to embryo transfer, whereas those with more than three waves per minute have significantly lower pregnancy rates [24].

Currently, EP waves are detected visually by transvaginal ultrasound, but the results are highly subjective and poorly reproducible, and the procedure is time-consuming, making it challenging to adopt in routine clinical practice. Therefore, more accurate testing equipment and analytical methods are needed to further explore this area.

6.3 Hemodynamic Markers for Evaluating ER by Ultrasound

Poor uterine perfusion was first identified by Goswamy in 1988 as a potential cause of female infertility. With the increasing demand for assisted reproduction, clinical studies evaluating uterine perfusion via ultrasound have become more widespread. Some researchers suggest that Doppler ultrasound assessment of uterine perfusion may be a useful ER marker. This evaluation includes using Doppler ultrasound to measure uterine arterial, endometrial, and sub-endometrial blood flows.

6.3.1 Anatomical Characteristics of Uterine Vessels

The uterine artery originates from the anterior trunk of the internal iliac artery and ascends along the lateral wall of the uterus, giving rise to the arcuate arteries. These arcuate arteries then branch into radial arteries within the myometrium, which further divide into basal arteries and spiral arteries in the basal and functional layers of the endometrium (Fig. 6.5). The uterine basal arteries supply the basal layer of the endometrium and are not influenced by hormonal fluctuations. In contrast, the

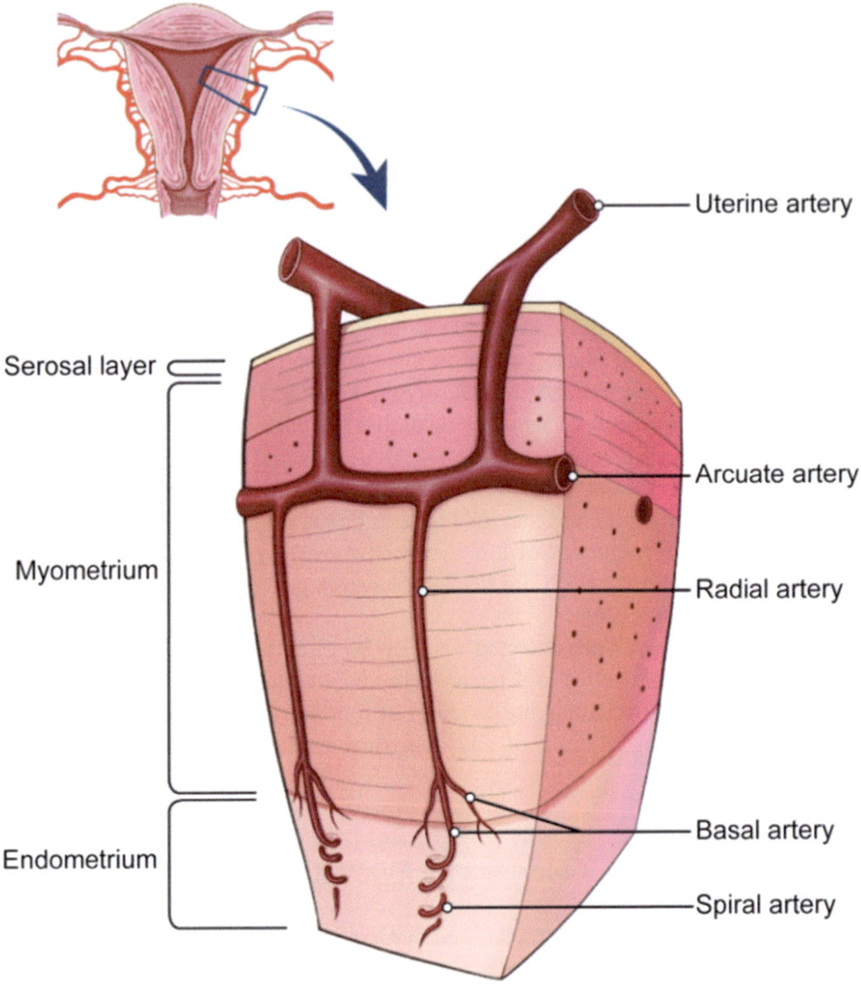

Fig. 6.5 Anatomical characteristics of uterine blood vessels

uterine spiral arteries extend deep into the functional layer of the endometrium, with their diameter varying in response to ovarian hormone levels. The uterine spiral arteries undergo physiological changes during pregnancy to support embryo growth.

6.3.2 Blood Flow in the Uterine Artery

1. Ultrasound scanning

   During transvaginal ultrasonography, position the transducer to obtain the midsagittal plane of the uterus. Place the color Doppler sampling frame at the junction of the cervix and uterus, and then move the transducer side to side to visualize the bilateral uterine arteries. Color Doppler will reveal bright, tortuous, tubular flow signals within the uterine arteries (Fig. 6.6).

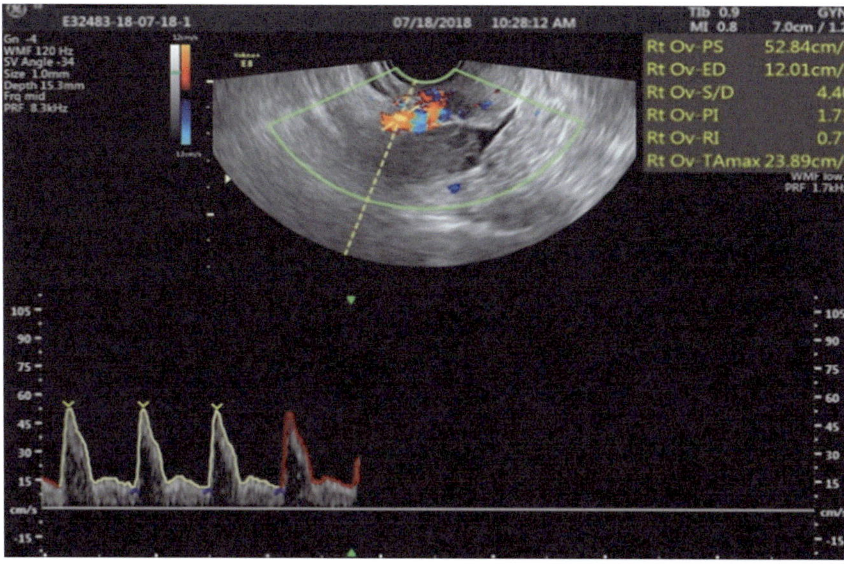

Fig. 6.6 Uterine artery blood flow

Fig. 6.7 Schematic of normal uterine artery blood flow waveform

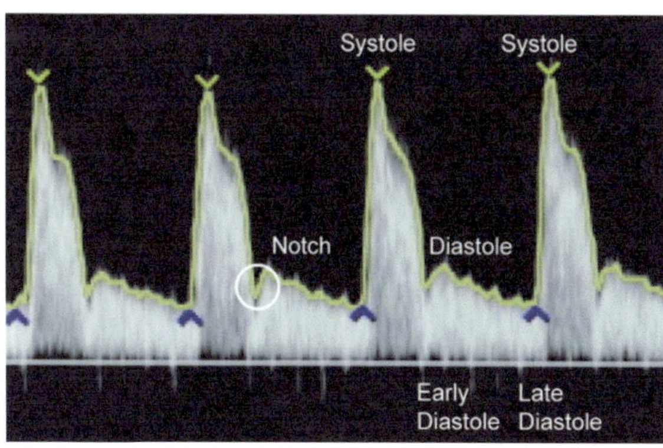

2. Waveforms of blood flow in the uterine artery

   Uterine artery blood flow waveforms are classified into four types based on reported literature (Figs. 6.7 and 6.8):

   - Type C: Continuous forward flow with an early diastolic notch
   - Type A: Presence of an early diastolic notch and loss of late diastolic flow
   - Type O1: Only systolic blood flow with no diastolic flow
   - Type O2: Presence of reverse early diastolic flow and absence of late diastolic flow

   Type C uterine artery waveforms are considered normal, with bilateral type C waveforms indicating favorable uterine perfusion. A combination of type C on one side and type A on the other suggests impaired, though still adequate, uterine perfusion. Any type O (O1 or O2, unilateral or bilateral) or bilateral type A

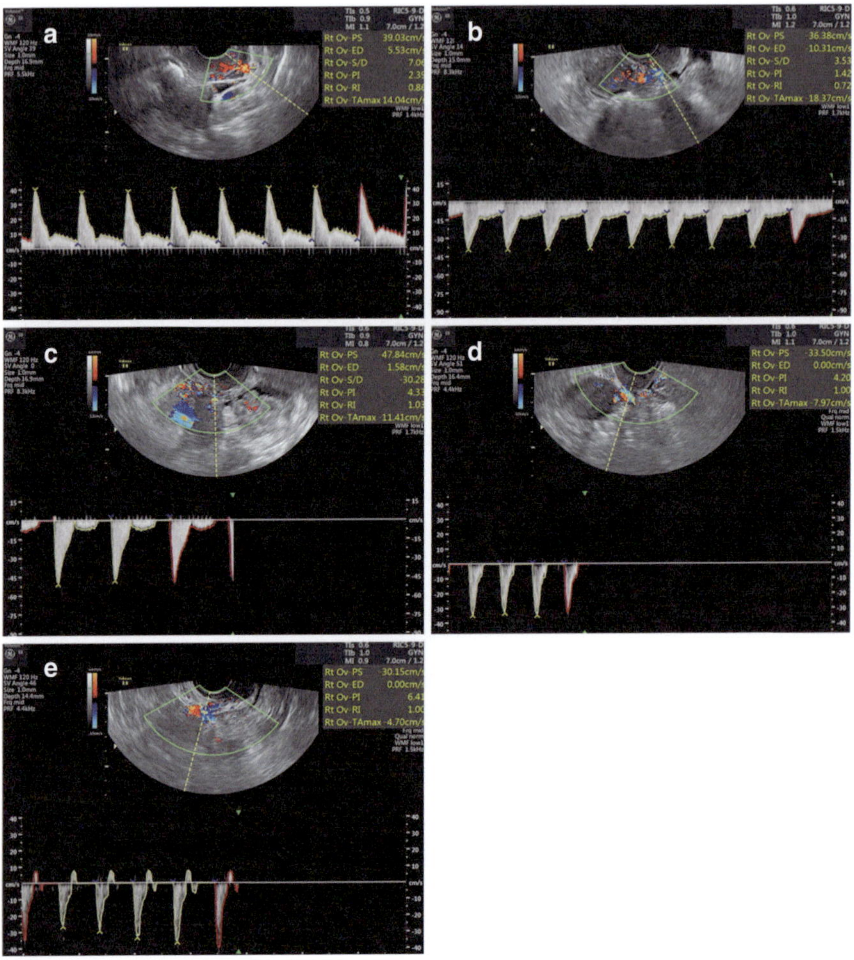

Fig. 6.8 (**a**) Type C uterine artery blood flow. (**b**) Type C uterine artery blood flow. (**c**) Type A uterine artery blood flow. (**d**) Type O1 uterine artery blood flow. (**e**) Type O2 uterine artery blood flow. Note: The direction of the wave represents the direction of blood flow—toward the ultrasound probe or away from it

waveforms indicate adverse blood flow, with the absence of late diastolic blood flow associated with high resistance in these vessels [25].

3. Parameters of uterine artery blood flow

   Uterine artery blood flow parameters include the pulse index (PI), resistance index (RI), systolic-diastolic ratio (S/D), peak systolic velocity (PSV), and end-diastolic velocity (EDV), defined as follows:

   - RI = (PSV − EDV)/PSV
   - PI = (PSV − EDV)/mean blood velocity
   - S/D = PSV/EDV

Table 6.1 Reference values of uterine artery blood flow parameters in nonpregnancy

Item	Menstrual period	Proliferative phase	Luteal phase
RI	0.86 ± 0.04	0.88 ± 0.05	0.84 ± 0.06
PI	<3.0	<3.0	2.08 ± 0.47
S/D value	<8.0	<3.0	5.73 ± 1.47

Table 6.2 Reference values for normal uterine artery blood flow parameters during pregnancy

Item	Early pregnancy	Midpregnancy	Late pregnancy
RI	<0.75	<0.73	<0.58
PI	<2.25	<1.5	<0.82
S/D value	<6.0	<3.6	<2.6

These parameters must be measured over three complete consecutive cardiac cycles to accurately evaluate resistance to uterine blood flow.

Theoretically, lower PI and RI values indicate reduced vascular resistance and better uterine perfusion [26]. Estrogen levels peak 2–3 days before ovulation, resulting in decreased vascular resistance. After ovulation, progesterone levels gradually rise during the midluteal phase, promoting smooth muscle relaxation. Together, estrogen and progesterone contribute to further reduced resistance to uterine blood flow (Table 6.1) [27].

The uterine artery blood flow waveform in nonpregnant women is typically characterized by high resistance and low diastolic flow, accompanied by an early diastolic notch. This early diastolic notch persists in approximately 50% of early pregnancies. Between 14 and 16 weeks of gestation, the high-resistance blood flow transitions to a low-resistance pattern with increased diastolic flow to meet the demands of fetal growth and development. Uterine artery vascular resistance continues to decline from early to midpregnancy, with minimal changes observed during late pregnancy (Table 6.2) [27].

4. Uterine artery blood flow parameters and ER

   Numerous studies have highlighted the predictive value of uterine artery parameters in assessing ER. The RI, calculated as RI = (PSV − EDV)/PSV, ranges from 0.0 to 1.0, except in cases of reversed diastolic blood flow (negative EDV), where RI exceeds 1. A higher EDV corresponds to a lower RI, indicating low-resistance blood flow, which is associated with better uterine perfusion. Conversely, low EDV results in higher RI, reflecting increased vascular resistance. Increased resistance to blood flow may also be indicated by a higher PI [28].

   Several clinical studies have demonstrated significantly lower PI and RI values in the pregnant group compared to the nonpregnant group [29, 30]. Additionally, immunohistochemical assays of tissue sections have shown correlations between uterine arterial resistance and biomarkers of ER [30]. Early studies categorized uterine artery PI into low (0–1.99), medium (2.00–2.99), and high (≥3.00) groups, with low PI values associated with better pregnancy outcomes [28, 31, 32]. Furthermore, pregnancy rates were significantly lower when PI exceeded 3.00, and RI surpassed 0.92, with the lowest rates observed when PI exceeded 3.30, and RI exceeded 0.95 on the day of embryo transfer. Notably, high impedance (PI > 3.30 and RI > 0.95) was detected in 9% of total cycles [33].

Despite these findings, the literature also contains studies with conflicting results. A meta-analysis revealed that a PI < 3 on the day of embryo transfer was associated with improved pregnancy outcomes. However, the differences in uterine artery PI and RI between pregnant and nonpregnant groups were not statistically significant [8].

6.3.3 Endometrial and Sub-endometrial Blood Flow

The uterine artery supplies blood not only to the endometrium but also to other adjacent tissues, including the myometrium, fallopian tubes, ovaries, and vagina. As a result, uterine artery flow parameters may not precisely reflect the localized perfusion of the endometrium. In contrast, the assessment of endometrial and sub-endometrial blood flow provides a more specific and objective profile of the blood supply directly related to the endometrium.

1. 2D color Doppler ultrasound of endometrium and sub-endometrium

   Two-dimensional (2D) color Doppler ultrasound is a widely utilized tool for visualizing the spiral arteries of the endometrium and measuring their spectral profiles. The parameters assessed include the following:

   (a) Endometrial blood flow type: A classification based on the distribution of blood flow signals.

   (b) Endometrial and sub-endometrial blood flow indices include PI, RI, S/D, PSV, and EDV.

   Endometrial and sub-endometrial blood flow classification often follows Applebaum's uterine scoring system, which categorizes blood flow into three types (Figs. 6.9, 6.10, 6.11, and 6.12):

   (a) Type I: Blood flow signals are observed outside the endometrium but not within it (i.e., present in the sub-endometrial area but absent in the basal and functional layers).

   (b) Type II: Blood vessels penetrate the outer hypoechoic region of the endometrium but do not enter its inner hypoechoic area (i.e., blood flow is present in the basal layer but absent in the functional layer).

   (c) Type III: Blood vessels reach the inner hypoechoic area of the endometrium, indicating blood flow in the functional layer.

   Studies have linked poor endometrial and sub-endometrial blood supply to adverse pregnancy outcomes. Research reports that the presence of blood flow signals in both the endometrium and sub-endometrium is associated with a pregnancy rate of 47.8%. In comparison, the pregnancy rate drops to 29.7% when blood flow signals are confined to the sub-endometrium and plummets to 7.5% in cases where blood flow signals are absent in both regions. Patients in the latter

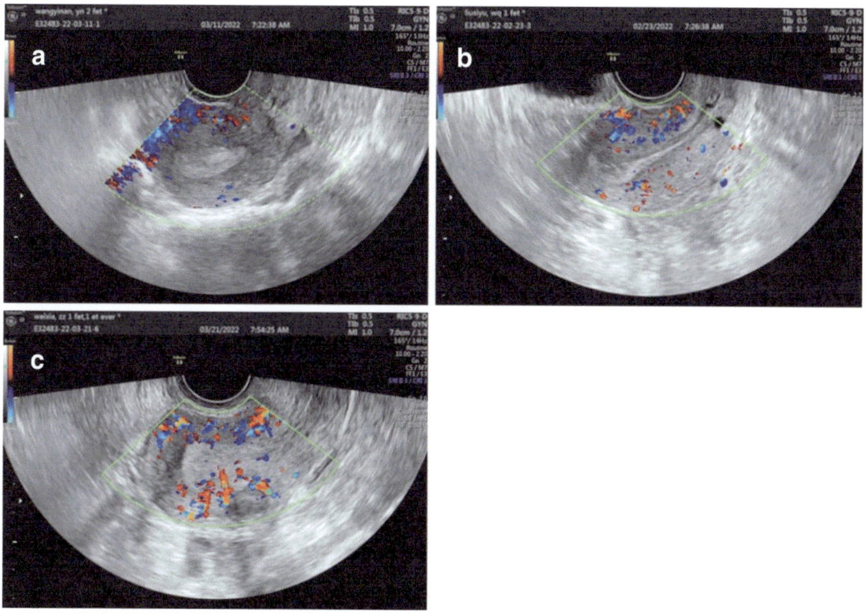

Fig. 6.9 (**a**) Type I. (**b**) Type II. (**c**) Type III

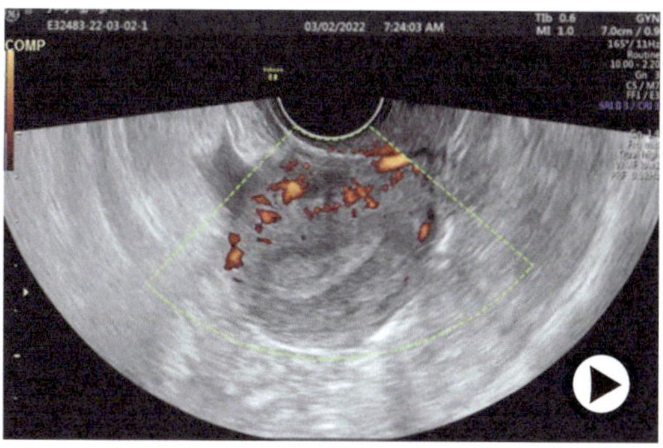

Fig. 6.10 Type I (▶ https://doi.org/10.1007/000-hrw)

group often exhibit advanced maternal age, thin endometrium, and elevated uterine artery resistance [34–36].

Research on the predictive value of endometrial spiral artery blood flow parameters has yielded mixed results. Studies by Battaglia and Kupesic demonstrated that PI values of the endometrial spiral arteries were significantly lower in the pregnant group compared to the nonpregnant group, indicating better blood perfusion as a potential factor for successful pregnancy [37, 38]. Meanwhile, a study by Seifeldin et al., using the Slowflow method to assess endometrial spiral arteries on embryo transfer day, reported higher RI values

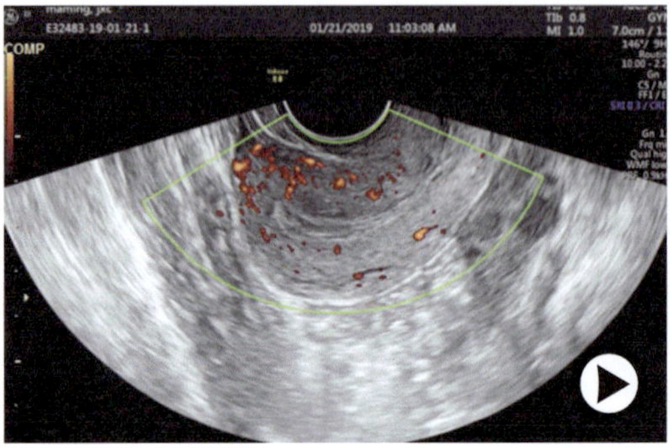

Fig. 6.11 Type II (▶ https://doi.org/10.1007/000-hrv)

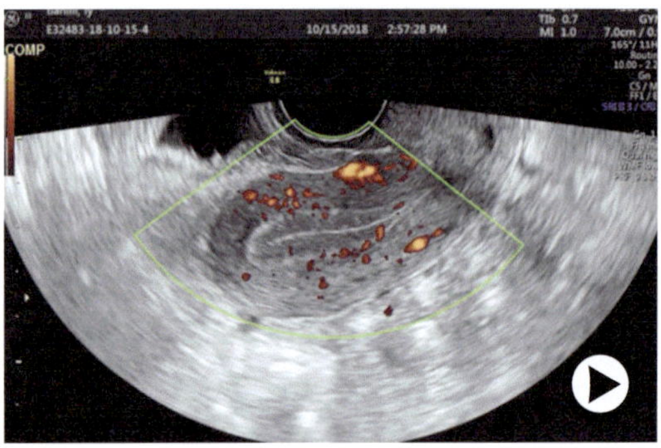

Fig. 6.12 Type III (▶ https://doi.org/10.1007/000-hry)

(0.68 vs. 0.65) and S/D ratio (3.91 vs. 3.17) in the pregnant group compared to the nonpregnant group [39]. This finding suggests that increased resistance might not necessarily preclude a successful pregnancy outcome. However, other studies have concluded that spectral ultrasound parameters of endometrial spiral arteries—such as PI, RI, and S/D—do not predict pregnancy outcomes after IVF treatment [40].

2. 3D power Doppler ultrasound parameters of the endometrium and sub-endometrium
   (a) Overview of 3D power Doppler ultrasound parameters

   Three-dimensional (3D) power Doppler ultrasound offers enhanced sensitivity compared to 2D Doppler, especially for detecting low-velocity blood flow and visualizing small blood vessels. This method quantitatively assesses signal intensity in both the endometrial and sub-endometrial regions, providing a detailed evaluation of vascularization and perfusion.

   The sub-endometrial region is the hypoechoic zone between the basal layer of the endometrium and the myometrium. In the literature, this region is typically measured within a 5 mm radius from the endometrial borders (Fig. 6.13) [41].

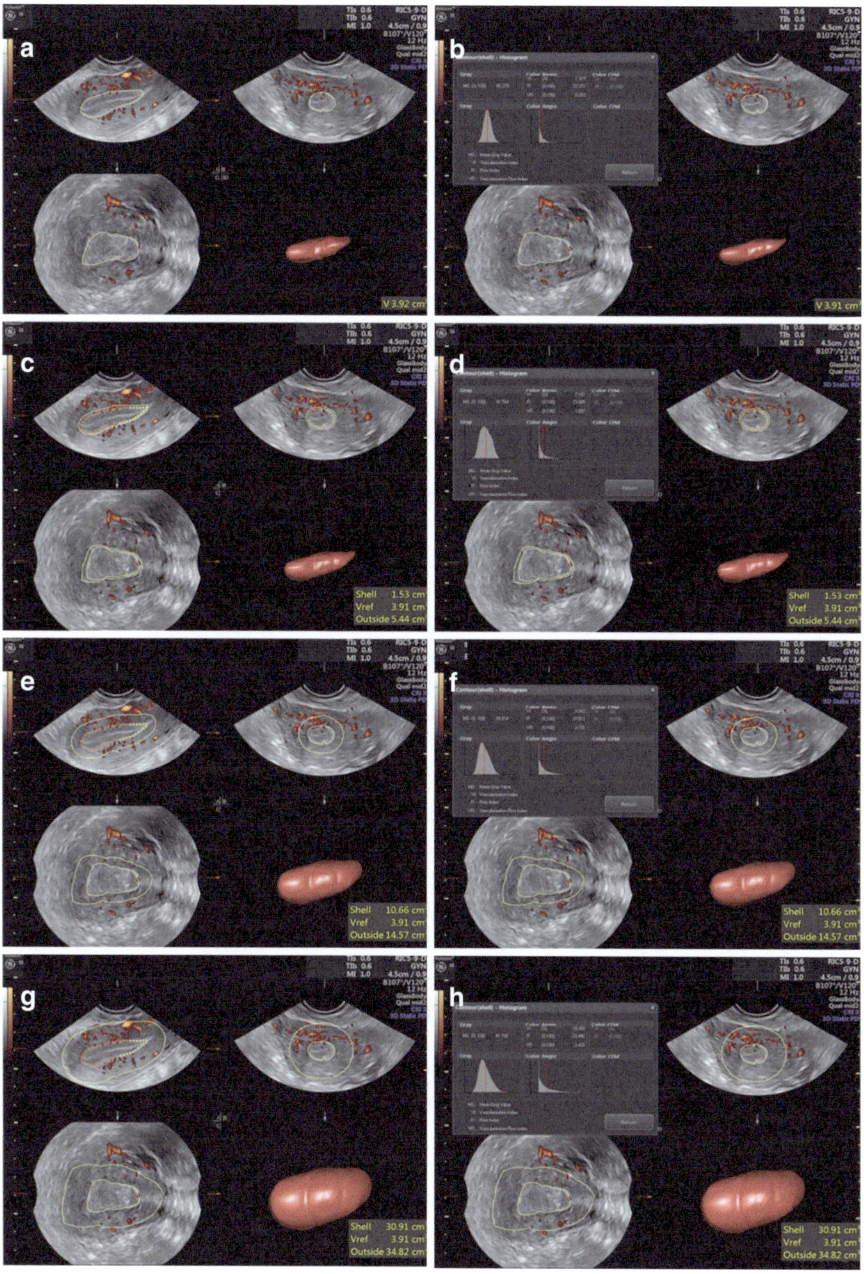

Fig. 6.13 (**a**) Measurement of endometrial blood flows by power Doppler. (**b**) Measurement of endometrial blood flows by power Doppler. (**c**) Measurement of endometrial and sub-endometrial (1 mm) blood flows (1 mm) by power Doppler. (**d**) Measurement of endometrial and sub-endometrial (1 mm) blood flows by power Doppler. (**e**) Measurement of endometrial and sub-endometrial (5 mm) blood flows by power Doppler. (**f**) Measurement of endometrial and sub-endometrial (5 mm) blood flows by power Doppler. (**g**) Measurement of endometrial and sub-endometrial (10 mm) blood flows by power Doppler. (**h**) Measurement of endometrial and sub-endometrial (10 mm) blood flows by power Doppler

The key parameters of 3D power Doppler ultrasound are as follows:

1. Vascularization Index (VI)
   - Definition: Represents the percentage of intravascular color-coded voxels within the area of interest
   - Significance: Indicates the density of blood vessels in the target tissue and reflects the vascular abundance or sparsity
2. Flow Index (FI)
   - Definition: Measures the average intensity of blood flow within the target volume, represented by the weighted mean color voxel
   - Significance: This reflects the number of red blood cells passing through the vessels during the 3D scanning
3. Vascularization Flow Index (VFI)
   - Definition: A composite measure derived by multiplying VI and FI
   - Significance: Combines information on both vascular density and flow intensity, providing a comprehensive assessment of blood supply

   Studies have demonstrated that endometrial and sub-endometrial blood flow parameters exhibit continuous changes throughout the menstrual cycle, closely corresponding to hormonal fluctuations:

   1. Proliferative phase: Blood flow gradually increases during this phase, in line with rising estrogen levels. Estrogen peaks approximately 3 days before ovulation, promoting enhanced vascularization and perfusion of the endometrium (Fig. 6.14).
   2. Post ovulation: About 5 days after ovulation, estrogen levels drop to their lowest point while progesterone levels rise.
   3. Late secretory phase: Despite the decline in both estrogen and progesterone after the midsecretory phase, blood flow parameters of the endometrium, as measured by power Doppler ultrasound, continue to increase.

   This sustained rise in blood flow may be attributed to the increased endometrial tissue density and spiral arterial curvature during the late secretory phase, as well as to the activity of the renin-angiotensin system in regulating menstruation [42].

(b) Measurement of endometrial and sub-endometrial blood flow using power Doppler ultrasound (GE Voluson E8 as an example)

1. Patient preparation and positioning
   - The patient should empty her bladder before the procedure and assume the lithotomy position.
   - Routine scanning of the uterus and bilateral adnexal regions is performed using an intracavitary volume transducer.
2. Imaging setup
   - Start by selecting the midsagittal plane of the uterus, which clearly shows the endometrial contour. This will serve as the starting point for the scan.
   - Keep both the patient and the ultrasound probe stationary.
   - Turn on the Power Doppler (PD) mode and the 3D imaging function.

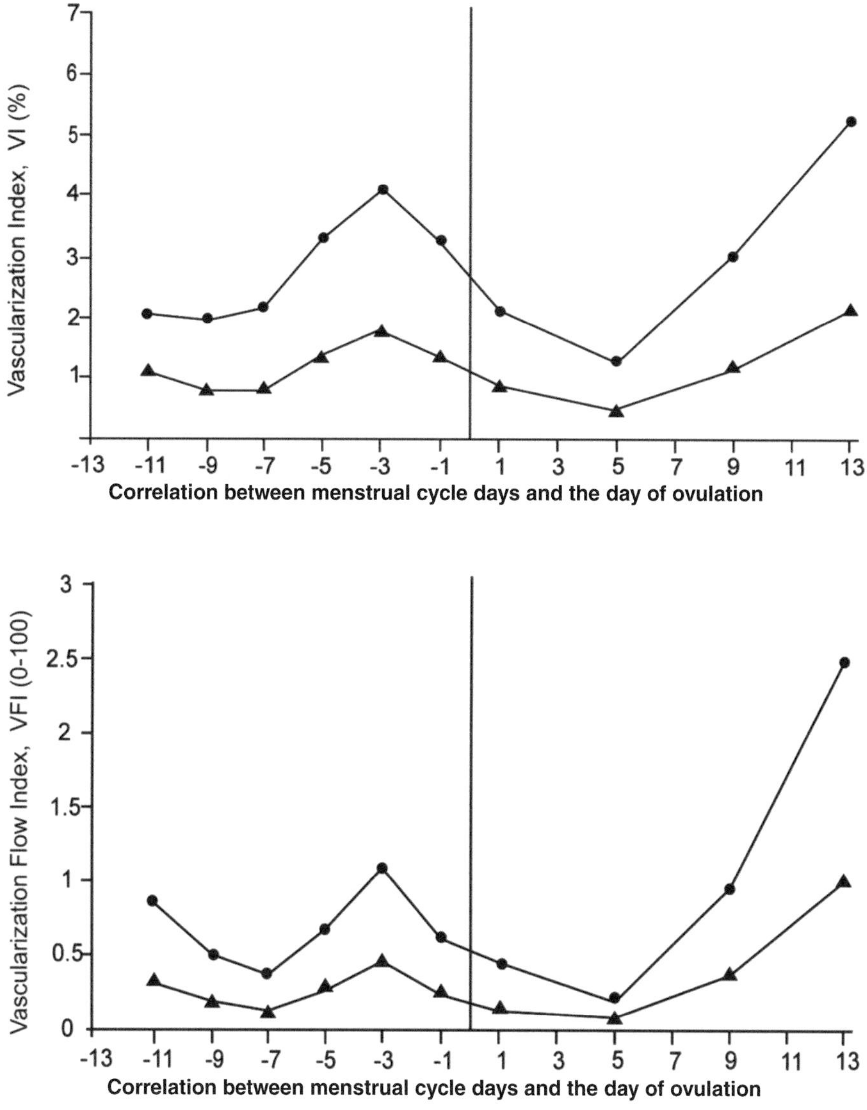

Fig. 6.14 Changes in endometrial and sub-endometrial 3D power Doppler parameters during the menstrual cycle. Note: The median line represents the "0" on the *x*-axis, corresponding to the day of ovulation. Curves marked with triangles indicate endometrial blood flow parameters, while circular points represent endometrial and sub-endometrial (5 mm) blood flow parameters

- Ensure the entire uterus is included in the sampling frame and proceed with performing a 3D scan of the uterus.

3. 3D imaging of the endometrium
   - Outline the 3D plane of the endometrial margin at the myometrial-endometrial interface, from the fundus to the internal cervical os,

across multiple parallel sections using the VOCAL (Virtual Organ Computer-Aided Analysis) function. This will automatically generate the endometrial volume.

- Use the "Histogram" function to extract the relevant endometrial blood flow parameters.

4. Sub-endometrial blood flow measurement
   - Based on the generated endometrial volume, select the "OUTSIDE" option.
   - Manually select an area between 1 and 10 mm in the sub-endometrial region to automatically calculate the flow parameters in that area.

(c) Power Doppler ultrasound parameters and ER

A study of 3D power Doppler ultrasound performed on the day of hCG administration in patients treated with IVF demonstrated a greater predictive value of the VFI of the endometrium, and better pregnancy outcomes were observed in patients with a VFI greater than 0.24 [41]. Similarly, higher VI, FI, and VFI values on the day of embryo transfer were linked to higher pregnancy rates, with specific cutoff values predicting pregnancy: VI > 0.95, FI > 12.94, and VFI > 0.15. However, the sub-endometrial blood flow parameters showed little predictive value [43].

A meta-analysis in 2018 showed that endometrial blood flow parameters, including VI, FI, and VFI, were significantly higher in the pregnant group compared to the nonpregnant group on the day of embryo transfer. However, no significant difference in these parameters was observed on the day of hCG administration. Additionally, sub-endometrial blood flow FI was higher in the pregnant group than in the nonpregnant group both on the day of hCG administration and on the day of embryo transfer. No significant differences between the two groups in freeze-thaw cycles were observed in sub-endometrial VI, FI, and VFI [44].

In contrast, a meta-analysis from 2019 found different conclusions. On the day of hCG administration, sub-endometrial VI was lower and sub-endometrial FI was higher in the pregnant group than in the nonpregnant group. On the day of embryo transfer, endometrial VI and VFI were higher in the pregnant group, whereas no significant difference in sub-endometrial blood flow parameters was found between the two groups [8]. Table 6.3 summarizes the findings of these two meta-analyses.

In conclusion, although 3D power Doppler ultrasound can provide a quantitative and high-resolution visualization of regional endometrial perfusion, the clinical significance of this test remains controversial. In addition to the influence of subjective and objective factors such as operator, equipment, and timing of the inspection, individualized patient uterine position and depth of endometrial detection have rarely been analyzed and discussed in extensive clinical studies. Different uterine positions can influence the results of blood flow parameters. Ultrasound attenuation due to increased depth of detection also significantly reduces the endothelial flow readings

Table 6.3 Differences in endothelial parameters measured by 3D power Doppler ultrasound at different timings and in different types of cycles between the pregnant and nonpregnant groups (2019 vs. 2018 meta-analysis)

	Meta-analysis 2019		Meta-analysis 2018			
	Day of hCG injection	Day of embryo transfer	Day of hCG injection	Day of embryo transfer	Fresh cycle	Freeze-thaw cycle
Endothelial VI	NS	+	NS	+	NS	+
Endothelial FI	NS	NS	NS	+	NS	+
Endothelial VFI	NS	+	NS	+	NS	+
Subendothelial VI	–	NS	NS	NS	NS	NS
Subendothelial FI	+	NS	+	+	+	NS
Subendothelial VFI	NS	NS	NS	NS	NS	NS

Note: NS (not significant) means no statistically significant difference in this blood flow parameter between the pregnant group and the nonpregnant group; "+" means that the value of this blood flow parameter in the pregnant group was significantly higher than that in the nonpregnant group; "–" means that the value of this blood flow parameter in the pregnant group was significantly lower than that in the nonpregnant group

measured by power Doppler—a confounding factor that has not been investigated in the available studies and may be one of the reasons for the controversy surrounding this test. The meta-analysis concluded that the accuracy of these indices in predicting pregnancy occurrence must be further evaluated in additional large-scale studies [44].

6.4 Ovulation Induction, Controlled Ovarian Hyperstimulation, and ER

Ovulation induction uses pro-ovulatory medications to stimulate the development and release of one or more eggs from the ovaries, commonly used to treat ovulatory dysfunction or during an intrauterine insemination (IUI) cycle. Controlled ovarian hyperstimulation (COH) involves administering exogenous gonadotropins to encourage the simultaneous development of multiple follicles. This approach is integral to the success of in vitro fertilization (IVF) cycles, significantly improving cumulative pregnancy rates. However, the hormonal changes induced by ovulation induction or COH may affect ER, potentially altering the timing and quality of endometrial development.

To comprehensively assess ER, clinicians must consider sonographic markers, the patient's medication history, COH regimen, and hormonal profile. A holistic evaluation of these factors will help tailor individualized treatment plans, optimizing the chances of a successful pregnancy.

6.4.1 Oral Ovulation-Inducing Drugs Affecting Endothelial Receptivity

Clomiphene citrate (CC) is a widely used ovulation-inducing drug. It competitively binds to estrogen receptors, creating a low estrogen environment that triggers negative feedback, stimulating the secretion of pituitary gonadotropins and inducing ovulation. However, due to CC's long half-life, its antiestrogenic effects can hinder endometrial growth and adversely affect the quality of cervical mucus, potentially impairing fertilization and implantation. To mitigate these effects, CC is often coadministered with estradiol valerate, which counteracts CC's restrictive impact on ovulation and improves pregnancy rates.

Letrozole (LE), an aromatase inhibitor, induces ovulation by inhibiting estrogen synthesis and reducing estrogen's negative feedback on the hypothalamic-pituitary-ovarian axis. Unlike CC, LE does not bind to estrogen receptors: it does not negatively affect endometrial thickness or morphology. As a result, LE has a lower impact on ER and has increasingly replaced CC as the first-line pro-ovulatory drug for ovulation induction.

6.4.2 Hormones and ER

Estrogen and progesterone, secreted by the ovaries, are the primary regulators of endometrial development. The impact of COH on ER is primarily due to the super-physiological levels of estrogen and progesterone, which disrupt the balance between these hormones, leading to an inappropriate estrogen-to-progesterone ratio. Elevated estrogen levels can impair trophoblast infiltration, contributing to adverse obstetric outcomes such as preeclampsia and small-for-gestational-age infants [45].

Furthermore, a progesterone level exceeding 1.5 ng/mL on the day of hCG administration signals a shift in the implantation window, which is a significant risk factor for poor IVF pregnancy outcomes [46]. To mitigate these risks, clinical guidelines recommend canceling fresh embryo transfers for patients with more than 15 retrieved eggs during COH cycles and/or a progesterone level above 1.5 ng/mL on the day of hCG administration. In such cases, a freeze-all strategy is advised to prevent ovarian hyperstimulation syndrome and reduce the risk of embryo loss [47, 48].

6.4.3 COH Regimen and ER

Commonly used drugs for COH include gonadotropin-releasing hormone (GnRH) analogs and gonadotropins. GnRH analogs are classified into GnRH agonists (GnRH-a) and GnRH antagonists (GnRH-ant), which are used in two main COH regimens: the agonist long protocol and the antagonist protocol.

GnRH agonists, available in long- and short-acting formulations, are typically used in long COH protocols. These formulations regulate the pituitary gland to inhibit an early LH peak by desensitizing it, allowing follicle development to be fully controlled by external gonadotropins. This synchronization helps to regulate the development of follicles. In contrast, GnRH-ant binds competitively to pituitary gonadotropin receptors to inhibit the secretion of gonadotropins, especially LH, without requiring the extended downregulation period of GnRH-a protocols. As a result, antagonist protocols are more flexible and convenient.

Studies have shown that GnRH-a protocols can enhance ER and improve live birth rates through various mechanisms, including regulating enzymes and cytokines and preventing premature luteinization [49–52]. Additionally, GnRH-a pretreatment in resuscitation cycles has been found to improve pregnancy outcomes in patients with repeat implantation failure [53]. On the other hand, the lower ongoing pregnancy rates with GnRH-ant protocols are thought to be due to insufficient suppression of endogenous LH, which can lead to premature progesterone rises, shifting the implantation window too early, and the more asynchronous development of follicles from endogenous FSH secretion during the early follicular phase [52].

While GnRH-a long protocols were once considered the most effective for COH, recent advancements in assisted reproductive technology (ART) and research findings have challenged this view. A recent meta-analysis found moderate-quality evidence that GnRH-ant protocols significantly reduce the incidence of ovarian hyperstimulation syndrome (OHSS) without compromising live birth rates compared to GnRH-a long protocols [54]. These protocols also involve shorter durations of gonadotropin use and lower doses, which have made them increasingly popular in clinical practice.

COH can alter ER in fresh cycles due to the supraphysiological steroid levels that affect endometrial maturation. However, the vitrification and thawing of embryos can prevent unnecessary embryo loss and increase the cumulative pregnancy rate per COH cycle while also reducing the risk of OHSS. Performing embryo transfer in a subsequent cycle, separate from ovarian stimulation, allows for resynchronization of the endometrium and embryos, further improving the chances of successful implantation [55].

6.4.4 Timing of Embryo Transfer in the Thawing Cycle and Endometrial Receptivity

After COH and egg retrieval, enlarged ovaries and luteinized cysts may be observed in patients for 1–2 months or even longer, especially in those with high ovarian responses (Fig. 6.15). To mitigate the adverse effects of COH, it has become routine practice to wait for at least one menstrual cycle after egg retrieval before proceeding with further treatments. However, this waiting period extends the overall duration of the IVF process and may heighten anxiety for some patients.

A meta-analysis published in 2021 suggested that immediate embryo transfer in the first menstrual cycle following egg retrieval was associated with higher clinical pregnancy and live birth rates. This finding challenges the conventional practice of postponed frozen embryo transfer, implying that waiting may not always be the

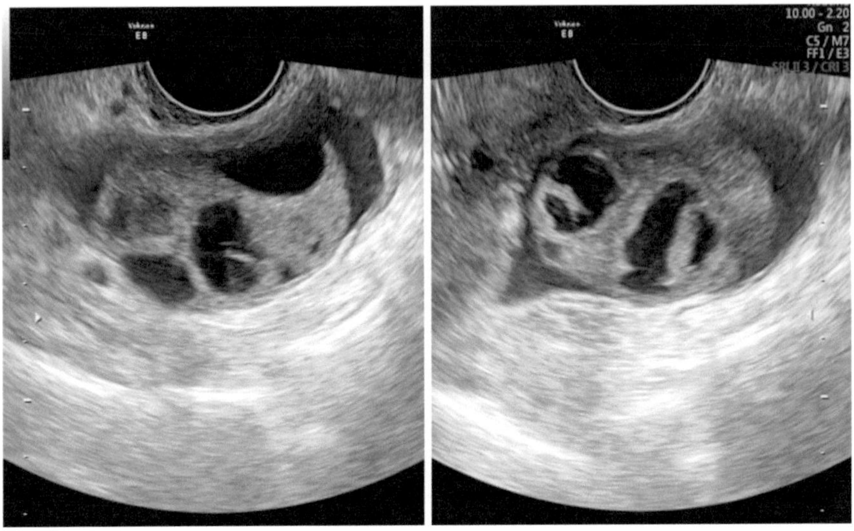

Fig. 6.15 Imaging of the bilateral ovaries following the first menstrual period after egg retrieval

most effective strategy [56]. Additionally, studies have shown that luteinized cysts formed after egg retrieval can increase the expression of relaxin in peripheral blood circulation [57], which may contribute to endometrial angiogenesis, promoting a more favorable environment for embryo implantation and potentially reducing the risk of miscarriage [58].

References

1. Lessey BA. Assessment of endometrial receptivity. Fertil Steril. 2011;96:522–9.
2. Ng EH, Chan CC, Tang OS, et al. The role of endometrial blood flow measured by three-dimensional power Doppler ultrasound in the prediction of pregnancy during in vitro fertilization treatment. Eur J Obstet Gynecol Reprod Biol. 2007;135:8–16.
3. Feng X, Zhu N, Yang S, et al. Transcutaneous electrical acupoint stimulation improves endometrial receptivity resulting in improved IVF-ET pregnancy outcomes in older women: a multicenter, randomized, controlled clinical trial. Reprod Biol Endocrinol. 2022;20:127.
4. Chinese Ultrasound Doctors Association. Guidelines for gynecological ultrasound examination in China. Bei Jing: People's Medical Publishing House; 2017. p. 1–192.
5. Noyes RW, Hertig AT, Rock J. Reprint of: dating the endometrial biopsy. Fertil Steril. 2019;112:e93–e115.
6. Achache H, Revel A. Endometrial receptivity markers, the journey to successful embryo implantation. Hum Reprod Update. 2006;12:731–46.
7. Hershko-Klement A, Tepper R. Ultrasound in assisted reproduction: a call to fill the endometrial gap. Fertil Steril. 2016;105:1394–402.e4.
8. Craciunas L, Gallos I, Chu J, et al. Conventional and modern markers of endometrial receptivity: a systematic review and meta-analysis. Hum Reprod Update. 2019;25:202–23.
9. Liu Y, Zhou Q, Peng B, et al. Automatic measurement of endometrial thickness from transvaginal ultrasound images. Front Bioeng Biotechnol. 2022;10:853845.

10. El-Toukhy T, Coomarasamy A, Khairy M, et al. The relationship between endometrial thickness and outcome of medicated frozen embryo replacement cycles. Fertil Steril. 2008;89:832–9.
11. Gao G, Cui X, Li S, et al. Endometrial thickness and IVF cycle outcomes: a meta-analysis. Reprod Biomed Online. 2020;40:124–33.
12. Liu KE, Hartman M, Hartman A, et al. The impact of a thin endometrial lining on fresh and frozen-thaw IVF outcomes: an analysis of over 40 000 embryo transfers. Hum Reprod. 2018;33:1883–8.
13. Buyalos RP, Hubert GD, Shamonki MI. The mystery of optimal endometrial thickness…never too thick, but when is thin…too thin? Fertil Steril. 2022;117:801–2.
14. Griesinger G, Trevisan S, Cometti B. Endometrial thickness on the day of embryo transfer is a poor predictor of IVF treatment outcome. Hum Reprod Open. 2018;2018:hox031.
15. Critchley HOD, Maybin JA, Armstrong GM, et al. Physiology of the endometrium and regulation of menstruation. Physiol Rev. 2020;100:1149–79.
16. Casper RF. Frozen embryo transfer: evidence-based markers for successful endometrial preparation. Fertil Steril. 2020;113:248–51.
17. Haas J, Smith R, Zilberberg E, et al. Endometrial compaction (decreased thickness) in response to progesterone results in optimal pregnancy outcome in frozen-thawed embryo transfers. Fertil Steril. 2019;112:503–9.e1.
18. Jin Z, Shi H, Lu M, et al. Endometrial thickness changes after progesterone administration do not affect the pregnancy outcomes of frozen-thawed euploid blastocyst transfer: a retrospective cohort study. Fertil Steril. 2021;116:1502–12.
19. Zollner U, Zollner KP, Specketer MT, et al. Endometrial volume as assessed by three-dimensional ultrasound is a predictor of pregnancy outcome after in vitro fertilization and embryo transfer. Fertil Steril. 2003;80:1515–7.
20. Zollner U, Specketer MT, Dietl J, et al. 3D-endometrial volume and outcome of cryopreserved embryo replacement cycles. Arch Gynecol Obstet. 2012;286:517–23.
21. Ijland MM, Evers JL, Dunselman GA, Hoogland HJ. Subendometrial contractions in the non-pregnant uterus: an ultrasound study. Eur J Obstet Gynecol Reprod Biol. 1996;70:23–4.
22. Ijland MM, Evers JL, Dunselman GA, et al. Endometrial wavelike movements during the menstrual cycle. Fertil Steril. 1996;65:746–9.
23. Huang Y, Rees C, Sammali F, et al. Characterization of uterine peristaltic waves by ultrasound strain analysis. IEEE Trans Ultrason Ferroelectr Freq Control. 2022;69:2050–60.
24. Zhu L, Che HS, Xiao L, et al. Uterine peristalsis before embryo transfer affects the chance of clinical pregnancy in fresh and frozen-thawed embryo transfer cycles. Hum Reprod. 2014;29:1238–43.
25. Tekay A, Martikainen H, Jouppila P. Comparison of uterine blood flow characteristics between spontaneous and stimulated cycles before embryo transfer. Hum Reprod. 1996;11:364–8.
26. Browne VA, Julian CG, Toledo-Jaldin L, et al. Uterine artery blood flow, fetal hypoxia and fetal growth. Philos Trans R Soc Lond Ser B Biol Sci. 2015;370:20140068.
27. Wan ST, Wang XT. Application of uterine artery blood flow monitoring in obstetrics. Chin J Pract Gynecol Obstet. 2022;38:403–6.
28. Friedler S, Schenker JG, Herman A, et al. The role of ultrasonography in the evaluation of endometrial receptivity following assisted reproductive treatments: a critical review. Hum Reprod Update. 1996;2:323–35.
29. Chien LW, Lee WS, Au HK, et al. Assessment of changes in utero-ovarian arterial impedance during the peri-implantation period by Doppler sonography in women undergoing assisted reproduction. Ultrasound Obstet Gynecol. 2004;23:496–500.
30. Steer CV, Tan SL, Dillon D, et al. Vaginal color Doppler assessment of uterine artery impedance correlates with immunohistochemical markers of endometrial receptivity required for the implantation of an embryo. Fertil Steril. 1995;63:101–8.
31. Steer CV, Campbell S, Tan SL, et al. The use of transvaginal color flow imaging after in vitro fertilization to identify optimum uterine conditions before embryo transfer. Fertil Steril. 1992;57:372–6.

32. Ivanovski M, Damcevski N, Radevska B, et al. Assessment of uterine artery and arcuate artery blood flow by transvaginal color Doppler ultrasound on the day of human chorionic gonadotropin administration as predictors of pregnancy in an in vitro fertilization program. Akush Ginekol (Sofiia). 2012;51:55–60.
33. Cacciatore B, Simberg N, Fusaro P, et al. Transvaginal Doppler study of uterine artery blood flow in in vitro fertilization-embryo transfer cycles. Fertil Steril. 1996;66:130–4.
34. Applebaum M. The uterine biophysical profile. Ultrasound Obstet Gynecol. 1995;5:67–8.
35. Wang L, Qiao J, Li R, et al. Role of endometrial blood flow assessment with color Doppler energy in predicting pregnancy outcome of IVF-ET cycles. Reprod Biol Endocrinol. 2010;8:122.
36. Chien LW, Au HK, Chen PL, et al. Assessment of uterine receptivity by the endometrial-subendometrial blood flow distribution pattern in women undergoing in vitro fertilization-embryo transfer. Fertil Steril. 2002;78:245–51.
37. Battaglia C, Artini PG, Giulini S, et al. Colour Doppler changes and thromboxane production after ovarian stimulation with gonadotrophin-releasing hormone agonist. Hum Reprod. 1997;12:2477–82.
38. Kupesic S, Bekavac I, Bjelos D, et al. Assessment of endometrial receptivity by transvaginal color Doppler and three-dimensional power Doppler ultrasonography in patients undergoing in vitro fertilization procedures. J Ultrasound Med. 2001;20:125–34.
39. Sadek S, Matitashvili T, Kovac A, et al. Assessment of uterine receptivity by endometrial and sub-endometrial blood flow using SlowflowHD in hormone prepared frozen embryo transfer cycles: a pilot study. J Assist Reprod Genet. 2022;39:1069–79.
40. Schild RL, Knobloch C, Dorn C, et al. Endometrial receptivity in an in vitro fertilization program as assessed by spiral artery blood flow, endometrial thickness, endometrial volume, and uterine artery blood flow. Fertil Steril. 2001;75:361–6.
41. Wu HM, Chiang CH, Huang HY, et al. Detection of the subendometrial vascularization flow index by three-dimensional ultrasound may be useful for predicting the pregnancy rate for patients undergoing in vitro fertilization-embryo transfer. Fertil Steril. 2003;79:507–11.
42. Raine-Fenning NJ, Campbell BK, Kendall NR, et al. Quantifying the changes in endometrial vascularity throughout the normal menstrual cycle with three-dimensional power Doppler angiography. Hum Reprod. 2004;19:330–8.
43. Kim A, Jung H, Choi WJ, et al. Detection of endometrial and subendometrial vasculature on the day of embryo transfer and prediction of pregnancy during fresh in vitro fertilization cycles. Taiwan J Obstet Gynecol. 2014;53:360–5.
44. Wang J, Xia F, Zhou Y, et al. Association between endometrial/subendometrial vasculature and embryo transfer outcome: a meta-analysis and subgroup analysis. J Ultrasound Med. 2018;37:149–63.
45. Imudia AN, Awonuga AO, Doyle JO, et al. Peak serum estradiol level during controlled ovarian hyperstimulation is associated with increased risk of small for gestational age and preeclampsia in singleton pregnancies after in vitro fertilization. Fertil Steril. 2012;97:1374–9.
46. Bosch E, Labarta E, Crespo J, et al. Circulating progesterone levels and ongoing pregnancy rates in controlled ovarian stimulation cycles for in vitro fertilization: analysis of over 4000 cycles. Hum Reprod. 2010;25:2092–100.
47. Dieamant FC, Petersen CG, Mauri AL, et al. Fresh embryos versus freeze-all embryos – transfer strategies: nuances of a meta-analysis. JBRA Assist Reprod. 2017;21:260–72.
48. Huang L, Huang S, Wen Y, et al. The impact of late follicular phase progesterone elevation on cumulative live birth rate and embryo quality in 4072 freeze-all cycles. J Clin Med. 2022;11:7300.
49. Li L, Liu L, Kou Z, et al. GnRH agonist treatment regulates IL-6 and IL-11 expression in endometrial stromal cells for patients with HRT regiment in frozen embryo transfer cycles. Reprod Biol. 2022;22:100608.
50. Ruan HC, Zhu XM, Luo Q, et al. Ovarian stimulation with GnRH agonist, but not GnRH antagonist, partially restores the expression of endometrial integrin beta3 and leukaemia-inhibitory factor and improves uterine receptivity in mice. Hum Reprod. 2006;21:2521–9.

51. Xu B, Geerts D, Hu S, et al. The depot GnRH agonist protocol improves the live birth rate per fresh embryo transfer cycle, but not the cumulative live birth rate in normal responders: a randomized controlled trial and molecular mechanism study. Hum Reprod. 2020;35:1306–18.
52. Lambalk CB, Banga FR, Huirne JA, et al. GnRH antagonist versus long agonist protocols in IVF: a systematic review and meta-analysis accounting for patient type. Hum Reprod Update. 2017;23:560–79.
53. Li X, Lin J, Zhang L, et al. Effects of gonadotropin-releasing hormone agonist pretreatment on frozen embryo transfer outcomes in artificial cycles: a meta-analysis. Arch Gynecol Obstet. 2023;308:675–83.
54. Al-Inany HG, Youssef MA, Ayeleke RO, et al. Gonadotrophin-releasing hormone antagonists for assisted reproductive technology. Cochrane Database Syst Rev. 2016;4:CD001750.
55. Bourdon M, Maignien C, Pocate-Cheriet K, Plu Bureau G, Marcellin L, Patrat C, et al. The freeze-all strategy after IVF: which indications? Reprod Biomed Online. 2021;42:529–45.
56. Bergenheim SJ, Saupstad M, Pistoljevic N, et al. Immediate versus postponed frozen embryo transfer after IVF/ICSI: a systematic review and meta-analysis. Hum Reprod Update. 2021;27:623–42.
57. Conrad KP, Baker VL. Corpus luteal contribution to maternal pregnancy physiology and outcomes in assisted reproductive technologies. Am J Physiol Regul Integr Comp Physiol. 2013;304:R69–72.
58. Chen X, Man GCW, Liu Y, et al. Physiological and pathological angiogenesis in endometrium at the time of embryo implantation. Am J Reprod Immunol. 2017;78:e12693.

Ultrasound Evaluation of Reproduction-Related Gynecologic Conditions

7

Da Li, Zhijing Na, and Xinlu Wang

Female infertility can result from various factors, with disorders of the reproductive system being among the most common causes. Ultrasonography has become the primary clinical tool for assessing female reproductive system conditions. Notably, three-dimensional (3D) ultrasound, which has advanced significantly in recent years, provides unique advantages in diagnosing and staging uterine malformations.

7.1 Malformations of the Reproductive System

Developmental abnormalities of the female reproductive system include those affecting the reproductive glands, ducts, and external genitalia, with uterine abnormalities being the most common.

7.1.1 Congenital Uterine Anomalies

Congenital uterine anomalies (CUAs), the most frequent developmental abnormalities of the female reproductive system, may adversely affect fertility. They are observed in up to 24.5% of infertile women who have experienced spontaneous abortions [1, 2].

D. Li (✉) · Z. Na · X. Wang
Shengjing Hospital of China Medical University, Shenyang, China
e-mail: wangxl1@sj-hospital.org

D. Li et al. (eds.), *Ultrasonography of the Female Reproductive System*, https://doi.org/10.1007/978-981-95-1373-4_7

1. Primordial uterus
   (1) Clinical overview:
   A primordial uterus arises from hypoplastic bilateral Müllerian ducts that fail to converge or from arrested development of the bilateral Müllerian ducts shortly after convergence [3]. It may present as a unilateral, bilateral, or fused muscular structure located behind the bladder. This primordial uterus is typically tiny, often lacks a uterine cavity, and is frequently associated with congenital vaginal agenesis.
   (2) Clinical manifestation:
   The primary clinical feature is primary amenorrhea [4].
   (3) Ultrasonographic features:
   On ultrasound, the uterus appears as a cord-like soft-tissue structure located medial to the pelvic wall (unilaterally or bilaterally) or posterior to the bladder. It measures 1–3 cm in length, lacks an endometrium, and shows no clear differentiation between the uterine body and cervix. Fibrous tissue may connect bilateral primordial uterine structures. The bilateral ovaries are typically visible. In cases associated with vaginal agenesis, the hyperechoic gas line within a normal vagina is absent on ultrasound (see Fig. 7.1).
   (4) Differential diagnosis:
   Refer to Table 7.1 for a detailed comparison.
   (5) Impact on fertility and treatment principles:
   The impact on fertility and treatment approach is consistent with that of congenital uterine agenesis.
2. Infantile uterus
   (1) Clinical overview:
   An infantile uterus, also referred to as uterine hypoplasia, results from arrested development of the bilateral Müllerian ducts shortly after their confluence. The uterus is smaller than normal, with a hypoplastic endometrium and a narrow uterine cavity.

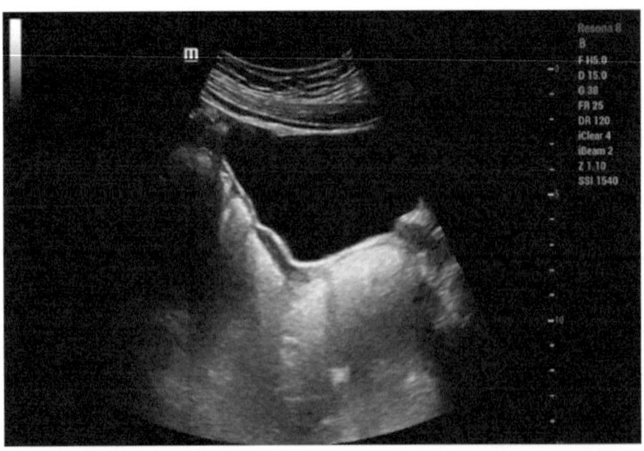

Fig. 7.1 An image of the uterus in a 16-year-old patient showing a cord-like soft tissue posterior to the bladder. The endometrium is absent, and the uterine body is indistinguishable from the cervix

Table 7.1 Key points for differential diagnosis of primordial uterus and infantile uterus

	Müllerian ducts development	Development of the uterus, vagina, and both ovaries	Clinical manifestations	Ultrasonographic features
Primordial uterus	Bilateral Müllerian ducts are hypoplastic and not confluent or bilateral Müllerian ducts stopped developing soon after confluence.	1. The uterus is tiny without a uterine cavity. 2. Often combined with congenital absence of vagina. 3. Bilateral ovaries may develop normally.	Primary amenorrhea	1. A cord-like soft tissue, 1–3 cm long, on the medial side of the pelvic wall (unilaterally or bilaterally) or posterior to the bladder. 2. The uterine body is poorly distinguished from the cervix. 3. Absence of endometrium.
Infantile uterus	Bilateral Müllerian ducts stopped developing soon after confluence.	1. The uterus is smaller than normal, with hypoplastic endometrium and narrow uterine cavity. 2. The vagina and bilateral ovaries may develop normally.	Delayed first menstrual period or low menstrual volume	1. The uterus is smaller than normal in all diameters, with its anterior-posterior diameter less than 2 cm. 2. Uterine length to cervix ratio = 2:3 or 1:1. 3. Thin and thread-like endometrium.

(2) Clinical manifestations:
The condition primarily presents as delayed onset of menstruation or low menstrual volume.

(3) Ultrasonographic features:
On ultrasound, the uterus is uniformly smaller than normal in all dimensions. The anterior-posterior diameter measures less than 2 cm, and the length of the uterine body is equal to or shorter than the length of the cervix. The uterine-to-cervical length ratio is 2:3 or 1:1. The endometrium is thin and often appears thread-like (see Fig. 7.2).

(4) Differential diagnosis: see Table 7.1.
Refer to Table 7.1 for a detailed differential diagnosis.

(5) Impact on fertility and treatment principles:
Endometrial or uterine dysplasia hinders fertilization and blastocyst implantation, resulting in infertility. Early treatment with low-dose estrogen and progesterone sequential therapy is recommended to stimulate uterine development.

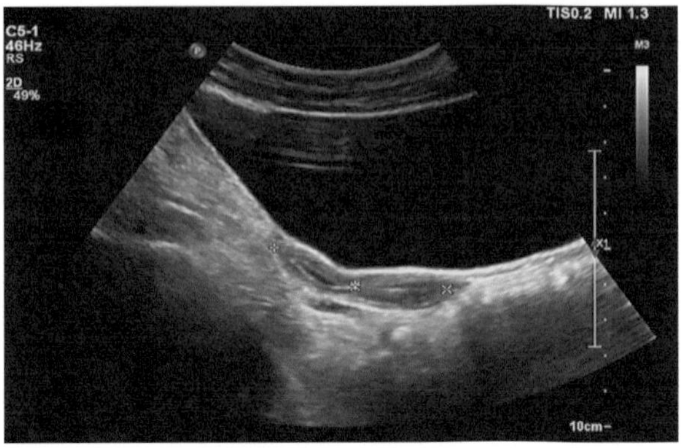

Fig. 7.2 An image of the uterus in a 17-year-old patient, demonstrating a smaller-than-normal size across all diameters. The length of the uterine body is equal to the length of the cervix, with a thin, thread-like endometrium

3. Unicornuate uterus and rudimentary horn of the uterus
   (1) Clinical overview:
   A unicornuate uterus consists of a fully developed Müllerian duct on one side and an underdeveloped or undeveloped rudimentary horn on the other.
   (2) Types and clinical manifestations:
   Patients with a unicornuate uterus commonly present with infertility, recurrent miscarriage, or preterm delivery. When accompanied by a rudimentary horn, the horn can be categorized based on its anatomical relationship to the unicornuate uterus [5]:
      (a) Type I (with endometrium and communicating with the uterine cavity): A rudimentary horn pregnancy is possible.
      (b) Type II (with endometrium and not communicating with the uterine cavity): Menstrual blood is unable to drain, potentially causing dysmenorrhea or endometriosis.
      (c) Type III (no endometrium): This is the most common type, usually presenting without significant clinical symptoms.
   (3) Ultrasonographic features:
   Ultrasonography is best performed during the endometrial secretory phase.
   A unicornuate uterus appears as a pike-shaped structure skewed toward the better-developed side with a reduced transverse diameter. Only the better-developed uterine horn is visible. The coronal view of the uterine cavity on 3D ultrasound shows a tubular pattern (see Fig. 7.3).
   Ultrasonographic features of the rudimentary horn [6]:
      (a) Type I: Appears as a small, solid, round structure adjacent to the unicornuate uterus with echogenicity similar to the myometrium and the hyperechoic endometrium in the center (see Fig. 7.4).
      (b) Type II: May show an anechoic cyst in the center of the solid structure or resemble the echogenicity of adenomyosis (see Fig. 7.5).
      (c) Type III: Presents as a solid structure with myometrial echogenicity and no endometrial echo in the center (see Fig. 7.6).

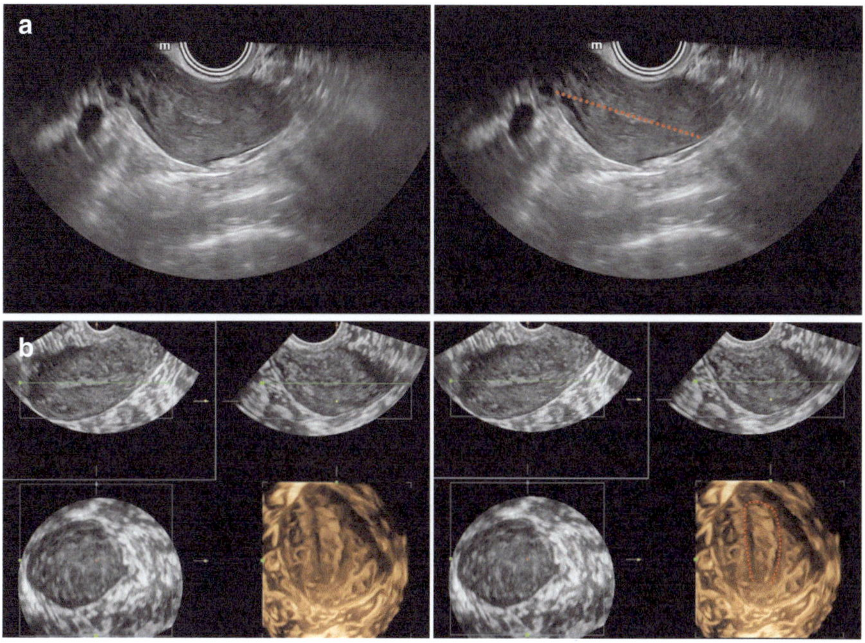

Fig. 7.3 (**a**) The uterus appears small in transverse diameter, with only one well-developed uterine horn. The transverse uterine diameter is highlighted in orange. (**b**) A coronal view of the uterine cavity in 3D ultrasound reveals a tubular shape. The tubular uterine cavity is outlined in orange

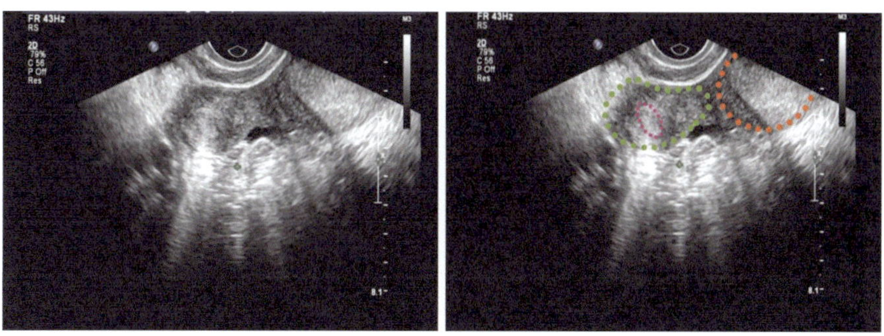

Fig. 7.4 Type I rudimentary horn of the uterus with endometrium communicating with the uterine cavity. Endometrial echoes are visible at the center of the rudimentary horn. The unicornuate uterus is outlined in orange; the rudimentary horn is outlined in green; the endometrium within the rudimentary horn is outlined in pink

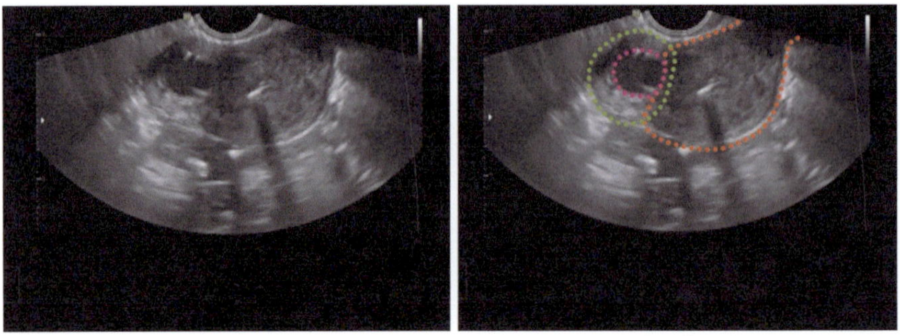

Fig. 7.5 Type II rudimentary horn of the uterus with endometrium that does not communicate with the uterine cavity, leading to retention of menstrual blood. The unicornuate uterus is circled in orange; the rudimentary horn of the uterus is circled in green; the fluid accumulated in the rudimentary horn is circled in pink

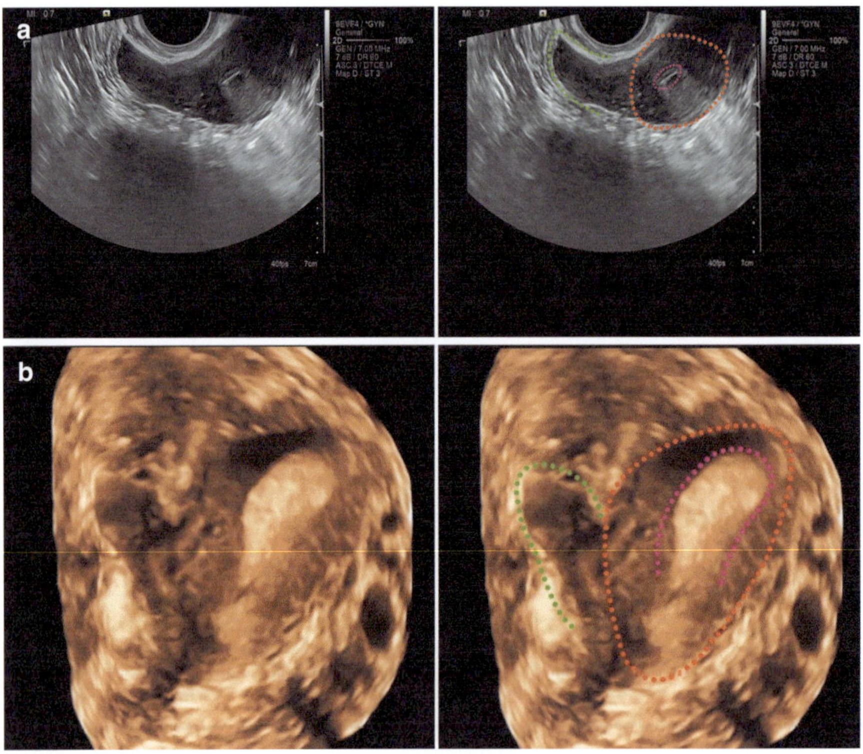

Fig. 7.6 (**a**) Type III rudimentary horn of the uterus on 2D ultrasound, located on the right side of a unicornuate uterus. It has the same echogenicity as the myometrium and shows no endometrial echoes. The unicornuate uterus is circled in orange; the rudimentary horn of the uterus is circled in green; the endometrium of the unicornuate uterus is circled in pink. (**b**) A 3D coronal view of the uterine cavity in a unicornuate uterus (on the left side of the rudimentary horn), which appears tubular in shape. The unicornuate uterus is circled in orange; the rudimentary horn is circled in green; the endometrium of the unicornuate uterus is circled in pink

(4) Differential diagnosis:
Unicornuate Uterus: Differentiate from a normal uterus, where both uterine horns are visible, and the uterine cavity appears as an inverted triangle on 3D ultrasound.

Rudimentary Horn: Differentiate from adnexal masses, which are distinctly separated from the uterus and demonstrate relative mobility.

(5) Impact on fertility and treatment principles:
Patients with a unicornuate uterus are at higher risk of miscarriage, preterm delivery, and other adverse pregnancy outcomes.

No treatment is necessary for a unicornuate uterus alone or a type III rudimentary horn [7].

For type I or type II rudimentary horns, progressively worsening dysmenorrhea and secondary endometriosis may occur. Pregnancy in these types can lead to uterine rupture during the second trimester. Upon confirmation of the diagnosis, laparoscopic resection of the rudimentary horn should be performed promptly.

4. Uterus didelphys

(1) Clinical overview:
Uterus didelphys, also known as a double uterus, is characterized by two uterine cavities, each with its cervix. The two cervixes may be completely separate or partially connected. Connected cervixes may present as a single cervix or one cervix with two cervical canals. In some cases, vaginal abnormalities such as a longitudinal or oblique vaginal septum are also present. Despite these anomalies, bilateral fallopian tubes and ovaries typically develop normally.

(2) Clinical manifestations:
Patients may present with one or more of the following:

- Heavy menstrual bleeding
- Prolonged menstruation
- Painful sexual intercourse (dyspareunia)
- Infertility
- Miscarriage
- Preterm labor
- Postpartum vaginal bleeding
- Incomplete abortion
- Conception while using an intrauterine device (IUD)

(3) Ultrasonographic features:

(a) Longitudinal view: Two uterine bodies of similar or differing sizes may be visualized, along with two cervices.

(b) Transverse view of the uterus: A pronounced concavity of the external uterine contour is observed, with endometrial echogenicity visible in the center of both uterine bodies.

(c) Transverse view of the cervix: Single cervix, double cervices, or a single cervix with two cervical canals may be seen.

(d) Coronal view on 3D ultrasound: Both uterine cavities appear tubular (see Fig. 7.7).

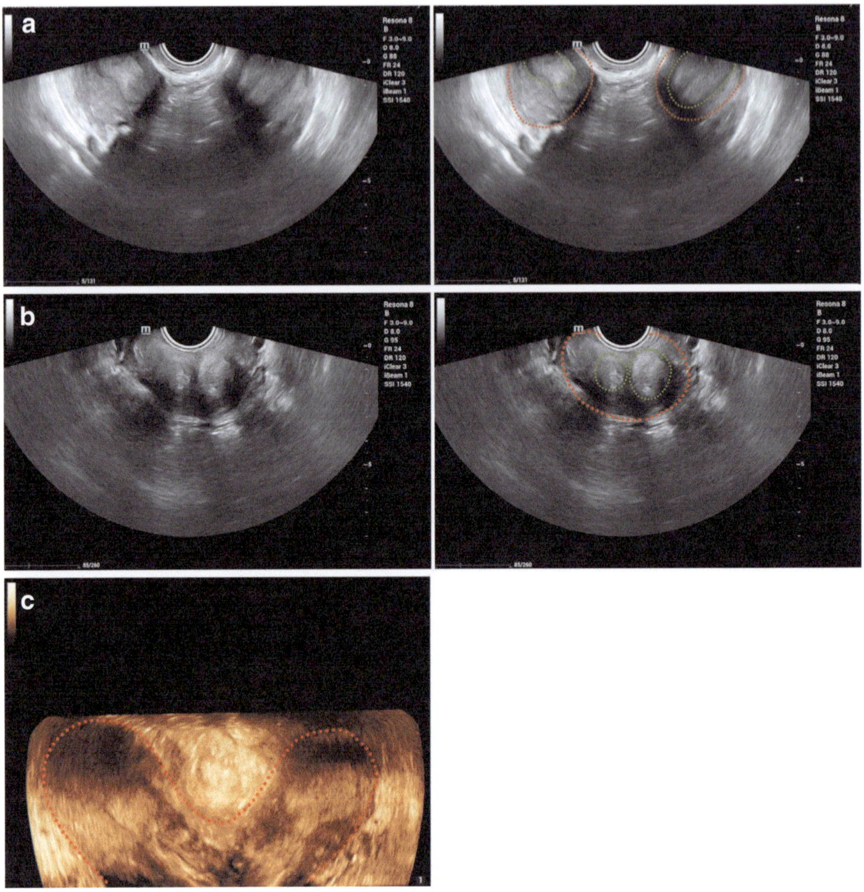

Fig. 7.7 (**a**) Transverse view of the uterus on ultrasound showing two similarly sized uterine bodies, each exhibiting endometrial echoes at the center. The two uterine bodies are circled in orange, with the endometrial echoes circled in green. (**b**) Transverse view of the cervix on ultrasound showing a single cervix with double cervical canals. The cervix is circled in orange; the cervical canals are circled in green. (**c**) Coronal view of the uterus on 3D ultrasound showing both uterine cavities with a tubular pattern

(4) Differential diagnosis:
Refer to Table 7.2 for detailed comparisons.

(5) Impact on fertility and treatment principles:
Patients with uterus didelphys are at increased risk for miscarriage, preterm labor, abnormal fetal positioning, and other adverse pregnancy outcomes. In cases with an associated oblique vaginal septum, surgical removal may be necessary to prevent menstrual blood retention and associated complications.

Table 7.2 Differential diagnosis of congenital uterine malformations by ultrasound

Uterine malformations	Outline of the uterine fundus	Endometrial profile at the uterine fundus	Endothelial morphology in the coronal plane of 3D ultrasound
Normal uterus	Outwardly protruding or flat	Outwardly protruding or flat	Upside-down triangle
Arcuate uterus	Convex, flat, or with a depression depth of ≤1 cm	Inwardly depressed with a depth of ≤1 cm; the angle between the two lateral endometrial folds >90°	Slightly "Y" shaped
Incomplete uterus septum	Convex, flat, or with a depression depth ≤1 cm	Inwardly depressed but not to the level of the internal cervical os; the angle between the two lateral endometrial folds ≤90°	"Y" shaped
Complete uterus septum	Convex, flat, or with a depression depth ≤1 cm	Inwardly depressed to the level of the internal cervical os, the angle between the two lateral endometrial folds ≤90°	"V" shaped
Incomplete bicornuate uterus	Inwardly depressed, with a depth of >1 cm but not to the level of the internal cervical os	Inwardly depressed but not to the level of the internal cervical os	"Y" shaped
Complete bicornuate uterus	Inwardly depressed to the level of the internal cervical os	Inwardly depressed to the level of the internal cervical os	"V" shaped
Uterus didelphys	Significant depression of the uterine fundus	Two separate endometriums	Two separated tubular endometriums

5. Bicornuate uterus
   (1) Clinical overview:
   A bicornuate uterus is classified as either complete or incomplete based on the extent of the confluence of the Müllerian ducts.
   (a) A complete bicornuate uterus divides below the internal cervical os.
   (b) An incomplete bicornuate uterus divides above the internal cervical os.
   (2) Clinical manifestations:
   Patients may experience the following symptoms:
   - Prolonged menstrual periods
   - Increased menstrual blood volume
   - Recurrent miscarriages
   - Premature labor
   - Postpartum vaginal bleeding [8]

(3) Ultrasonographic features:
  (a) Large fundal cleft: A significant fundal cleft (>1 cm deep) is observed.
  (b) Transverse view: Ultrasound reveals the endometrium divided into right and left components, with the uterus resembling a "butterfly-wing-like" pattern.
  (c) Coronal View on 3D Ultrasound:
    - In a complete bicornuate uterus, the endometrium appears as a "V-shape."
    - In an incomplete bicornuate uterus, the endometrium forms a "Y-shape" (see Figs. 7.8 and 7.9).

(4) Differential diagnosis:
Refer to Table 7.2 for a detailed differential diagnosis.

(5) Impact on fertility and treatment principles:
Patients with a bicornuate uterus are at risk for adverse pregnancy outcomes, including miscarriage, preterm labor, and abnormal fetal positioning. Surgical reconstruction of the uterus is recommended for patients experiencing recurrent miscarriages or preterm deliveries.

6. Septate Uterus
(1) Clinical overview:
A septate uterus, also known as a uterine septum, is classified into two types:
  (a) Complete uterine septum: Extends to the cervix
  (b) Incomplete uterine septum: Does not extend to the cervix [2]

(2) Clinical manifestations:
Patients with a septate uterus may experience the following:
- Infertility
- Premature labor
- Recurrent miscarriage
- Retained placenta [9]

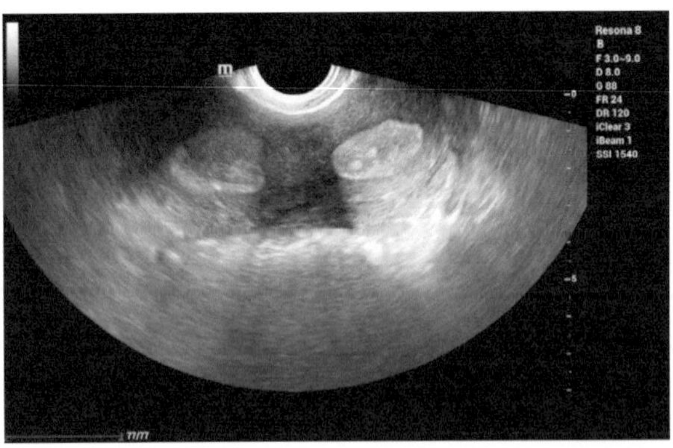

Fig. 7.8 Transverse view of the uterus on ultrasound showing a widened uterus with separated endometrium, creating a "butterfly-wing-like" appearance

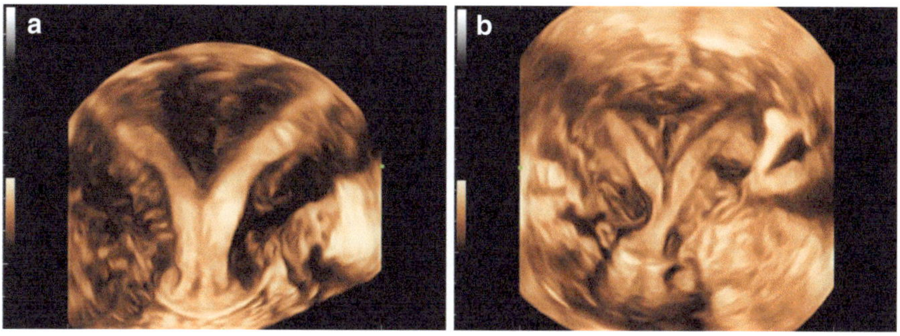

Fig. 7.9 (**a**) Coronal view of the endometrium in an incomplete bicornuate uterus on 3D ultrasound, showing a "Y-shaped" endometrium. (**b**) Coronal view of the endometrium in a complete bicornuate uterus on 3D ultrasound, showing a "V-shaped" endometrium

(3) Ultrasonographic features:
   (a) External uterine contour: May appear slightly widened and can be convex, flat, or mildly concave, with a depression depth of ≤1 cm.
   (b) Transverse view of the uterus: The endometrium is divided into right and left segments, with an angle of ≤90° between the two segments [2].
   (c) Coronal view on 3D Ultrasound:
      - A complete septum forms a "V" pattern.
      - An incomplete septum forms a "Y" pattern (see Figs. 7.10, 7.11, and 7.12).
(4) Differential diagnosis:
   Refer to Table 7.2 for detailed comparisons.
(5) Impact on fertility and treatment principles:
   Uterine septa can cause adverse pregnancy outcomes, including recurrent miscarriage, infertility, and preterm labor [10]. For patients with such manifestations, hysteroscopic resection of the septum is recommended.

7. Arcuate uterus
   (1) Clinical overview:
   An arcuate uterus results from incomplete resorption of the uterine septum during embryological development [11].
   (2) Clinical manifestations:
   Most patients with an arcuate uterus are asymptomatic and do not exhibit noticeable clinical symptoms.
   (3) Ultrasonographic features:
      (a) External uterine contour: Normal in appearance.
      (b) Fundal segment of the endometrium: A broad, smooth indentation is observed, with a depression depth of ≤1 cm.
      (c) Transverse plane: The indentation may appear as a subtle, focal, superior duplication of the endometrial echogenic complex.
      (d) Endometrial angle: The angle between the two endometrial "folds" is >90° (see Fig. 7.13).

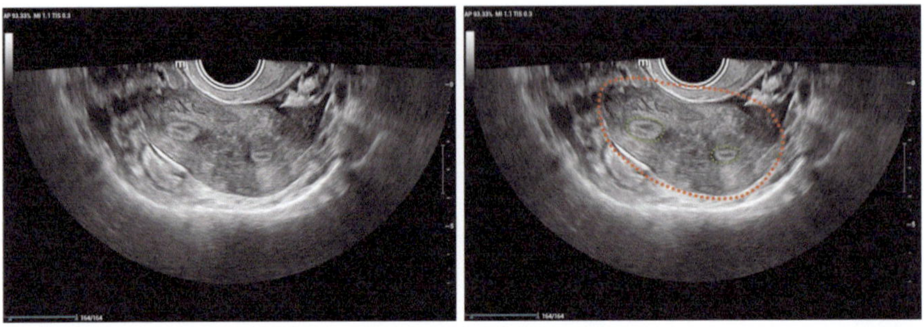

Fig. 7.10 Transverse view of the uterus showing a slightly widened uterine fundus with separated endometrium. The uterus is circled in orange; the two green circles indicate the separated endometrium

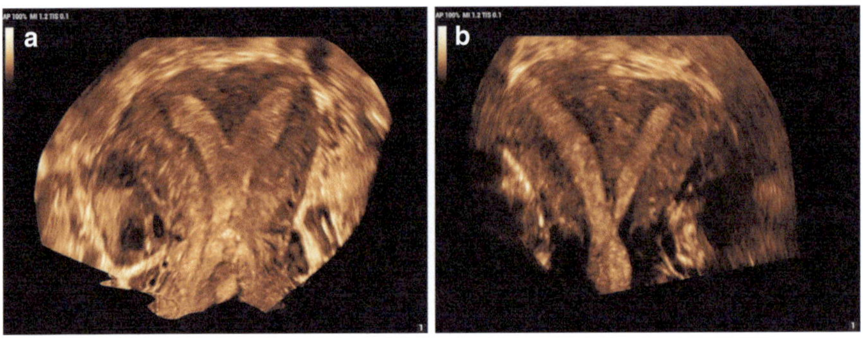

Fig. 7.11 (**a**) Coronal view on 3D ultrasound showing a "Y-shaped" endometrium in an incomplete uterine septum. (**b**) Coronal view on 3D ultrasound showing a "V-shaped" endometrium in a complete uterine septum

(4) Differential diagnosis:
Refer to Table 7.2 for detailed differential diagnosis.

(5) Impact on fertility and treatment principles:
While an arcuate uterus often has no significant impact on fertility, in cases of recurrent miscarriage, infertility, or preterm labor without an identifiable cause, hysteroscopic metroplasty may be considered [12].

8. T-shaped uterus

(1) Clinical overview:
A T-shaped uterus is characterized by a narrow uterine cavity with thickened lateral walls. This condition may be associated with diethylstilbestrol (DES)-related etiology and secondary causes such as intrauterine adhesion syndrome, tuberculosis, or adenomyosis [13, 14].

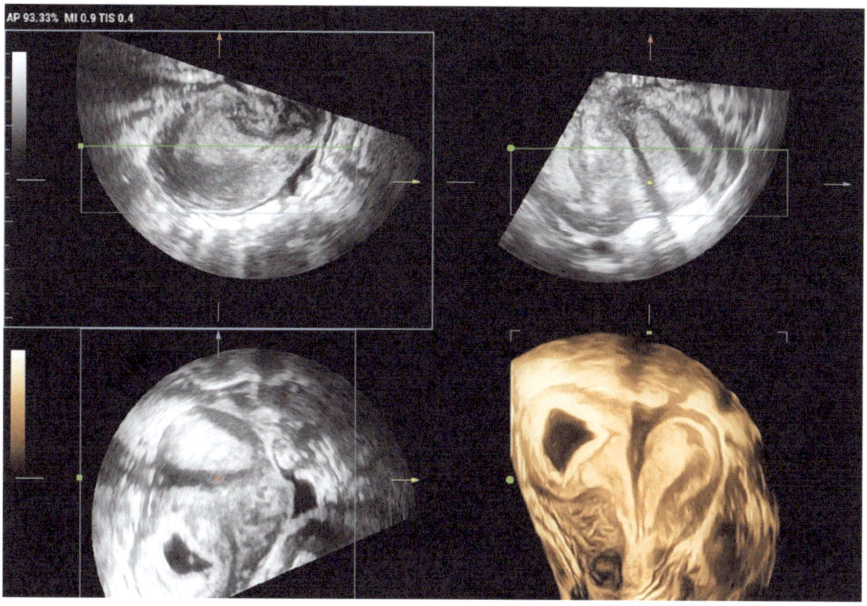

Fig. 7.12 Coronal view of a completely septated uterus with a gestation sac visible in the right uterine cavity on 3D ultrasound

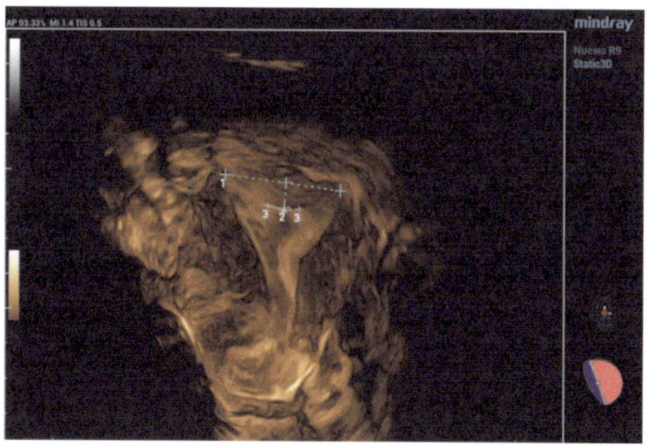

Fig. 7.13 3D coronal view of an arcuate uterus, showing an angle greater than 90° between the two endometrial folds

(2) Clinical manifestations:
Patients typically present with the following:
- Infertility
- Recurrent miscarriage
- Premature labor

(3) Ultrasonographic features:
   (a) 2D ultrasound: The endometrium appears thin and may lack cyclic changes.
   (b) 3D coronal plane: The uterine cavity is flattened at the fundus, forming a wide top and narrow bottom, creating the characteristic "T" shape (see Fig. 7.14) [14].
   (c) Diagnostic challenges: Ultrasound has significant limitations in detecting T-shaped uteruses, making precise imaging crucial.

(4) Impact on fertility and treatment principles:
   Patients are at risk for adverse pregnancy outcomes, including recurrent miscarriage and preterm labor. For those with severe symptoms, hysteroscopic metroplasty is recommended to reshape the uterine cavity. Patients with a history of miscarriage or preterm labor may benefit from cervical cerclage in subsequent pregnancies.

7.1.2 Conditions Associated with Abnormal Vaginal Development

1. Imperforate hymen
   (1) Clinical overview:
   An imperforate hymen results from the failure of the hymenal membrane to perforate, thereby preventing a connection between the vaginal canal and the vestibule.
   (2) Clinical manifestations:
   Patients with an imperforate hymen typically present with the following:
   - Absence of menstruation (amenorrhea) at puberty.
   - Progressive, cyclic lower abdominal pain.

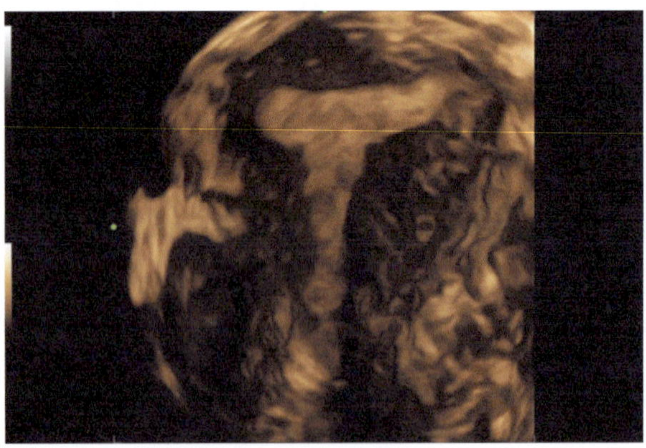

Fig. 7.14 T-shaped uterus in the coronal plane of 3D ultrasound, characterized by a flat base of the uterine cavity, creating a "T" shape with a wide upper part and a narrow lower part

  - Severe cases may present with difficulty in urination or defecation due to blood accumulation in the vagina (hematocolpos).
  - Physical examination reveals a bulging, bluish hymenal membrane at the vaginal opening [15–17].

(3) Ultrasonographic features:

Ultrasound imaging reveals an enlarged, sac-like vagina filled with a large volume of fluid displaying dense, fine dot-like echoes. As fluid accumulation progresses, it may extend into the uterine cavity and vagina, connected via the narrow cervical canal. Further progression can lead to bilateral tubal dilatation with fluid accumulation (see Fig. 7.15).

(4) Differential diagnosis:

Refer to Table 7.3 for conditions to be distinguished from an imperforate hymen.

(5) Impact on fertility and treatment principles

If untreated, an imperforate hymen can lead to damage to the endometrium and fallopian tubes, potentially causing infertility. Once diagnosed, a hymenotomy should be performed promptly to prevent complications [18].

2. Congenital absence of vagina

(1) Clinical overview

Most female patients with a congenital absence of a vagina also exhibit either an absent uterus or a rudimentary uterus, and a minority may have a functional endometrium. This condition is also referred to as Mayer-Rokitansky-Küster-Hauser (MRKH) syndrome.

(2) Clinical manifestations

  - Primary amenorrhea and dyspareunia
  - Associated anomalies such as:
    - Urinary malformations
    - Skeletal malformations
    - Cardiac malformations

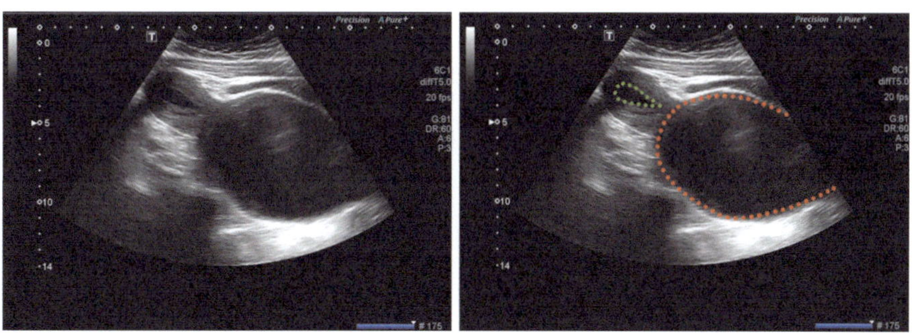

Fig. 7.15 The vagina appears enlarged in a sac-like pattern, with the uterine cavity above it filled with fluid. The two are connected by the fluid-filled, relatively narrow cervical canal. The orange circle highlights the enlarged sac-like vagina and the cervical canal, while the green circle indicates the fluid-filled uterine cavity

Table 7.3 Differential diagnosis of congenital vaginal abnormalities

Congenital vaginal abnormalities	Mechanisms	Clinical manifestations	Physical examination	Uterine development	Combined other malformations	Ultrasonographic features
Imperforate hymen	Failure of perforation to make a connection between the vestibule and the vaginal canal.	Primary amenorrhea, cyclic lower abdominal pain.	No vaginal opening, with bulging, bluish hymenal membrane; a mass in the vagina.	May develop normally.	Mostly without.	1. The vagina dilates into a sac-like shape. 2. Blood accumulation in the uterine cavity and cervical canal. 3. Continued progression may result in bilateral tubal dilatation.
Congenital absence of the vagina	Caused by dysplasia of bilateral Müllerian ducts	Primary amenorrhea and dyspareunia.	The hymen is visible, with no vaginal opening or with a vestibular indentation.	Mostly combined with the absence of a uterus or rudimentary uterus.	May also have urinary, skeletal, and cardiac malformations.	1. No uterus or a rudimentary uterus 2. No vaginal gas lines 3. May cause blood accumulation in the uterine cavity due to functional endometrium 4. Most often combined with urological malformations

Vagina atresia	The urogenital sinus did not take part in the formation of the lower end of the vagina.	Primary amenorrhea, periodic lower abdominal pain, dysuria, pelvic mass.	No vaginal opening; the mucosa at the atresia is normal; the mass of the vagina is higher than that caused by the imperforate hymen.	In lower vaginal atresia, the uterus develops normally; in complete vaginal atresia, it is frequently combined with congenital uterine anomalies.	It may be combined with uterine malformations.	Blood may accumulate in the vagina, cervix, and uterine cavity above the atresia site.
Longitudinal vaginal septum	Unabsorbed or incompletely absorbed longitudinal septum after the convergence of bilateral Müllerian ducts.	Most patients are asymptomatic, and some have dyspareunia and/or dysmenorrhea.	A longitudinal muscular structure in the vagina.	Most often combined with double cervixes and double uteruses.	Mostly without.	1. Double uteruses and double cervixes can be observed. Double vaginas are usually poorly visualized. 2. A few cases have an accumulation of blood in the vagina, cervix, or uterine cavity.

(continued)

Table 7.3 (continued)

Congenital vaginal abnormalities	Mechanisms	Clinical manifestations	Physical examination	Uterine development	Combined other malformations	Ultrasonographic features
OVSS	Bilateral Müllerian ducts with incomplete resorption of the septum.	Complete vaginal obstruction causes periodic lower abdominal pain and pelvic mass. Incomplete vaginal obstruction may be asymptomatic or have varying degrees of dysmenorrhea, prolonged menstrual periods, irregular vaginal bleeding, and purulent discharge.	A bulging oblique vaginal septum or a hole in the septum with bloody secretion; a cystic mass on one side of the vaginal wall; double uteruses and double cervixes; the uterus may enlarge when combined with intrauterine blood accumulation.	Most often combined with double cervixes and double uteruses.	It may be combined with urinary malformations, with renal agenesis being the most common.	1. Double uteruses and double cervixes. 2. A large amount of blood in the vagina; in severe cases, blood may accumulate in the cervix and even in the uterine cavity. 3. In a few cases, a hyperechogenic band is observed connecting the vaginal walls on both sides. 4. The kidney on the oblique septum side may be absent.

- Hearing abnormalities
- Neurological abnormalities

- Patients with functional endometrium may experience cyclic lower abdominal pain.
- Physical signs:
  - Normal vulvar and secondary sexual development.
  - The presence of the hymen but the absence of a vaginal opening or a 1–2 cm or more profound depression in the vaginal vestibule when gently pressed is termed vestibular recess.

(3) Ultrasonographic features

- Absence or rudimentary development of the uterus, with rudimentary uterine structures often presenting as spindle-shaped or elongated muscular echoes without visible cervix or endometrium.
- No vaginal structures are visible between the urethra and rectum, replaced by hypoechoic connective tissue without gas lines.
- In most cases, the bilateral fallopian tubes and ovaries are normal, with both ovaries close to the ipsilateral rudimentary uterus.
- In cases with functional endometrium, blood accumulation may occur in the uterine cavity.
- Associated urological malformations, such as horseshoe kidneys, ectopic kidneys, or unilateral renal agenesis (see Fig. 7.16).

(4) Differential diagnosis:
Refer to Table 7.3 for detailed differential diagnosis.

(5) Impact on fertility and treatment principles:
These patients do not have normal reproductive function. For those seeking a sexual life, vaginoplasty is recommended.

3. Vaginal atresia

(1) Clinical overview
Vaginal atresia is primarily a developmental abnormality caused by the failure of the urogenital sinus in forming the lower end of the vagina [19, 20]. The uterus and cervix are usually unaffected due to normal development of the Müllerian ducts [21].

(2) Clinical manifestations
Typical symptoms include the following:

- Primary amenorrhea
- Cyclic lower abdominal pain
- Dysuria
- Pelvic masses

The timing and severity of symptoms depend on the function of the endometrium.

Physical signs include the following:

- Normal female secondary sexual characteristics and absence of vaginal opening.
- The mucosal surface at the site of vaginal atresia is normal in color and does not bulge outward.

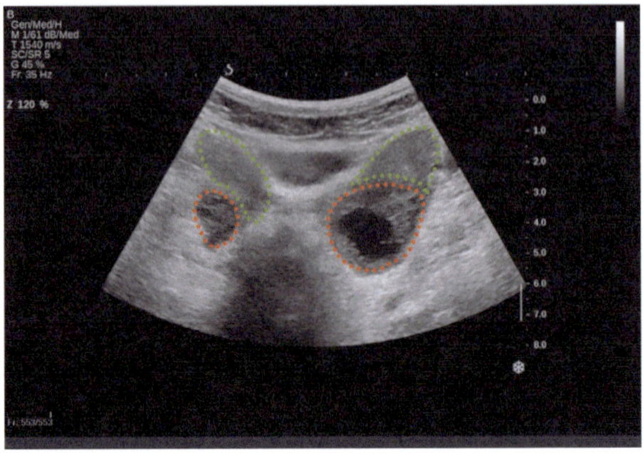

Fig. 7.16 The myxoid structures located anterior to the bilateral ovaries represent the bilateral rudimentary uteruses. The ovaries are circled in orange, and the rudimentary uteruses are circled in green

- The palpable mass on anal examination is higher in position than that caused by imperforate hymen.

(3) Ultrasonographic features

Fluid may accumulate in the vagina, cervix, and uterine cavity above the site of atresia, which can be visualized as dense and tiny light spots, moving and tumbling when pressure is applied. The degree of effusion is inversely correlated with the duration of the atresia, meaning that the greater the amount of effusion, the shorter the duration. In severe cases, tubal effusion may also be observed (see Fig. 7.17).

(4) Differential diagnosis:

Refer to Table 7.3.

(5) Impact on fertility and treatment principles

- Patients with vaginal atresia typically do not have normal reproductive function.
- Lower vaginal atresia can be treated surgically with favorable outcomes.
- Patients with complete vaginal atresia and a well-developed uterus, and no endometriosis in the pelvis, may be candidates for vaginoplasty and cervicoplasty.
- These patients require persistent postoperative cervical dilation and may be considered for in vitro fertilization and embryo transfer (IVF-ET) treatment.

4. Longitudinal vaginal septum

(1) Clinical overview

A vaginal septum occurs due to an unabsorbed or incompletely absorbed partition following the fusion of the bilateral Müllerian ducts [22]. This condition is classified into the following types:

(a) Complete longitudinal septum:

- Divides the vagina into two separate canals
- Often associated with double cervices and double uteruses

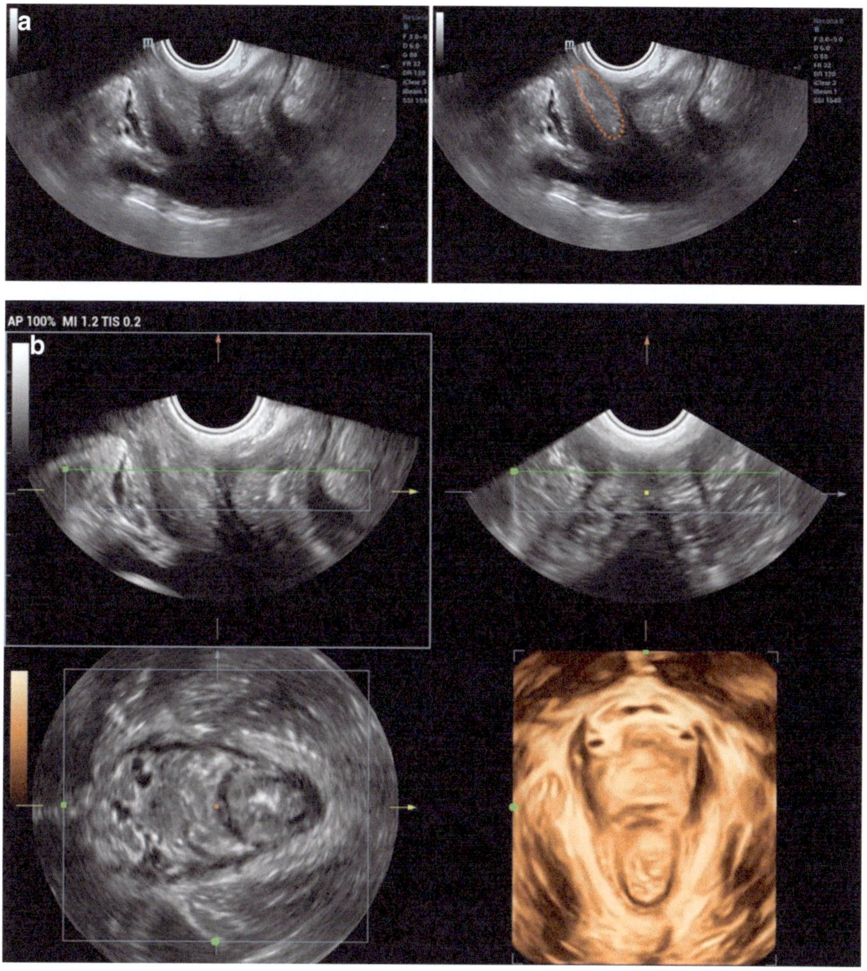

Fig. 7.17 (**a**) Transperineal ultrasound reveals the absence of vaginal gas lines, with hypoechoic muscular structures visible. The area of vaginal atresia is circled in orange. The area of vaginal atresia is circled in orange. (**b**) A 3D ultrasound image shows the absence of vaginal gas lines

(b) Partial longitudinal septum:
- Typically located in the upper part of the vagina
- Results from the partition between the fused Müllerian ducts disappearing from below upward [23]

(2) Clinical manifestations

Patients with a vaginal septum may experience the following symptoms:
- Dyspareunia: Painful intercourse
- Dysmenorrhea: Painful menstruation due to poor drainage of menstrual blood [24]

Physical examination findings:

- A longitudinal structure divides the vagina into two channels.
- This structure extends from the cervix or upper vagina down to the vaginal opening.
- Double cervices and double uteruses may be palpable.

(3) Ultrasonographic features:

(a) Complete longitudinal septum:

- Double uteruses and double cervices may be visualized.
- The vaginal septum itself is usually poorly visualized.

(b) Partial longitudinal septum:

- No distinctive ultrasound features are typically present.
- Blood accumulation may be visible in cases of poor menstrual drainage in the vagina, cervix, or uterine cavity (see Fig. 7.18).

(4) Differential diagnosis:

For conditions that should be considered in the differential diagnosis, refer to Table 7.3.

(5) Impact on fertility and treatment principles

Surgical excision is recommended for patients experiencing sexual dysfunction. A complete longitudinal septum is associated with an increased risk of preterm labor during pregnancy. A partial septum may obstruct fetal delivery and should be removed before pregnancy or, at the latest, before delivery.

5. Oblique vaginal septum syndrome (OVSS)

(1) Clinical overview:

OVSS is characterized by the following features:

- Double uteruses
- Double cervixes
- Double vaginas
- Complete or partial atresia of one vagina

It is often associated with urinary malformations on the atretic side, with renal agenesis being the most common. OVSS is also known as Herlyn-Werner-Wunderlich syndrome.

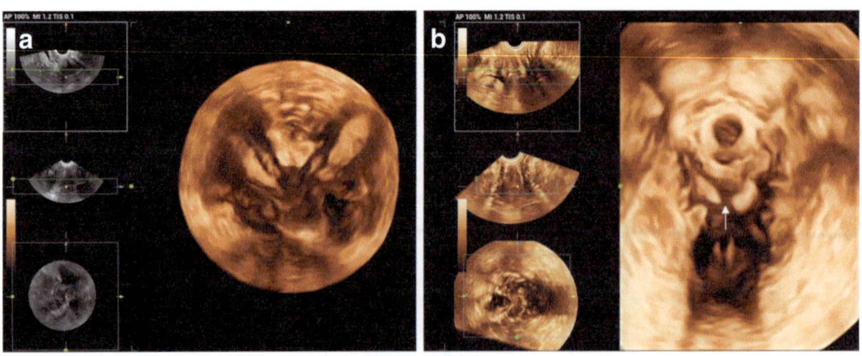

Fig. 7.18 (**a**) A 3D ultrasound image of the uterus reveals the presence of two uteruses and two cervixes. (**b**) A 3D ultrasound image of the vagina shows an interrupted vaginal gas line, indicated by an arrow

(2) Classification
Based on their anatomical characteristics, OVSS can be classified into three types [25] (see Fig. 7.19).
(a) Type I (imperforated type):
- One side of the vagina is completely blocked.
- The uterus behind the septum is completely separated from the outside and the contralateral uterus.
- There is no passage between the two uteruses or vaginas.
- Menstrual blood accumulates in the cavity behind the septum.

(b) Type II (perforated type):
- One side of the vagina is incompletely blocked, with a small hole in the oblique septum.
- The uterus behind the septum is isolated from the contralateral uterus.
- Vaginal secretions or menstrual blood drain from the small hole in the septum.
- Accumulation of pus or blood may occur due to poor drainage.

(c) Type III (imperforated with cervical fistula):
- One vagina is completely blocked, and the two vaginas are not connected.
- A fistula exists between the two cervices or between the posterior septal cavity and the contralateral cervix.
- Pus or blood often accumulates due to poor drainage.
- This type is relatively rare.

(3) Clinical manifestations
(a) Type I OVSS:
Presents with complete obstruction and severe symptoms such as periodic lower abdominal pain and pelvic masses during puberty

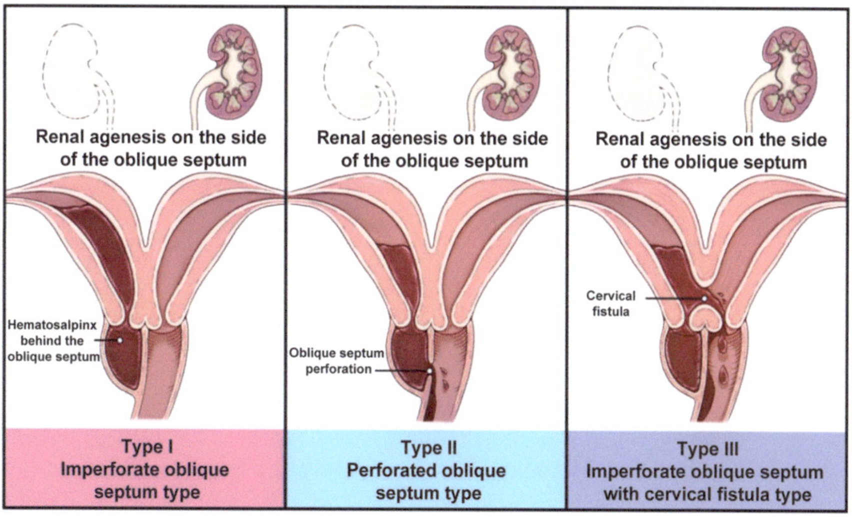

Fig. 7.19 OVSS classification

(b) Types II and III OVSS:
Present with incomplete obstruction and may be characterized by the following:
- Dysmenorrhea (painful menstruation)
- Prolonged menstrual periods
- Irregular vaginal bleeding
- Purulent discharge [25]

(c) Physical examination findings:
- A bulging or perforated oblique vaginal septum with bloody discharge.
- A cystic mass may be palpated on one side of the vaginal wall.
- Two uteruses and two cervices may be palpated.
- The uterus may be enlarged due to blood accumulation.

(4) Ultrasonographic features:
Double uteruses and double cervices can be visualized.

Intravaginal blood accumulation may be seen, with or without cervical or uterine blood accumulation.

- Type I: Shows a large amount of blood in the vagina, often accompanied by cervical and/or uterine blood accumulation. The contralateral uterus may shift due to compression.
- Types II and III: Exhibit milder intravaginal blood accumulation than Type I.

In a few cases, a strap-like echogenicity may be seen connecting the vaginal walls on both sides. Renal agenesis may be detected on the side of the vaginal oblique septum (see Figs. 7.20 and 7.21).

(5) Differential diagnosis:
For a list of conditions to be considered in the differential diagnosis, refer to Table 7.3.

(6) Impact on fertility and treatment principles:
Patients with a double uterus may experience infertility, preterm labor, and miscarriages. Once diagnosed, the septum should be surgically removed as soon as possible to prevent complications.

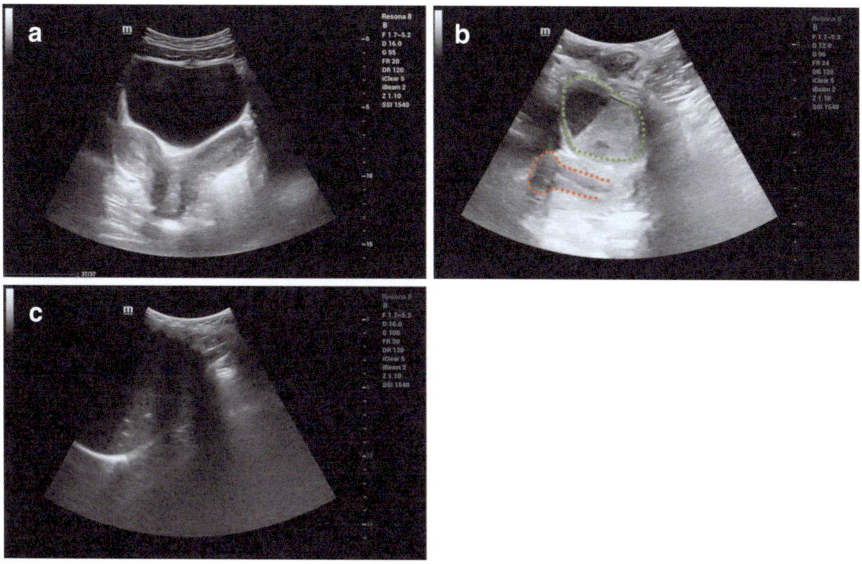

Fig. 7.20 (**a**) Double uteruses and double cervixes. (**b**) Intravaginal area with massive fluid and fine dot-like echoes. The uterus is circled in orange, and the fluid area is circled in green. (**c**) Absence of one kidney

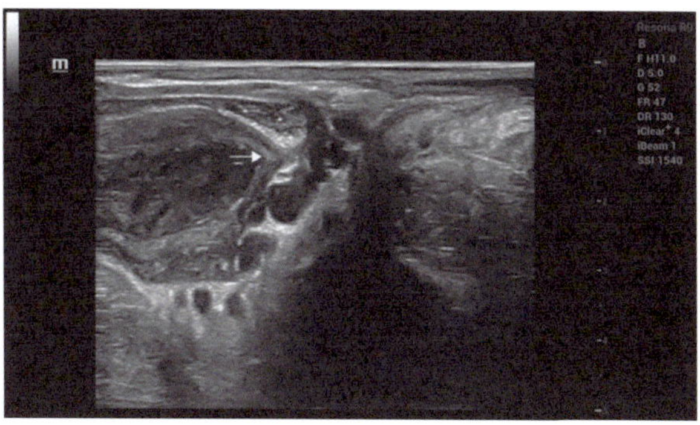

Fig. 7.21 This patient has two uteruses and two cervixes. Transrectal ultrasound reveals an oblique septum attached to one side of the vaginal wall at one end after saline injection, with a fluid area above the septum and dense, fine dot-like echoes. The arrow indicates the septum

7.2 Uterus-Related Diseases

Any factor that interferes with the transport of sperm, fertilized eggs, and embryo implantation can cause infertility.

7.2.1 Endometrial Diseases

1. Endometrial hyperplasia (EH)
   (1) Clinical overview:
   Endometrial hyperplasia (EH) is a nonphysiological, noninvasive overgrowth of the endometrium. It is characterized by
   - Alterations in glandular structure
   - Changes in the ratio of glands to interstitium [26]
   In 2014, the WHO classified EH into two categories [7]:
   (a) Endometrial Hyperplasia without Atypical Hyperplasia:
   Considered a benign condition with a cancer risk of less than 5% [8]
   (b) Endometrial Hyperplasia with Atypical Hyperplasia:
   A precancerous condition that may progress to endometrial cancer
   (2) Clinical manifestations:
   The most common symptom of EH is abnormal uterine bleeding, which can present as
   - Disturbed menstrual cycles.
   - Irregular or prolonged menstrual periods.
   - Increased or heavy menstrual flow.
   - Note: Abdominal pain or discomfort is usually absent during menstrual bleeding.
   (3) Ultrasonographic features:
   (a) Evenly thickened endometrium:
   - Thickness ≥12 mm before menopause.
   - Thickness ≥4 mm after menopause.
   - The thickened endometrium is well-demarcated from the myometrium.
   (b) Echogenicity:
   - It may be homogeneous, or
   - May present a honeycomb-like pattern with scattered small fluid areas
   - Can also appear heterogeneous
   (c) Doppler Ultrasound:
   - Color and spectral Doppler ultrasound can detect dot-like blood flow signals within the thickened endometrium.
   - High resistance arterial flow may also be seen (see Fig. 7.22).
   (4) Differential diagnosis:
   For a list of differential diagnoses, refer to Table 7.4.

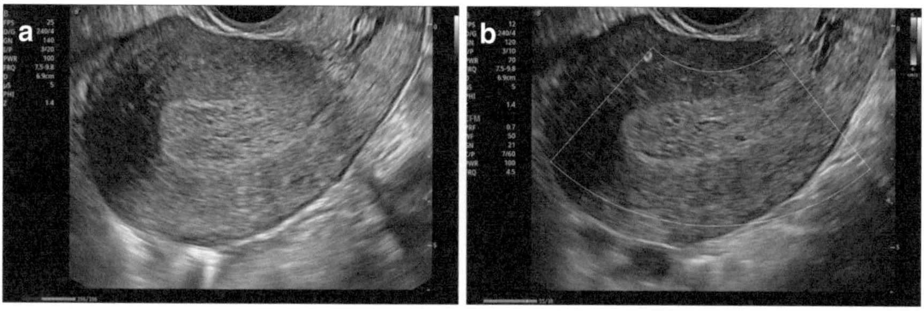

Fig. 7.22 (**a**) B-mode ultrasound shows a honeycomb pattern of the thickened endometrium in the longitudinal view of the uterus. (**b**) Color Doppler ultrasound shows dot-like blood flow within the endometrium

(5) Impact on fertility and treatment principles:

Patients with EH often experience significantly impaired fertility.

Pharmacological therapy is the first-line treatment to control abnormal uterine bleeding and restore the endometrium. In cases where endometrial cancer risk is low, treatment aims to prevent progression to cancer [27]. For patients with a desire for children, pro-ovulation therapy may be used after restoring the endometrium to help with conception.

2. Endometrial polyps (EMPs)

(1) Clinical overview:

Endometrial polyps (EMPs) are a common cause of abnormal uterine bleeding. They are frequently diagnosed in women of childbearing age. Most solitary polyps occur at the uterine fundus, while some may develop near the openings of the fallopian tubes. Multiple polyps tend to affect various areas of the uterus.

(2) Clinical manifestations:

- Asymptomatic cases are common.
- The most frequent symptom is abnormal uterine bleeding, which may include the following:
  - Excessive menstrual blood flow
  - Prolonged menstrual periods
  - Irregular vaginal bleeding (especially after menopause) [28]
- Some patients may also experience infertility or miscarriage.

(3) Ultrasonographic features:

(a) Single polyp:

- Appears as a teardrop-shaped hyperechoic mass with clear boundaries from the normal endometrium.
- The mass may contain a dark fluid area.
- When combined with intrauterine effusion, the polyp is more clearly visualized.

Table 7.4 Differential diagnosis of endometrial pathologies by ultrasound

	Morphology	Boundaries between endometrium and myometrium	Endometrial midline	Ultrasonic echogenicity	Color Doppler ultrasound findings
EH	Homogeneous thickening of the endometrium.	Well-defined endometrium.	The endometrial midline may be deviated or poorly displayed.	The ultrasonic echoes can be homogeneous, heterogeneous, or honeycomb-like.	Punctate blood flow signals may be visualized.
EMP0	On ultrasonography, a solitary polyp appears as a teardrop or clump; multiple polyps appear as regular clusters.	A single polyp is well-defined from the surrounding normal endometrium; multiple polyps are poorly defined from the normal endometrium surrounding them.	The endometrial midline may be deviated.	Hypoechoic, may be accompanied by dark fluid areas.	A single dominant vessel in the polyp.
Submucous fibroids (FIGO classification type 0 to type 2)	A short or absent tumor pedicle results in a regular-shaped fibroid, while a long pedicle causes the fibroid to appear irregular or protrude into the cervical canal or vagina.	The tumor pedicle can be observed in the myometrium or endometrium.	The endometrial midline may be deviated or poorly displayed.	Fibroids appear homogeneously hypoechoic when small; as they grow, they may become unevenly echogenic and undergo degeneration.	Stripes of blood flow originating from the myometrium and endometrium may be visualized at the tumor's pedicle.
EC	The endometrium is diffusely or focally thickened.	The endometrial-myometrial junction is regular when the cancer has not infiltrated the myometrium and irregular when infiltration occurs.	Poorly defined.	Primarily mixed low-to-moderate echoes with heterogeneous echogenicity.	Abundant punctate, streaky, or clustered blood flow around and within the EC, with a low-resistance arterial spectrum

(b) Multiple polyps:
- Characterized by thickened and unevenly echogenic endometrium.
- There may be clusters of irregular hyperechoic patterns, often poorly demarcated from the normal endometrium.
- Some patients also present with cervical polyps.
- Shift of the uterine lining may be observed, particularly in large or multiple polyps.

(c) Doppler ultrasound findings:
- Under color Doppler and spectral Doppler ultrasound, a single dominant vessel can be observed in the polyp, often displaying a "stellate" pattern.
- A high-resistance arterial spectrum may also be detected with a resistance index (RI) >0.50 (see Figs. 7.23, 7.24, and 7.25).

(4) Differential diagnosis:
For a comprehensive list of differential diagnoses, refer to Table 7.4.

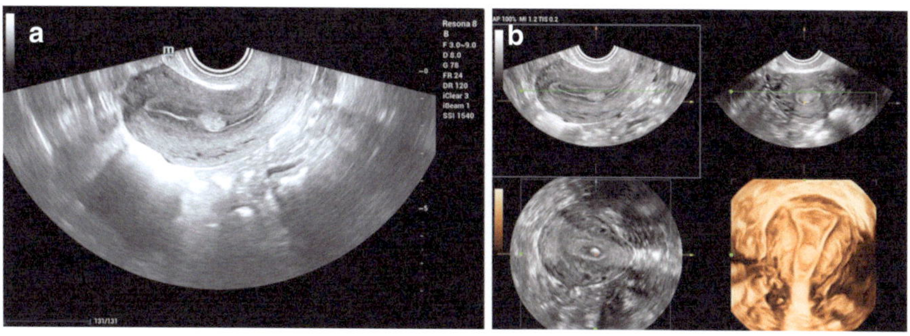

Fig. 7.23 (**a**) On 2D ultrasound, an endometrial polyp demonstrates a well-defined, teardrop-shaped hyperechoic mass. (**b**) A 3D coronal view shows an endometrial polyp

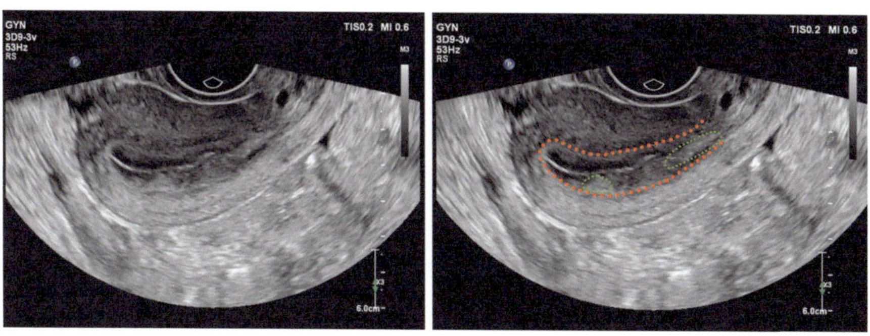

Fig. 7.24 Multiple endometrial polyps are observed with a thickened endometrium and uneven echogenicity on ultrasound. The uterine cavity is circled in orange; the polyps are circled in green

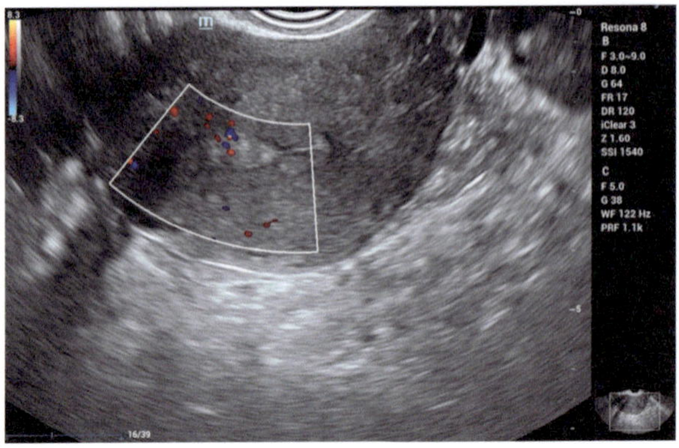

Fig. 7.25 Color Doppler shows short streaks of blood flow within an endometrial polyp

(5) Impact on fertility and treatment principles:

Endometrial polyps can obstruct the ostium function, hinder sperm migration, and cause biochemical effects that negatively impact implantation or embryo development [29].

Treatment:

- Asymptomatic, single polyps that are <1 cm in diameter may be left untreated.
- Larger or multiple polyps with wider bases should be treated with surgical resection.
- For infertile patients, hysteroscopic examination and surgical removal of the polyps are safe and cost-effective [30].

3. Endometrial carcinoma (EC)

(1) Clinical overview:

The clinical staging of endometrial cancer follows the International Federation of Gynecology and Obstetrics (FIGO) criteria [31].

(2) Clinical manifestations:

Abnormal menstruation and irregular vaginal bleeding are the first signs in many patients. Some patients may also experience abnormal vaginal discharge and bleeding during sexual intercourse. In advanced stages, systemic symptoms, including anemia, weight loss, and cachexia, may develop.

(3) Ultrasonographic features of mid- to late-stage EC:

(a) Endometrial changes:

- The endometrium appears diffusely or focally thickened, with uneven echogenicity (typically low-moderate mixed echogenicity).
- When cancerous tissue blocks the cervical internal os, uterine effusion occurs, which may appear as tiny bright echo spots within an otherwise echo-less intrauterine area.

(b) Myometrial changes:

- Infiltration of cancerous tissue into the myometrium results in an irregular endometrial–myometrial junction.
- The affected myometrium may show uneven hypoechoicity and poor demarcation from the surrounding normal myometrium.

(c) Cervical changes:
When the cervix is affected by EC, it becomes thickened, with messy echogenicity and poor visualization of the cervical canal structures.

(d) Pelvic invasion:
As the tumor metastasizes outside the uterus in advanced stages, it may present as
- Para-uterine masses
- Ascites
- Lymph node metastasis
- Signs of distant metastasis

(e) Doppler ultrasound findings:
- Abundant point-like, strip-like, or mass-like blood flows may be detected in the periphery and interior of the EC.
- Low-resistance arterial flow may also be seen.
- When EC infiltrates the myometrium, increased blood flow signals within the affected myometrium can be detected (see Figs. 7.26, 7.27, and 7.28).

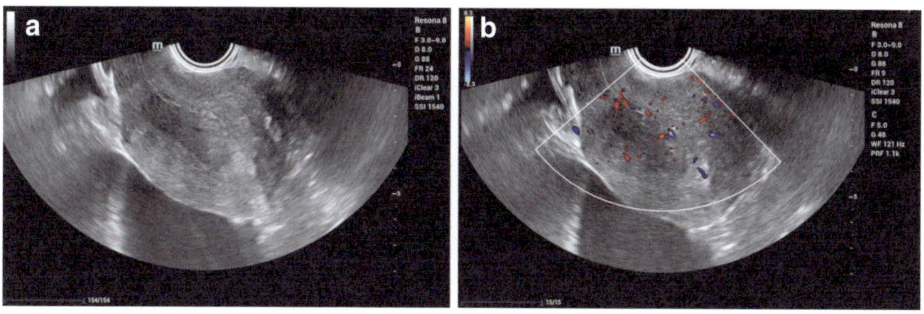

Fig. 7.26 (**a**) Ultrasound shows diffuse thickening of the endometrium with mixed low to moderate echogenicity. (**b**) Color Doppler shows abundant blood flow signals within and around the endometrium. This patient's pathology revealed severe atypical hyperplasia of the endometrium with focal malignant changes

Fig. 7.27 EC and intrauterine effusion are circled in orange

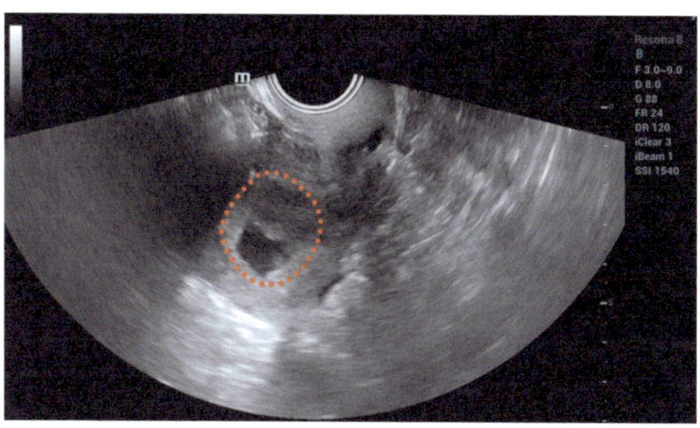

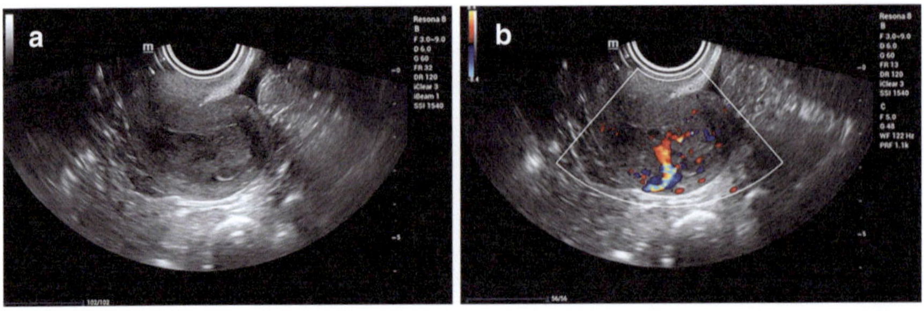

Fig. 7.28 (**a**) Ultrasound shows a thickened endometrium with uneven echogenicity and the absence of a clear boundary between the endometrium and the myometrium of the anterior wall. (**b**) Color Doppler shows abundant blood flows within the endometrium, predominantly derived from the myometrium of the anterior uterine wall. Pathological examination confirmed EC with myometrial infiltration

(4) Differential diagnosis:
For a comprehensive list of differential diagnoses, refer to Table 7.4.

(5) Impact on fertility and treatment principles:
Fertility preservation:

- High-dose progesterone treatment is recommended for young patients with early-stage, well-differentiated EC who wish to bear children.
- Pathological biopsy should be performed every 3 months to monitor disease progression.
- If disease reversal occurs, treatment can continue for 6–12 months, with continuous follow-up after discontinuation.
- If the disease progresses or persists, a hysterectomy should be considered.
- Once pathological results confirm complete remission, trying to conceive should be initiated.

For patients with risk factors: Women with a history of infertility or risk factors (e.g., obesity, polycystic ovary syndrome (PCOS), diabetes mellitus, or anovulatory disorders) are advised to complete childbearing as soon as possible, with the aid of IVF-ET [32].

4. Intrauterine adhesions (IUA)

(1) Clinical overview:
Intrauterine adhesions (IUA), also known as Asherman syndrome, is a pathological condition resulting from

- Damage to the basal layer of the endometrium due to intrauterine mechanical manipulation or infection.
- Poor endometrial repair leads to adhesion zones that reduce the uterine cavity volume.

In severe cases, the uterine cavity may become partially or completely obliterated, significantly reducing its functional volume [33].

(2) Clinical manifestations:
Common symptoms include the following:
- Hypomenorrhea or amenorrhea
- Pelvic pain
- Infertility
- Recurrent spontaneous abortion

(3) Ultrasonographic features:
In clinical practice in China, IUA is classified into four types based on ultrasound findings:
(a) Type I (mild adhesion):
- The endometrium is clearly displayed but partly discontinuous.
- Irregular hypoechoic bands can be visualized at discontinuities and are connected to the myometrium, affecting ≤1/2 of the uterine cavity's longitudinal diameter (see Fig. 7.29).

(b) Type II (moderate adhesion):
- Mild separation of the uterine cavity, with an internal diameter of ≤1 cm.

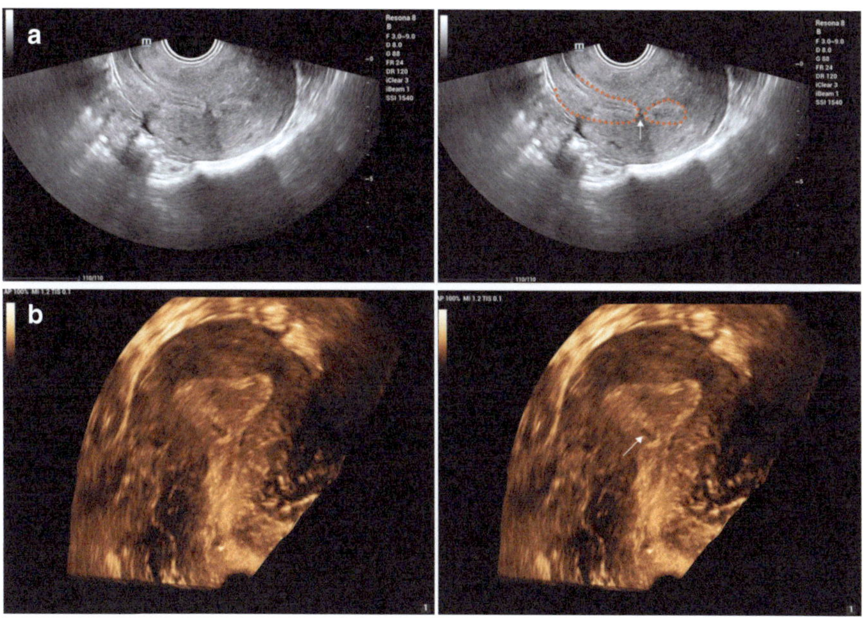

Fig. 7.29 (**a**) Type I IUA, showing discontinuous endometrial echogenicity and an irregular hypoechoic band at the site of the discontinuity. The endometrium is circled in orange, and the arrow points to the hypoechoic zone. (**b**) A case of Type I IUA, with adhesion bands visualized on the coronal plane of 3D ultrasound. The arrow indicates an adhesive band

    - A slightly echogenic band connecting the anterior and posterior walls of the uterus can be visualized (see Fig. 7.30).

  (c) Type III (severe adhesion):
    - The endometrium is thin (<0.2 cm) and poorly displayed with an irregular endometrial–myometrial junction.
    - Multiple irregular hypoechoic areas can be visualized.
    - The adhesion affects >1/2 of the uterine cavity's longitudinal diameter (see Fig. 7.31).

  (d) Type IV (complete adhesion):
    - Severe separation within the uterine cavity with an internal diameter >1 cm due to complete adhesion at the internal cervical os.
    - Blood accumulation in the uterine cavity (see Fig. 7.32).

      3D ultrasound findings:

      The coronal plane may show damage to the junctional zone:
    - In mild injury: The hypoechoic halo appears poorly defined and irregularly arranged.
    - In severe injury: The junctional zone disappears completely.

(4) Differential diagnosis:

IUA should be differentiated from congenital uterine abnormalities, such as:

- Unicornuate uterus
- Uterus septum

Key differentiating features include the following:

- Patients with congenital abnormalities tend to have normal or slightly increased menstrual blood flow.
- The endometrium may be abnormal in shape but usually has normal thickness.
- The endometrial–myometrial junction remains regular.

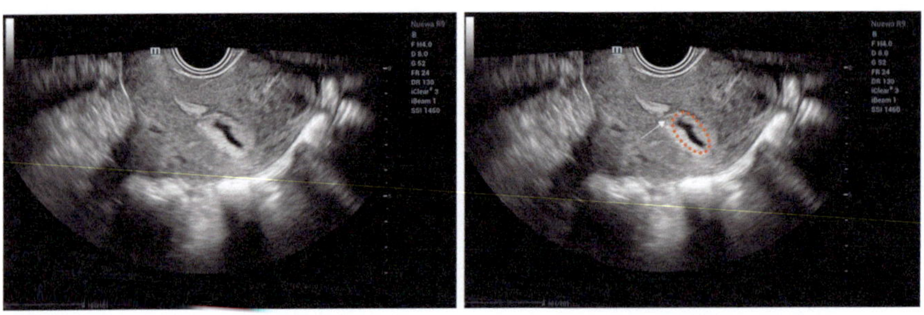

Fig. 7.30 Type II IUA, with an irregular hypoechoic band in the mid-lower part of the uterine cavity and a small amount of fluid above the band. The orange circle shows intrauterine fluid; the arrow indicates the irregular hypoechoic band

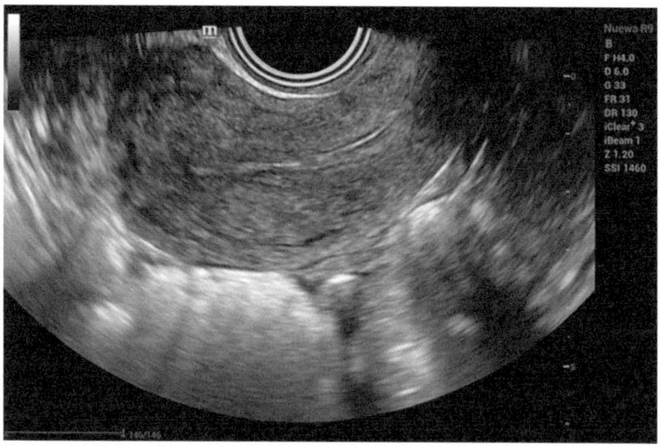

Fig. 7.31 Type III IUA, with an endometrium <2 mm thick, poorly demarcated from the myometrium

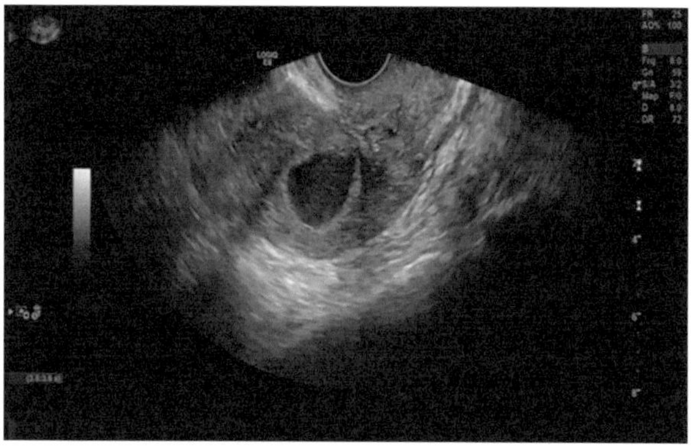

Fig. 7.32 Type IV IUA, with a completely adherent endocervical os and blood in the uterine cavity

(5) Impact on fertility and treatment principles:

Patients with IUA often experience infertility, difficulty in conceiving, or recurrent miscarriages. In mid-pregnancy, inadequate blood supply or abnormal placental implantation can occur, leading to complications such as placenta praevia and placenta accreta.

Treatment strategy:

- Surgical restoration of normal uterine cavity anatomy
- Prevention of re-adhesions
- Promotion of endometrial growth and improvement of its function
- Comprehensive postoperative evaluation to ensure success and reduce recurrence

7.2.2 Fibroids (Uterine Myomas)

1. Clinical overview:
   Fibroids, composed of smooth muscle and connective tissue, are among the most common female reproductive system benign tumors [34].
2. Classification:
   Fibroids are classified based on their location and relationship to the uterine anatomy. By site:
   Uterine fibroids: Account for approximately 90% of cases.
   Cervical fibroids: Constitute the remaining 10%.
   By relationship to the myometrium [35, 36]:
   (1) Intramural Fibroids:
   - The most common type, comprising 60–70% of cases.
   - Fibroids are embedded within the myometrium.

   (2) Subserosal fibroids:
   - Originate from intramural fibroids and develop toward the serosa, protruding beyond the uterine surface.
   - Often attached to the uterus via pedicles.
   - Represent about 20% of cases and have minimal impact on menstruation.

   (3) Submucosal fibroids:
   - Grow inward toward the intrauterine cavity, covered only by the mucosal layer.
   - Account for 10–15% of fibroids.
   - Commonly associated with enlarged and deformed intrauterine cavities, heavy menstrual flow, irregular bleeding, and occasional pain.
   - In severe cases, fibroids with long pedicles may protrude into the cervix or vagina.

   In 2011, the International Federation of Gynecology and Obstetrics (FIGO) introduced a nine-type classification system for fibroids to guide the assessment of surgical complexity and the choice of surgical approach [37] (see Fig. 7.33).
3. Clinical manifestations:
   Symptoms vary based on the fibroid's size, location, and degeneration status:
   (1) Menstrual changes:
   - The most common symptom, including increased menstrual flow, prolonged periods, shortened cycles, and irregular bleeding.
   - Frequently observed in patients with large intramural fibroids, multiple fibroids, or submucosal fibroids.
   - Chronic heavy bleeding may result in anemia.

   (2) Lower abdominal mass:
   It is mostly seen in patients with large or multiple fibroids.
   (3) Compression symptoms:
   - Bladder compression: This leads to urinary retention or frequency.
   - Rectal compression: Causes constipation.

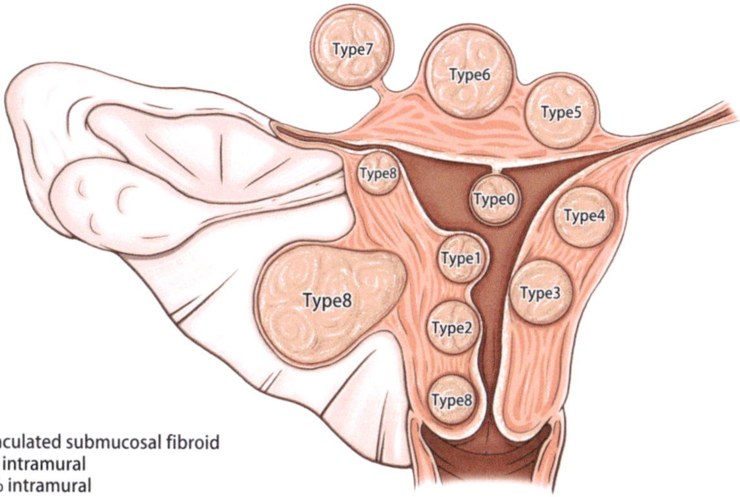

Type 0: Pedunculated submucosal fibroid
Type 1: <50% intramural
Type 2: ⩾50% intramural
Type 3: 100% intramural; contacts endometrium
Type 4: intramural (neither protruding towards the serosal layer nor the mucosal layer)
Type 5: subserosal, ⩾50% intramural
Type 6: subserosal, <50% intramural
Type 7: subserosal and pedunculated
Type 8: Other types (e.g., fibroids in special locations such as the cervix, uterine horn, broad ligament)

Fig. 7.33 FIGO classification of fibroids

(4) Other symptoms:
- Acute abdominal symptoms: May occur due to red degeneration or torsion of fibroids.
- Reproductive issues: Submucosal fibroids can lead to infertility or miscarriage.

4. Ultrasonographic features of fibroids:

The uterus appears enlarged and morphologically irregular in cases of large or multiple fibroids. The echogenicity of the fibroid varies depending on the fibrous tissue content and the presence or absence of degeneration. Fibroids without degeneration typically appear uniformly hypoechoic or hypoechoic masses with posterior acoustic shadowing [38].

(1) Ultrasonographic features by type:

(a) Intermural fibroids:

These appear as round nodules with regular morphology and well-defined peripheral boundaries due to the formation of a pseudocapsule.

(b) Subserosal fibroids:
- Manifest as intramural nodules protruding over the uterine surface.
- Often attached to the uterus by a pedicle when completely projecting out.

(c) Submucosal fibroids:
- Characterized by hypoechoic nodules in the myometrium that protrude into the uterine cavity.

- When entirely within the uterine cavity, a slit-like space can be seen between the fibroid and the uterine lining, with the fibroid's pedicle visible in the slit.
- Fibroids with long pedicles may extend into the cervical canal or vagina (see Fig. 7.34).

  Images corresponding to the FIGO classification are illustrated in Figs. 7.35, 7.36, 7.37, 7.38, 7.39, 7.40, 7.41, 7.42, and 7.43.

(2) Doppler ultrasound features:

  (a) Small fibroids: Exhibit short linear blood flow inside and around the tumor

  (b) Large intramural fibroids: Surrounded by a pseudocapsule with circumferential or semicircular blood flow, which branches into the tumor

  (c) Pedunculated fibroids: Display striated blood flow signals within the pedicle

  Spectral Doppler ultrasound detects high-resistance arterial spectra in most cases (See Fig. 7.44).

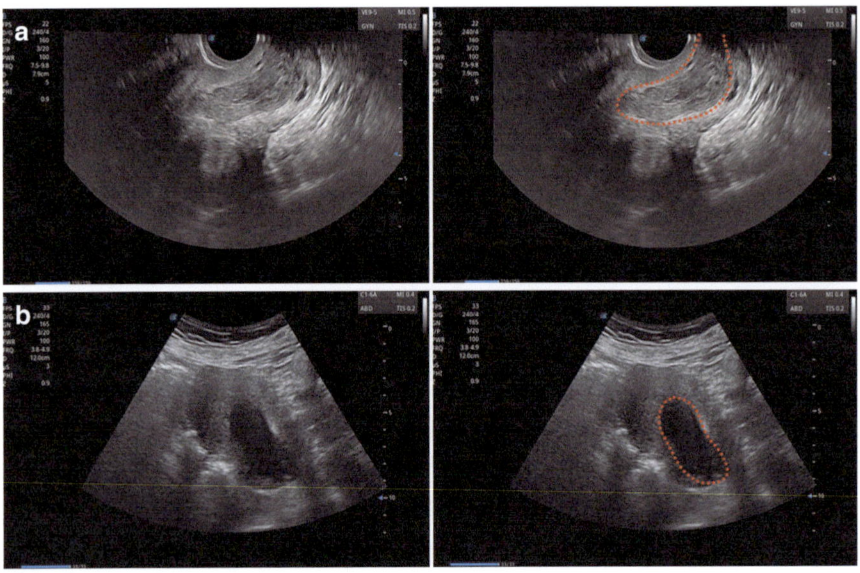

Fig. 7.34 (**a**) A submucosal fibroid hanging into the cervical canal, as shown on transvaginal ultrasound. The fibroid is circled in orange. (**b**) A submucosal fibroid hanging into the cervical canal, as shown on transabdominal ultrasound. The fibroid is circled in orange

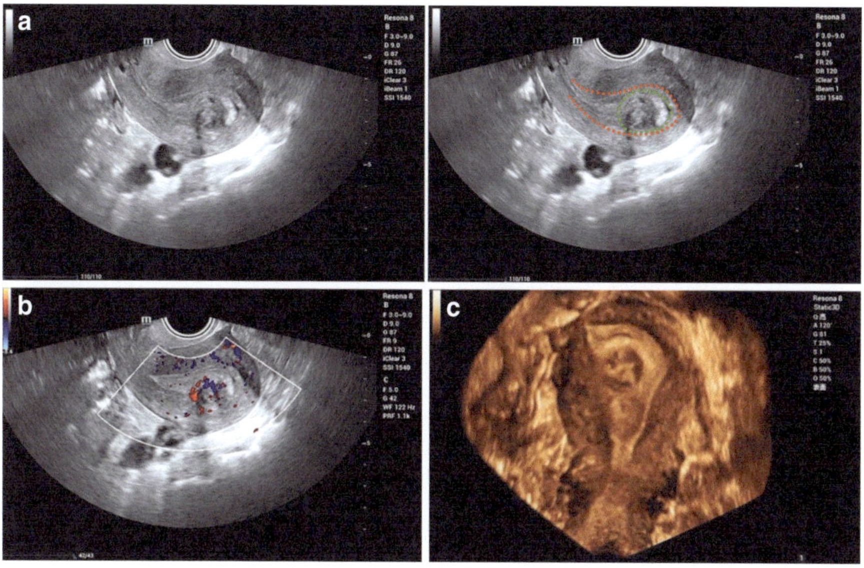

Fig. 7.35 (**a**) Type 0 fibroid: B-mode ultrasound shows a submucosal fibroid that protrudes from the myometrium and completely emerges into the uterine cavity. The endometrium is marked in orange; the fibroid is circled in green. (**b**) Type 0 fibroid: Color Doppler ultrasound shows abundant blood flows in the fibroid pedicle. (**c**) Type 0 fibroid: Coronal plane of the uterus on 3D ultrasound shows that the fibroid is completely within the uterine cavity

5. Ultrasonographic features of degenerated fibroids:
   (1) Hyaline degeneration:
   - The most common type of degeneration [38]
   - Swirling structures within the fibroid disappear, replaced by homogenous hyaline-like tissue
   - Minimal or no significant changes on ultrasound, with slightly reduced and heterogeneous echogenicity

   (2) Cystic degeneration:
   - Occurs due to necrosis and liquefaction of myocytes [39].
   - Appears as irregular nonechoic areas of varying sizes within the tumor.
   - Multiple cavities may coalesce into larger cystic spaces (see Fig. 7.45).

   (3) Red degeneration:
   - Specific to pregnancy or oral contraceptive use, involving necrosis of the fibroid.
   - The fibroid enlarges rapidly, with associated pressure pain [40].
   - Ultrasound shows increased fibroid size, reduced echogenicity, and a fine-patterned echogenic structure without attenuation.

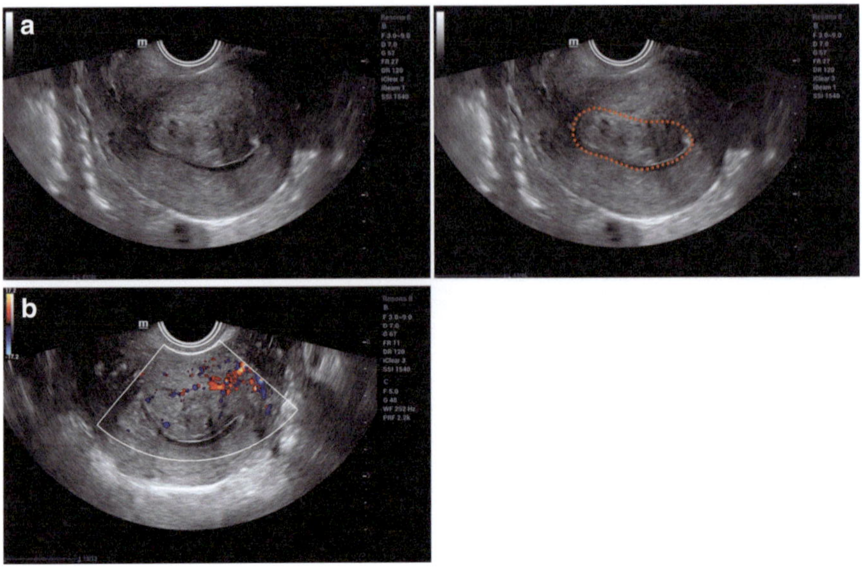

Fig. 7.36 (**a**) Type 1 Fibroid: B-mode ultrasound shows a fibroid in the posterior wall of the uterus, with most of it inside the uterine cavity. The fibroid is circled in orange. (**b**) Color Doppler shows the blood supply to the fibroid, originating from the posterior wall of the uterus

- Color Doppler shows decreased blood flow within the tumor (see Fig. 7.46).

(4) Fatty degeneration and calcification:
- Fatty degeneration: Deposition of fat globules within the fibroid, seen as hyperechoic areas on ultrasound.
- Calcification: Presents as ring-like or speckled strong echoes with posterior sound attenuation and reduced blood flow on Doppler (see Fig. 7.47).

(5) Sarcomatous degeneration:
- Mainly occurs in postmenopausal women and is associated with malignant transformation, leading to rapid growth, pain, and bleeding.
- Tumor tissue appears soft, brittle, and grayish-yellow, with poorly defined boundaries.
- Ultrasound shows a rapidly enlarging mass with unclear borders and heterogeneous echogenicity.
- Doppler reveals increased blood flow signals and a marked reduction in the resistance index (see Fig. 7.48).

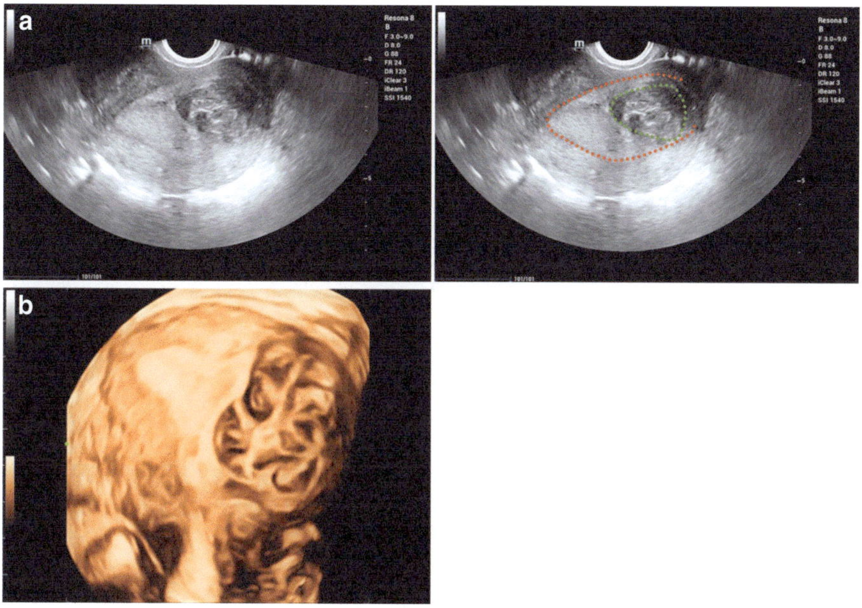

Fig. 7.37 (**a**) Type 2 intramural fibroid protruding into the submucosa: 2D ultrasound shows a fibroid in the left wall of the uterus, most of which lies intramurally, with a localized protrusion into the mucosa. The orange dotted line marks the endometrium; the green circle marks the fibroid. (**b**) Type 2 fibroid: The coronal plane of the uterus on 3D ultrasound provides a stereoscopic visualization of the fibroid in relation to the endometrium and shows the protrusion of the fibroid into the lower segment of the uterine cavity

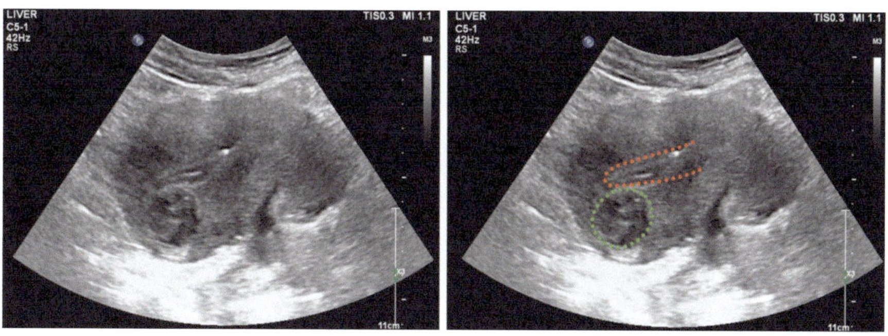

Fig. 7.38 Type 3 fibroid: This fibroid is entirely located in the muscular layer of the uterine wall, closely adjacent to the mucosa. The endometrium is marked in orange; the fibroid is circled in green

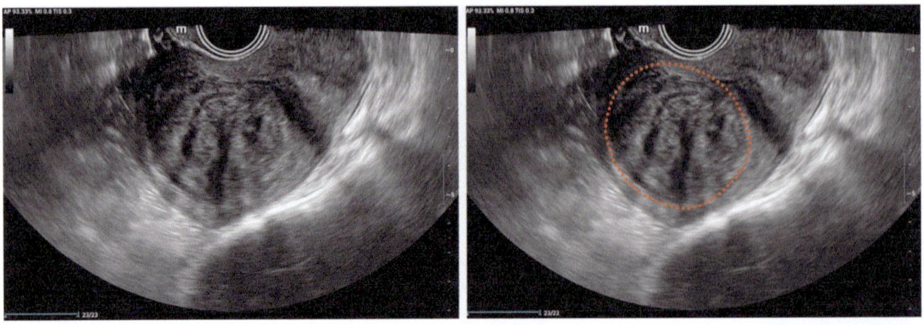

Fig. 7.39 Type 4 fibroid: The fibroid is confined to the muscular layer of the uterine wall, neither close to the serosa nor protruding into the mucosa. The fibroid is circled in orange

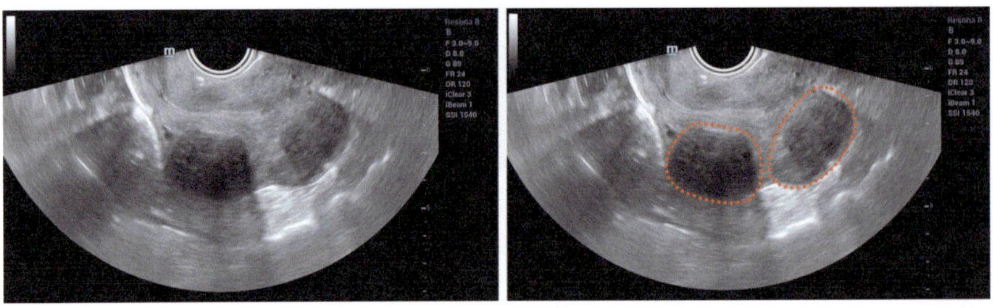

Fig. 7.40 Type 5 fibroid: This fibroid extends into the serosa, but ≥50% of it remains embedded in the muscular layer of the uterine wall. The fibroid is outlined in orange

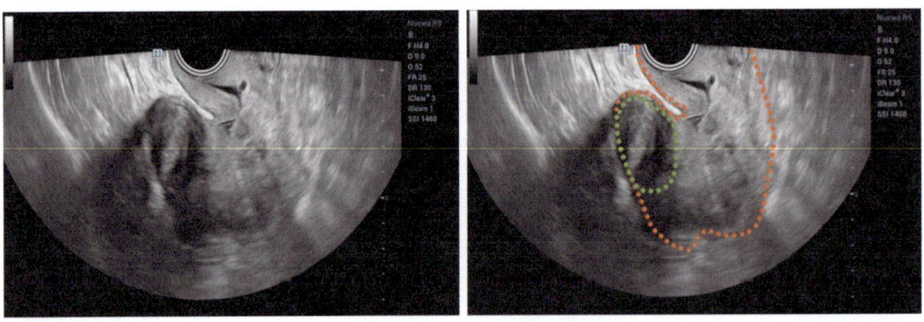

Fig. 7.41 Type 6 fibroid: This fibroid protrudes into the serosa, with <50% of it embedded in the muscular layer of the uterine wall. The uterus is marked in orange; the fibroid is circled in green

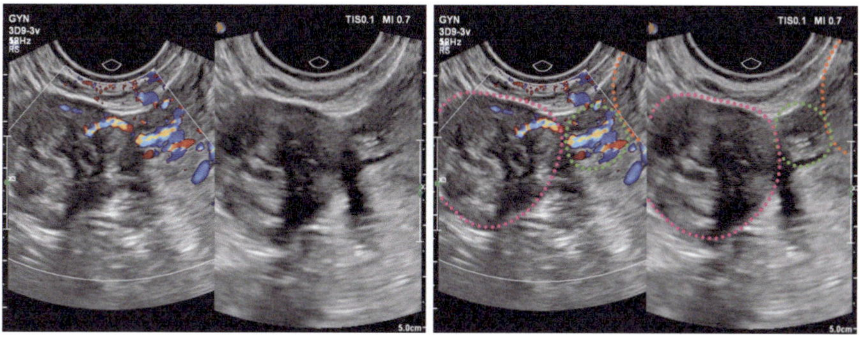

Fig. 7.42 Type 7 fibroid—Left: color Doppler ultrasound shows blood flow from the uterus at the pedicle of the subserosal fibroid. Right: B-mode ultrasound shows the pedicle of the fibroid. The uterus is outlined in orange; the fibroid is circled in pink; the fibroid pedicle is circled in green

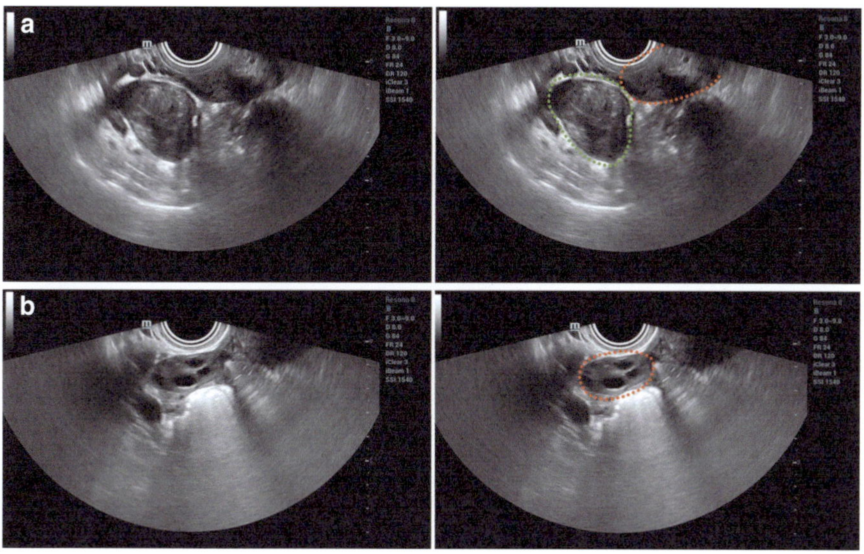

Fig. 7.43 (**a**) Type 8 broad ligament fibroid: This ultrasound image shows that the fibroid is located on the right side of the uterus and is not visibly connected to the uterus. The uterus is outlined in orange; the broad ligament fibroid is circled in green. (**b**) Type 8 broad ligament fibroid: An image of the ovary ipsilateral to the fibroid. The right ovary is circled in orange

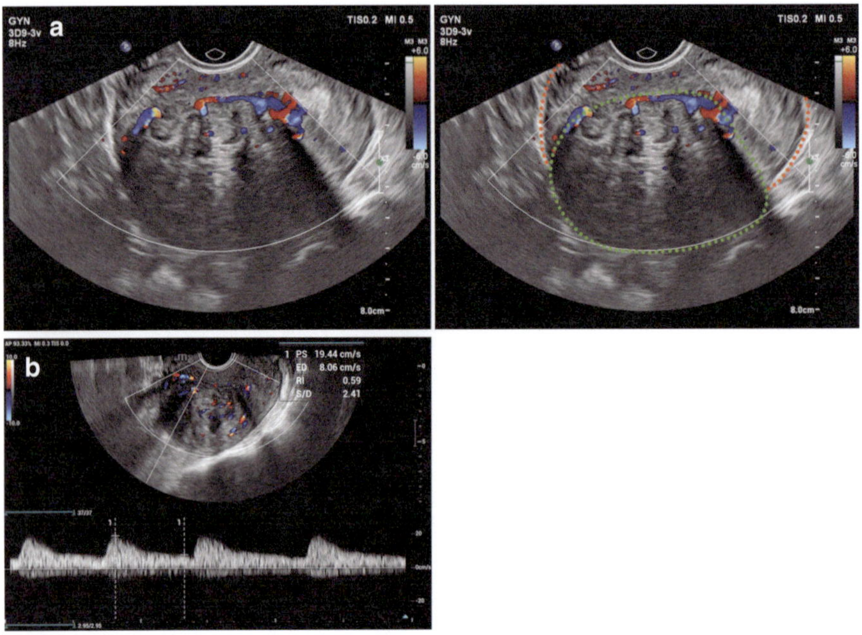

Fig. 7.44 (**a**) Color Doppler ultrasound reveals semicircular blood flow signals surrounding the fibroid, with branching into the tumor. The uterus is outlined in orange; the fibroid is circled in green. (**b**) High-resistance arterial flow detected on Doppler ultrasound

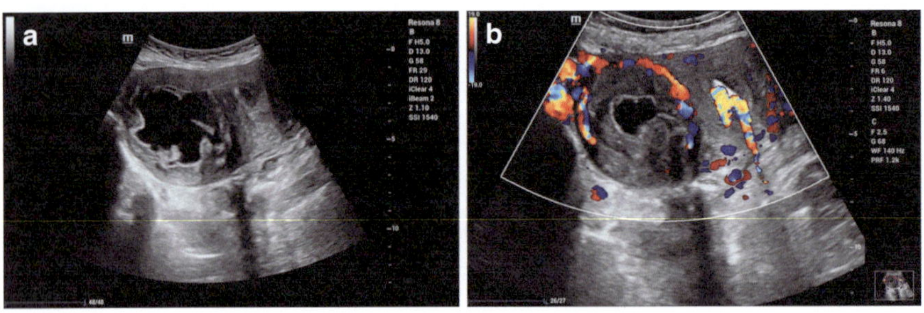

Fig. 7.45 (**a**) A fibroid with cystic degeneration, characterized by an irregular fluid area within the fibroid. (**b**) A fibroid with cystic degeneration, showing semicircular blood flow around the fibroid on color Doppler ultrasound

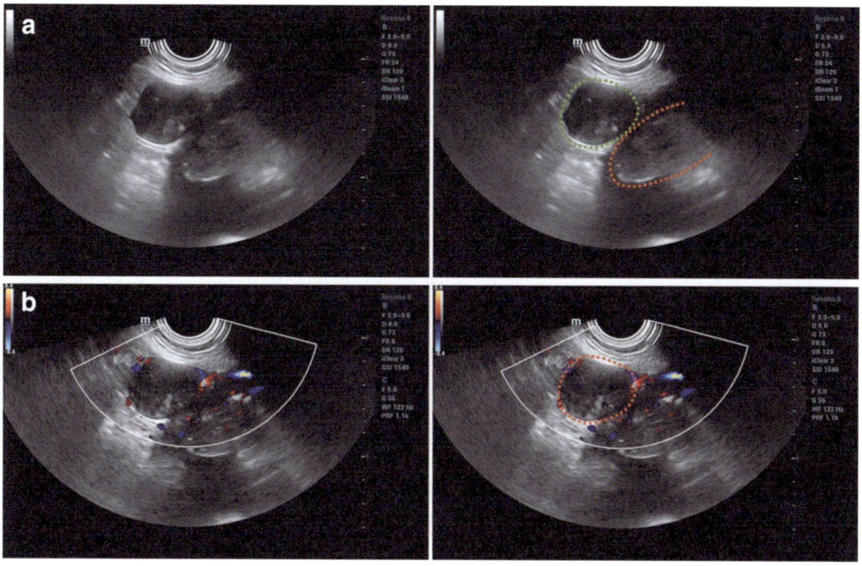

Fig. 7.46 (**a**) Red degeneration of the fibroid: A subserosal fibroid in the lateral wall of the uterus with decreased echogenicity internally and no attenuation of echogenicity in the posterior area. The placenta is outlined in orange; the fibroid is circled in green. (**b**) Red degeneration of the fibroid: Color Doppler ultrasound shows no significant blood flow within the fibroid (the patient was pregnant and experienced significant abdominal pain). The fibroid is circled in orange

6. Differential diagnosis:
   (1) Submucosal fibroids:
   Must be differentiated from
   - Endometrial hyperplasia
   - Endometrial polyps
   - Endometrial cancer

   Refer to Table 7.4 for detailed comparisons.

   (2) Subserosal fibroids:
   Need to be differentiated from solid ovarian tumors:
   - A subserosal fibroid is likely if the tumor is connected to the uterus via a pedicle and the ipsilateral normal ovary is visualized.
   - Distinguishing the two becomes challenging when the pedicle is too delicate to identify and the ipsilateral ovary is poorly visualized.
7. Impact on fertility and treatment principles:
   Uterine fibroids are a significant cause of infertility. Pregnant patients with fibroids face an increased risk of miscarriage and obstetric complications. Surgical removal of submucosal fibroids is strongly advised after diagnosis to improve fertility outcomes and reduce complications [41].

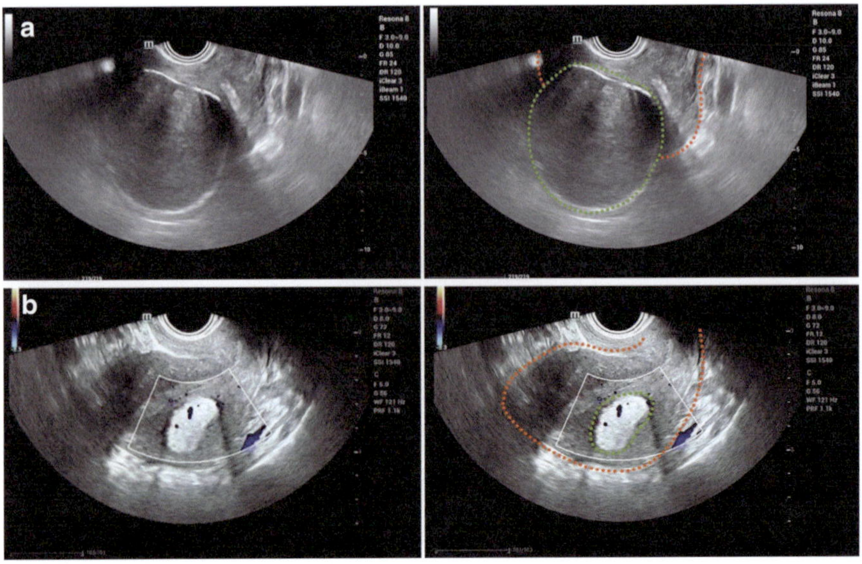

Fig. 7.47 (**a**) A calcified fibroid, showing ring-like strong echoes around the fibroid. The uterus is marked in orange; the fibroid is circled in green. (**b**) A fibroid with fatty degeneration, appearing as a hyperechoic mass within the fibroid, with punctate blood flow inside the tumor on CDFI. The uterus is marked in orange; the fibroid is circled in green

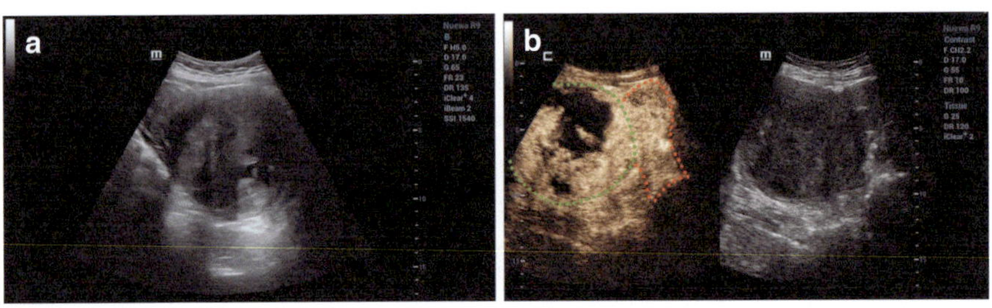

Fig. 7.48 (**a**) B-mode ultrasound shows a solid mass within the uterus with poorly defined borders, heterogeneous hypoechoic patterns, and irregular fluid areas. (**b**) The contrast-enhanced ultrasound image shows that the tumor is heterogeneously hyper-enhanced, with nonenhanced areas. The tumor is circled in green; the uterus is outlined in orange.

7.2.3 Uterine Adenomyosis

1. Clinical overview:
   Adenomyosis is characterized by the diffuse or localized presence of endometrial glands and stroma within the myometrium, leading to uterine enlargement and dysfunction [42].
2. Clinical manifestations:
   (1) Abnormal uterine bleeding:
   - Often presents as increased menstrual flow (menorrhagia) and/or prolonged menstrual periods.
   - Severe cases may lead to anemia.

   (2) Abdominal pain:
   - Includes progressive secondary dysmenorrhea and chronic pelvic pain

   (3) Other symptoms:
   - Infertility
   - Recurrent miscarriage
   - Painful intercourse and others

   (4) Physical signs:
   Gynecological examination may reveal:
   - A uniformly enlarged uterus or focal nodular elevations
   - Uterine stiffness with tenderness
   - Poor uterine mobility
3. Ultrasonographic features:
   (1) Sonographic features of adenomyosis lesions
   Adenomyosis is classified into diffuse and focal types based on lesion extent and echogenic characteristics [43, 44]:
   (a) Diffuse type:
   - The uterus is symmetrically enlarged in a spherical shape with a centralized endometrial stripe.
   - The myometrium is thickened with heterogeneous echogenicity, often showing coarse granular echoes and fan-shaped shadowing.
   - Asymmetric thickening of the anterior and posterior uterine walls is common, especially in the posterior wall and fundus, with displacement of the endometrial stripe (see Fig. 7.49).

   (b) Focal type (see Figs. 7.50 and 7.51):
   Focal adenomyosis is further classified into adenomyoma and cystic adenomyosis:
   Adenomyoma:
   - Nodular lesions in the myometrium with heterogeneous hypoechogenicity, often accompanied by fan-shaped shadowing
   - Poorly demarcated from normal myometrium

   Cystic adenomyosis: Appears as single or multiple fluid-filled areas within the myometrium containing fine punctate echoes of old hemorrhage

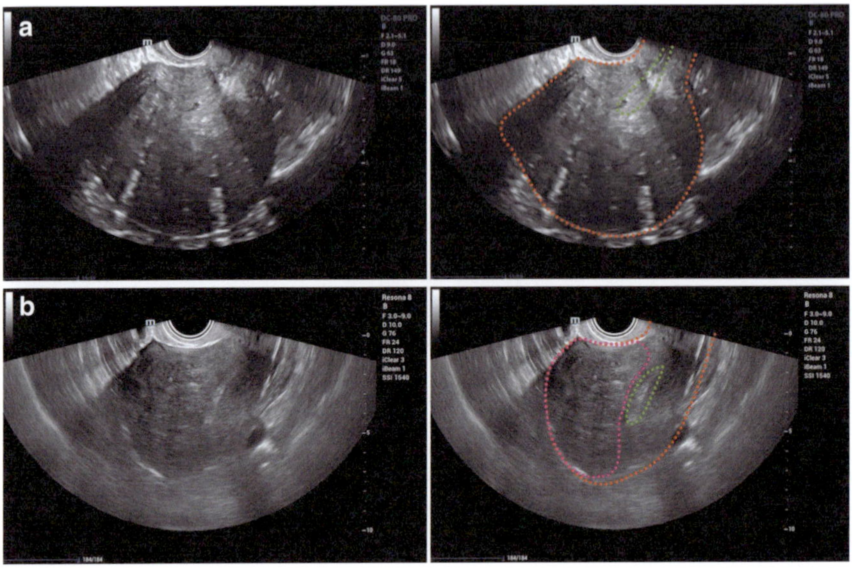

Fig. 7.49 (**a**) Diffuse adenomyosis: The uterus is spherically enlarged, with the posterior wall being most prominent. The endometrium is poorly visualized, and multiple small fluid areas are identified within the affected myometrium. The uterus is circled in orange; the endometrium is circled in green. (**b**) This ultrasound image shows adenomyosis confined to the anterior wall of the uterus, with posterior displacement of the endometrium and multiple small fluid areas within the affected myometrium. The uterus is outlined in orange; the endometrium is circled in green; the adenomyosis is circled in pink

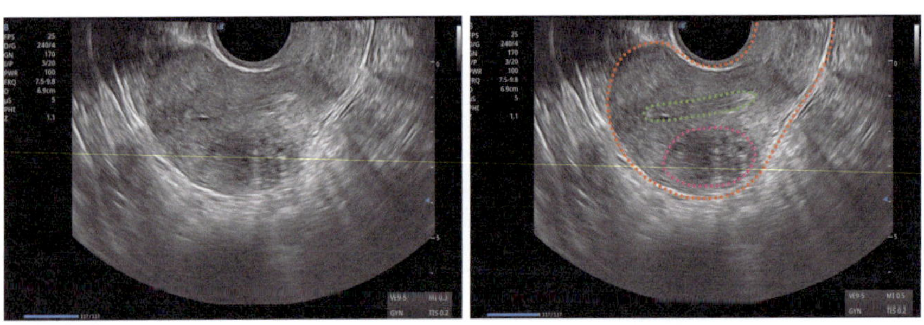

Fig. 7.50 Focal adenomyosis located in the posterior wall of the uterus, with poorly defined borders within the myometrium. Multiple small fluid areas are visualized. The uterus is circled in orange; the endometrium is circled in green; the adenomyoma is circled in pink

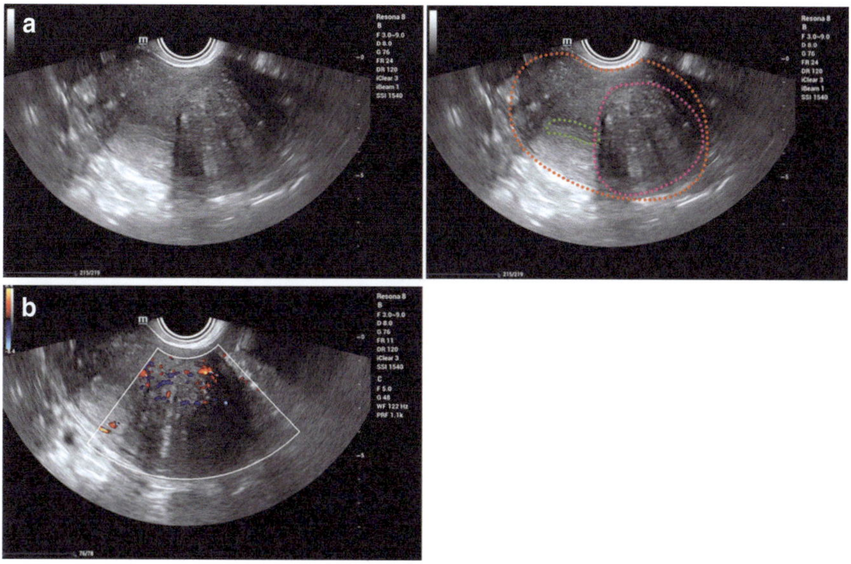

Fig. 7.51 (**a**) Focal adenomyosis located in the left wall of the uterus, with poorly defined borders between the adenomyosis, the myometrium, and the endometrium. The uterus is circled in orange; the endometrium is circled in green; the adenomyoma is circled in pink. (**b**) Color Doppler ultrasound shows increased blood flow in the affected myometrium, without peripheral circumferential blood flow

(2) Key features:
- Small fluid areas within the myometrium representing cystic dilatation of ectopic glands.
- Poorly defined endometrial–myometrial junction, often thickened, irregular, or interrupted.
- Hyperechogenic lines, buds, or islands under the endometrium indicate basal endometrial tissue invasion (see Fig. 7.52).

(3) "Question Mark Sign" [45] (see Fig. 7.53):
- Uterine morphology resembles a "question mark" in cases combined with posterior pelvic endometriosis.
- The uterus flexes backward, with the fundus oriented toward the posterior pelvis and the cervix toward the bladder.
- Negative uterine sliding sign.

(4) Color Doppler and spectral Doppler ultrasound (see Fig. 7.51):
- Increased blood flow within the affected myometrium, with vessels running perpendicular to the uterine cavity/serosa.
- Moderate resistance arterial spectra are often detected.

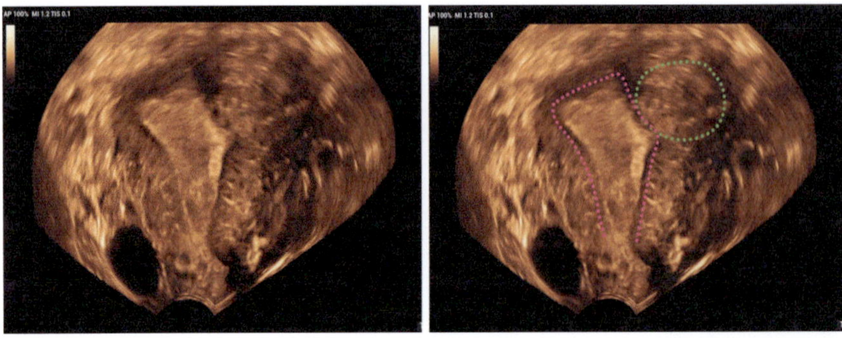

Fig. 7.52 Coronal plane of the uterus on 3D ultrasound shows an adenomyoma in the left wall, in close proximity to the uterine fundus, where the junctional zone is interrupted. The adenomyoma is circled in green; the hypoechoic junctional zone surrounding the endometrium is circled in pink

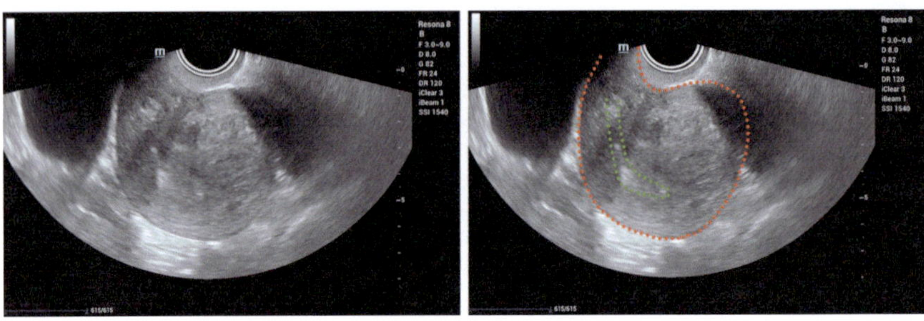

Fig. 7.53 Uterine morphology exhibiting the "question mark sign." The uterus is circled in orange; the endometrium is circled in green

4. Differential diagnosis:
   Uterine adenomyosis must be differentiated from uterine sarcoma, which primarily occurs in middle-aged and elderly women and often arises from sarcomatous degeneration of a fibroid. Key distinguishing features of uterine sarcoma include the following:
   - Rapid growth: A sudden and significant increase in the size of a fibroid over a short period
   - Color Doppler: Abnormally abundant blood flow
   - Spectral Doppler: Low-resistance arterial spectra within the tumor
5. Impact on fertility and treatment principles:
   Adenomyosis is associated with infertility and increased risks of adverse pregnancy outcomes, including preterm labor and miscarriage. For patients seeking to preserve fertility, hormonal therapy with GnRH antagonists followed by IVF-ET is recommended. For those without fertility needs, options include hysterectomy, localized lesion removal, or placement of a levonorgestrel-releasing intrauterine system to manage symptoms.

7.2.4 Cervical Diseases

1. Cervical polyp(s)
   (1) Clinical overview:
   Cervical polyps are benign growths formed by localized hyperplasia of endocervical glands and fibrous interstitium [46].
   (2) Clinical manifestations:
   Common symptoms include abnormal vaginal bleeding, increased leukorrhea, or bloody discharge. Some cases are asymptomatic and incidentally detected during routine examinations.
   (3) Ultrasonographic features:
   Detecting cervical polyps via ultrasound can be challenging in cases of a completely closed cervical canal, small polyps, or polyps near the external cervical os; however, when visible, they typically present with the following features:
   - Single or multiple droplet-shaped hyperechoic masses within the cervical canal, exhibiting regular morphology and clear boundaries, often surrounded by fluid in the cervical canal. Liquefaction may occur in rare cases.
   - Polyps may have either a broad base or a stalk connecting them to the cervical mucosa.
   - Color Doppler and Spectral Doppler ultrasound: A single feeding vessel is often seen centrally in the polyp, with high-resistance arterial spectra (see Figs. 7.54, 7.55, and 7.56).

   (4) Differential diagnosis:
   Endometrial hyperplasia extending into the cervical canal can mimic a polyp but is distinguishable by its unclear borders, extension from the endometrium, and internal echoes resembling the endometrium, especially in late proliferative or secretory phases. Repeat scanning during the early proliferative phase can aid differentiation.
   (5) Impact on fertility and treatment principles:
   Chronic cervical inflammation associated with polyps may alter the uterine environment, potentially affecting fertility. Large polyps can obstruct the cervical canal, hindering sperm entry. Hysteroscopic removal is recommended for large polyps to restore normal function.
2. Cervical cyst
   (1) Clinical overview:
   Cervical cysts, or Nabothian cysts, can be single or multiple and vary in size. They can develop at any location within the cervix.
   (2) Clinical manifestations:
   In some cases, cervical cysts may lead to an increase in vaginal discharge, especially when accompanied by infection. Large cysts may cause symptoms related to compressions, such as frequent or urgent urination, dysuria, dyspareunia, and rectal tenesmus [47].

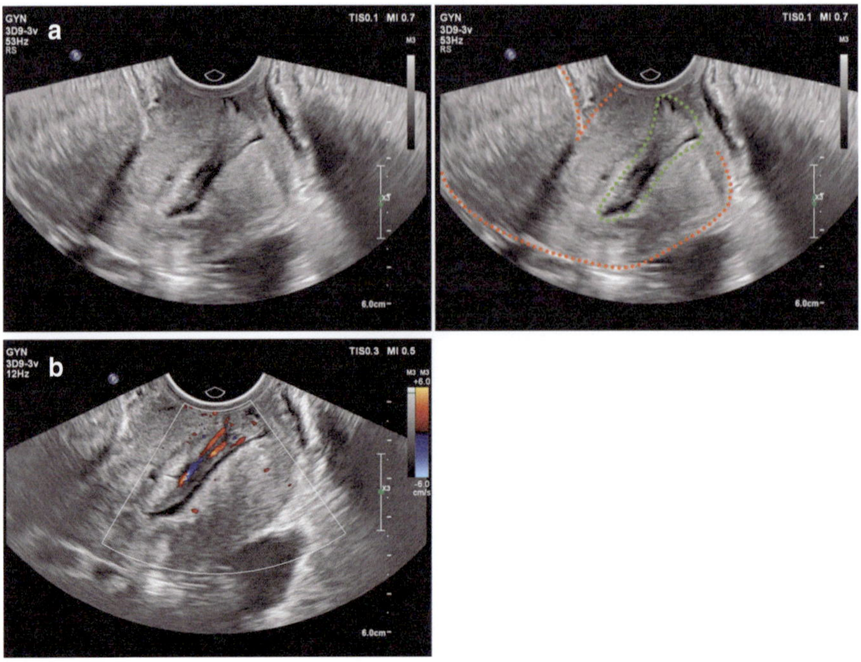

Fig. 7.54 (**a**) B-mode ultrasound shows a large cervical polyp protruding through the external cervical os, surrounded by a fluid-filled area (cervical canal effusion). The uterus and cervix are circled in orange; the cervical polyps is circled in green. (**b**) Blood flow within the polyp is demonstrated using color Doppler ultrasound

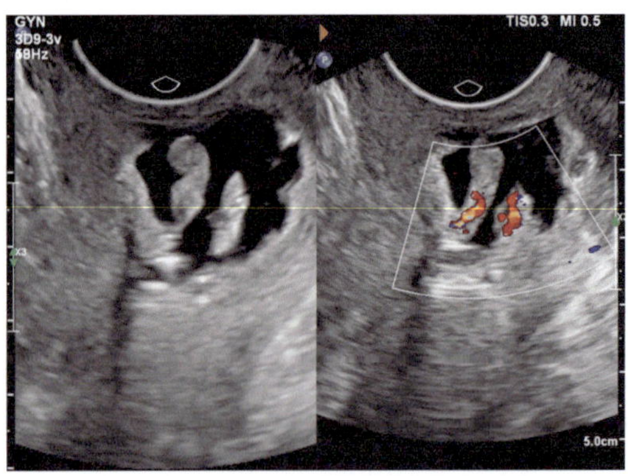

Fig. 7.55 Left: multiple cervical polyps visualized on B-mode ultrasound. Right: color Doppler ultrasound shows feeding blood flow connecting to the basal layer of the cervical mucosa

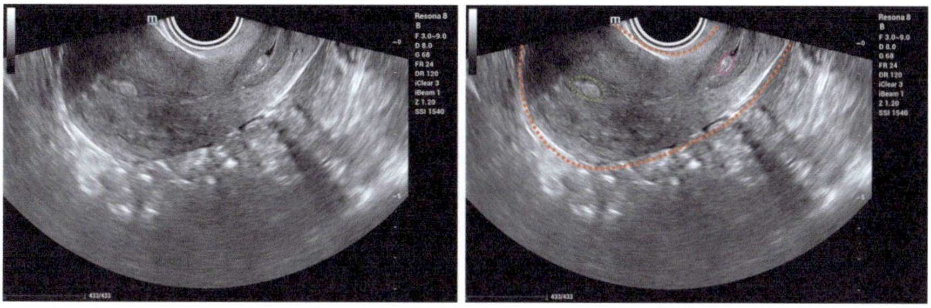

Fig. 7.56 A cervical polyp combined with an endometrial polyp. The uterus and cervix are circled in orange; the endometrial polyp is circled in green; the cervical polyp is circled in pink

(3) Ultrasonographic features:
Cervical cysts typically appear as single or multiple round or oval anechoic areas with well-defined borders and posterior acoustic enhancement. In the presence of infection or hemorrhage, fine dot-like or floccular echoes may be observed within the cyst (see Fig. 7.57).

(4) Differential diagnosis:
If infection or bleeding is present, the internal echoes of the cervical cyst may change, showing multiple tiny punctate echoes. When slight pressure is applied with the transducer, these echoes may float within the cyst. Color Doppler ultrasound will not detect any blood flow within the cyst.

(5) Impact on fertility and treatment principles:
The impact on reproductive function is similar to that of cervical polyps. Aspiring the fluid via puncture may be considered for symptomatic large cysts.

3. Cervical fibroid (cervical myoma)

(1) Clinical overview:
Cervical fibroids are classified into intramural, subserosal, and submucosal types based on their relationship to the cervical muscle wall. Intramural fibroids are the most prevalent.

(2) Clinical manifestations:
Large cervical fibroids may cause compression symptoms, including
- Frequent and/or urgent urination
- Difficulty in urination (dysuria)
- Difficulty in defecation (dyspareunia)
- Rectal tenesmus

Obstruction of the cervical canal may result in blockage of menstrual flow.

(3) Ultrasonographic features (see Figs. 7.58 and 7.59):

(a) General characteristics:
- Clear borders and regular morphology (typically round or oval)
- Internal echoes that are mostly homogeneous or heterogeneous hypoechoic

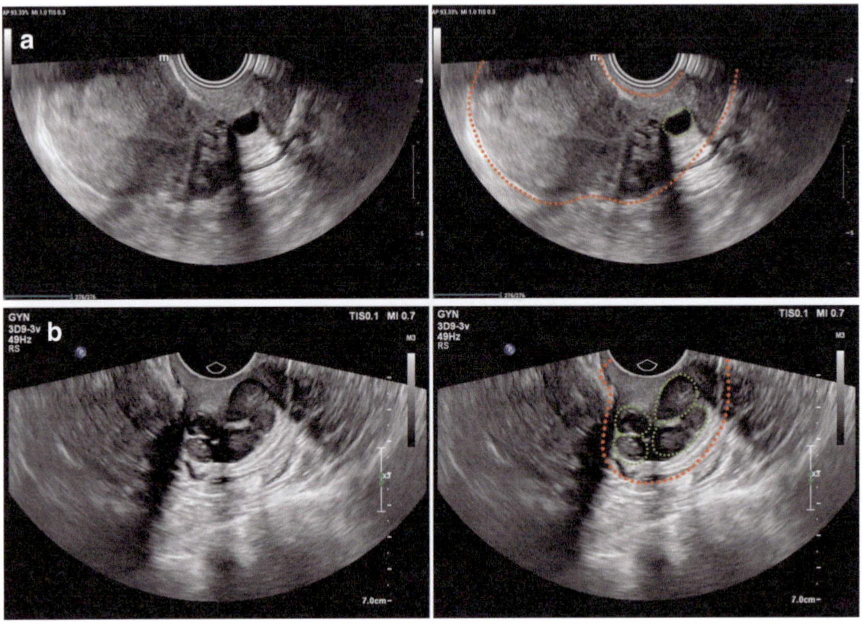

Fig. 7.57 (**a**) Single cervical cyst a round, well-defined anechoic area. The uterus and cervix are circled in orange; the cervical cyst is circled in green. (**b**) Multiple cervical cysts with fine punctate echoes. The cervix is circled in orange; the cervical cysts are circled in green

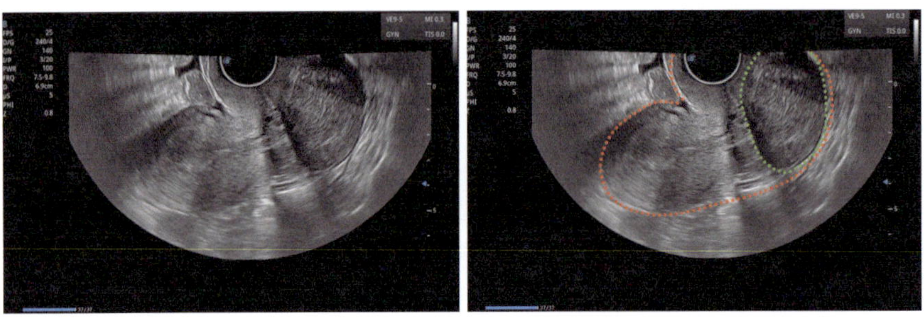

Fig. 7.58 A fibroid located in the posterior lip of the cervix, appearing oval, well-defined, and hypoechoic, with clearly visualized structures of the cervical canal. The uterus and cervix are circled in orange; the fibroid is circled in green

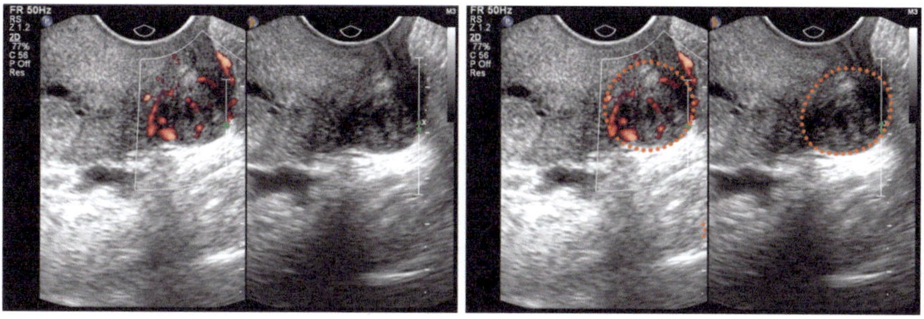

Fig. 7.59 Left: Power Doppler ultrasound demonstrates circumferential blood flow surrounding a cervical fibroid. Right: B-mode ultrasound shows a fibroid in the posterior lip of the cervix. The fibroid is circled in orange

(b) Intramural cervical fibroids:
- These are the most common type.
- Large fibroids or submucosal fibroids within the cervix may obscure the structure of the cervical canal on ultrasound.

(c) Degenerated cervical fibroids:
- Degeneration may alter the ultrasonographic appearance, as detailed in the section on uterine fibroid degeneration.

(d) Color Doppler and spectral Doppler ultrasound:
- Circumferential or semicircumferential blood flow is often detected around the fibroid, with branches penetrating its interior.
- High-resistance arterial spectra may also be observed.

(4) Differential diagnosis:

(a) Submucosal fibroids vs. prolapsing fibroids:
- A prolapsing submucosal fibroid may exhibit a long stalk attached to the uterus. Color Doppler ultrasound often shows feeding blood flow within the stalk.
- Submucosal cervical fibroids are rarer and typically have a shorter pedicle, which is usually continuous with the cervical mucosa or muscular wall.

(b) Cervical fibroids vs. cervical cancer:

Cervical fibroids:
- More common in women of childbearing age.
- Typically asymptomatic or present with minimal clinical symptoms.
- Ultrasound features include the following:
  - Clear borders and regular shapes
  - Clear visualization of the cervical canal structure
  - Color and spectral Doppler show annular or semiannular blood flow around the fibroid and high-resistance arterial spectra

Cervical cancer:

- More prevalent in middle-aged and elderly women
- Commonly associated with abnormal vaginal bleeding
- Ultrasound features include the following:
  - Indistinct borders and irregular shapes.
  - Poorly visualized cervical canal structure.
  - Color and spectral Doppler reveal abnormally abundant dendritic blood flow signals and low-resistance arterial spectra within the mass.

(5) Impact on reproductive function and treatment principles:

Large cervical fibroids can obstruct sperm passage into the uterine cavity, negatively affecting fertility. Surgical excision is recommended for fibroids compromising reproductive function [36].

4. Cervical cancer

(1) Clinical overview:

Cervical cancer can be classified into the following types based on gross visual characteristics:

(a) Exophytic: The most common type, characterized by outward growth.
(b) Endophytic: Growth infiltrating deeper tissues.
(c) Ulcerative: Lesions appear as ulcers.
(d) Cervical canal type: Cancer confined to the cervical canal.

The clinical staging of cervical cancer follows the International Federation of Gynecology and Obstetrics (FIGO, 2018) criteria [48].

(2) Clinical manifestations:

Symptoms progress with disease advancement and include the following:

(a) Vaginal bleeding: Most commonly, contact bleeding, irregular bleeding, prolonged menstrual periods, or heavy menstrual flow.
(b) Vaginal discharge: Thin, watery, whitish, or bloody discharge, often with a fishy odor.
(c) Advanced symptoms: Depend on invasion extent and may include the following:
  - Frequent or urgent urination
  - Constipation
  - Swelling or pain in the lower limbs
  - Ureteral obstruction, hydronephrosis, uremia
  - Anemia

(3) Ultrasonographic features:

Ultrasound findings vary with disease progression:

(a) Cervix:
  - Enlarged, barrel-shaped cervix.
  - Solid heterogeneous hypoechoic mass with indistinct borders and irregular morphology within the cervix.
  - The cervical canal may remain visible or become obscured.
  - Bright echogenic spots or patches may be observed within the mass (see Fig. 7.60).

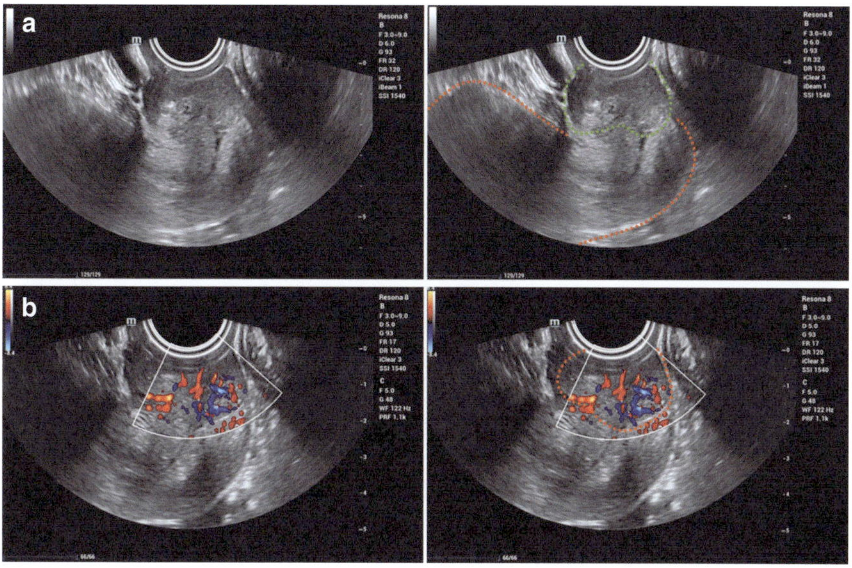

Fig. 7.60 (**a**) B-mode ultrasound shows a hypoechoic mass at the external cervical os (exophytic type) with poorly defined borders and irregular morphology. The structure of the cervical canal remains intact. The uterus and cervix are circled in orange; the tumor is circled in green. (**b**) Color Doppler ultrasound demonstrates abnormally abundant and branching blood flow signals within the cervical cancer. The tumor is circled in orange

(b) Infiltration into the uterus:
   - Poorly defined boundary between the cervix and the lower uterine segment
   - Hypoechoic lower uterine segment with poorly visualized endometrium (see Fig. 7.61)

(c) Para-uterine invasion:
   - Markedly dysmorphic cervix with unclear boundaries from surrounding tissues
   - Bladder invasion: Inhomogeneous bladder wall thickening with disrupted serosal echogenicity
   - Ureteral invasion: Leads to dilated ureter and hydronephrosis
   - Rectal invasion: Inhomogeneous rectal wall thickening [49–51]

(d) Color Doppler and Spectral Doppler:
   - Abundant branching blood flow signals within the mass.
   - Low-resistance arterial spectra are detectable (see Fig. 7.62).

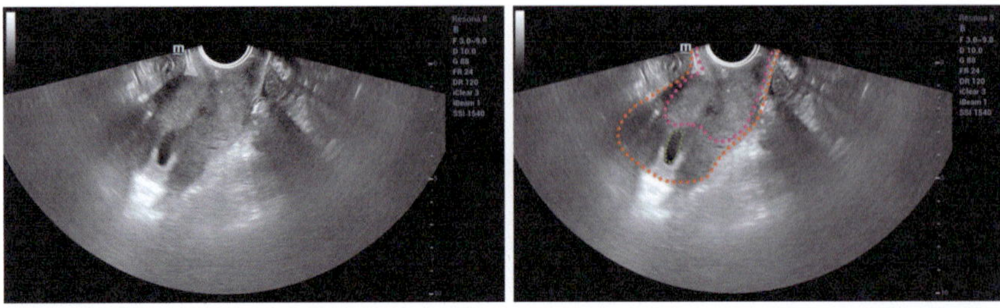

Fig. 7.61 Cervical cancer infiltrating the uterus, with cancerous tissue obstructing the cervical canal and causing intrauterine effusion. The uterus is circled in orange; the intrauterine effusion is circled in green; the tumor is circled in pink

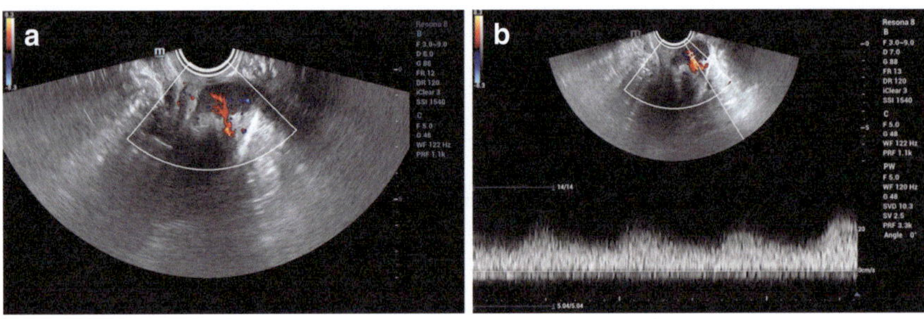

Fig. 7.62 (**a**) Color Doppler ultrasound image of cervical cancer demonstrating abundant blood flow in a dendritic pattern. (**b**) Spectral Doppler ultrasound showing a low-resistance arterial spectrum

(4) Differential diagnosis:

Cervical cancer must be differentiated from endometrial cancer infiltrating the cervix, especially in advanced cases where their presentations overlap.

Endometrial cancer is typically confined to the endometrium or invades the uterine muscular layer but may mimic cervical cancer when it extends into the cervix. Pathological examination is essential for distinguishing between the two conditions accurately.

(5) Impact on fertility and treatment principles:

For patients with stage IA1 or IA2 cervical cancer and strong fertility desires, fertility-preserving surgery is an option.

7.3 Ovary-Related Diseases

The ovaries, as the female gonads, perform critical reproductive and endocrine functions. Factors that disrupt ovarian ovulation can lead to infertility.

7.3.1 Ovarian Endometrial Cyst

1. Clinical overview:
   Endometriosis refers to the presence of endometrial tissues (glands and stroma) outside the uterus. Ovarian endometriotic lesions are categorized as microfoci in the early stages, which can progress into single or multiple cysts termed endometriotic ovarian cysts or ovarian chocolate cysts due to their characteristic contents of stale, chocolate-like blood [52].
2. Clinical manifestations:
   - Dysmenorrhea: Progressive secondary dysmenorrhea is the hallmark symptom.
   - Infertility: A common complication associated with ovarian endometriotic cysts.
   - Deep dyspareunia: Pain during deep penetration during intercourse.
   - Menstrual abnormalities: Increased menstrual flow and/or prolonged menstruation.
   - Ruptured cysts: Sudden, severe lower abdominal pain, often accompanied by nausea, vomiting, and a sensation of rectal fullness.
3. Ultrasonographic features:
   The visibility of normal ovarian tissue diminishes as the cyst size increases. Echogenicity varies with the disease's progression and menstrual cycle phases.
   (1) Simple cysts:
   - Round or oval anechoic areas with well-defined borders.
   - Slightly thickened walls and tiny bright internal echoes (see Fig. 7.63).

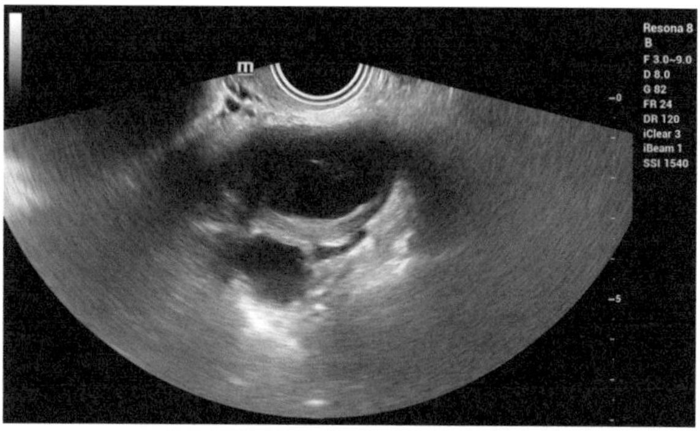

Fig. 7.63 A simple cyst presenting as a slightly thick-walled anechoic area with a few bright echoes inside

(2) Polycystic ovarian endometriosis:
   - Multiple round or irregular anechoic areas separated by septa of varying thickness
   - Thickened walls, rough inner lining, and fine bright echoes within the cyst (see Fig. 7.64)

(3) Homogeneous bright spot type:
   - Cysts filled with uniform, fine, bright echoes
   - Thickened, irregular inner walls [53] (see Fig. 7.65)

(4) Stratified cystic fluid type:
   - Thickened cyst wall with a rough inner surface
   - A fluid plane with dense bright spots on one side and an anechoic area on the other [54] (see Fig. 7.66)

(5) Intracystic mass type:
   - Thickened cyst wall with rough inner lining
   - Scattered tiny bright echoes and a hyperechoic mass along the posterior wall or center (see Fig. 7.67)

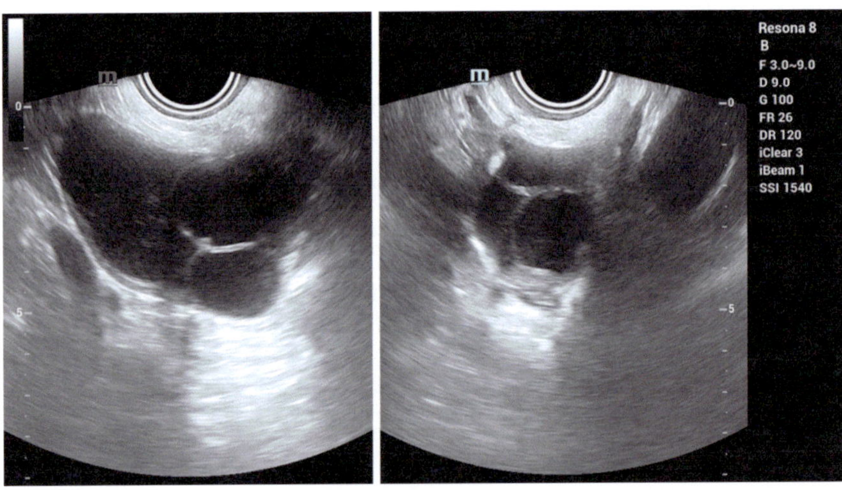

Fig. 7.64 Multicystic ovarian endometriosis, characterized by variably thick septations within the cyst

Fig. 7.65 A homogeneous bright spots-type cyst, filled with fine, homogeneous dot-like echoes

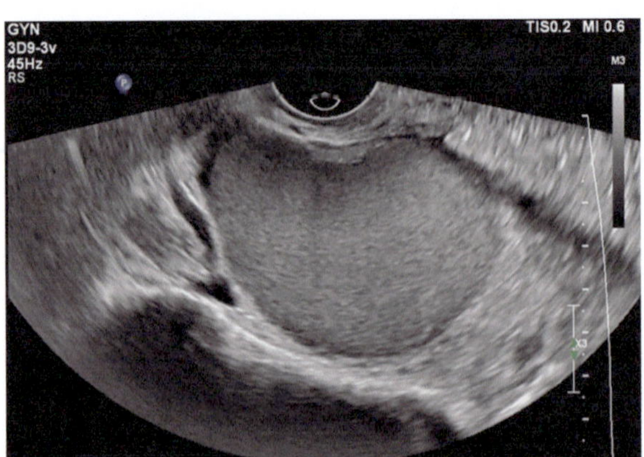

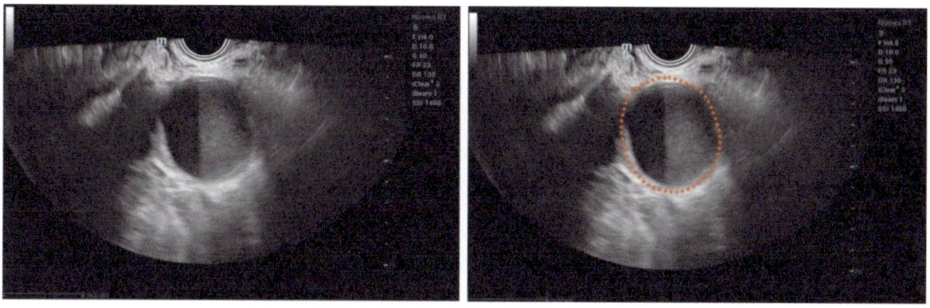

Fig. 7.66 A cyst exhibiting the sign of stratified cystic fluid, with dense bright spots deposited on one side and an anechoic area on the opposite side. The cyst is circled in orange

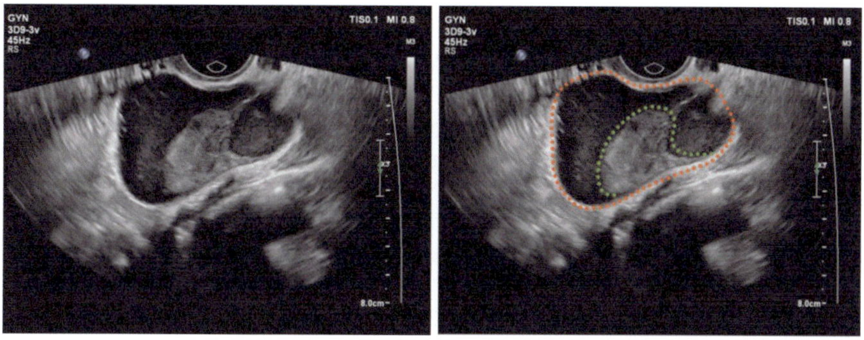

Fig. 7.67 Intracystic mass type: A hyperechoic mass is visualized on one side of the cyst wall. The cyst is circled in orange; the hyperechoic mass on the lateral wall of the cyst is circled in green

(6) Mixed type:
- Overlapping and intersecting features from the above types.

(7) Color Doppler and spectral Doppler ultrasound features:
- No blood flow signals within the cyst.
- Limited blood flow may be observed in the cyst wall or septa.
- Low-velocity, moderate-resistance blood flow spectra can be detected (see Fig. 7.68).

4. Differential diagnosis:

(1) Tubal abscess or tubo-ovarian abscess:
These conditions feature unevenly thickened walls and duct-like structures on ultrasound. A follow-up scan after anti-infective treatment can help confirm the diagnosis.

(2) Ovarian malignant tumor:
Distinguishing an ovarian chocolate cyst with irregular walls, solid echoes, and septa of varying thickness from a malignant tumor can be challenging.

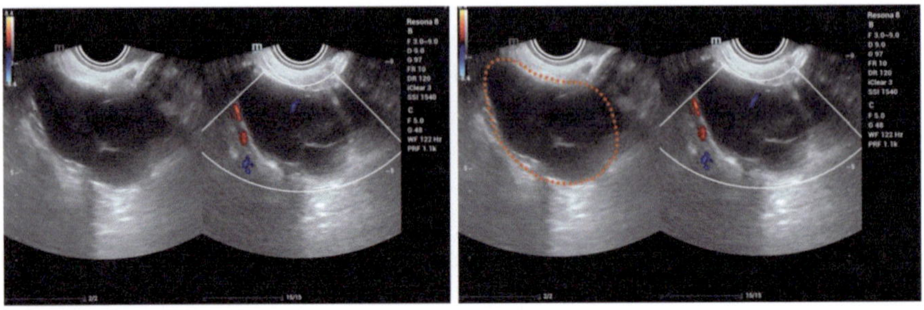

Fig. 7.68 Left: A gray-scale ultrasound image of a multicystic chocolate cyst; Right: A color Doppler ultrasound image showing blood flow signals in the cyst wall and its septa. The cyst is circled in orange

Malignant tumors typically show abundant blood flow signals in solid areas and septa. A high-velocity, low-resistance blood flow spectrum is indicative of malignancy.

5. Impact on fertility and treatment principles:
   Endometriosis can significantly impact fertility through mechanisms such as:
   - Anatomical abnormalities: Pelvic and tubal distortions.
   - Immune dysregulation: Aberrant cytokines and altered intra-abdominal environment.
   - Ovarian dysfunction: Decreased ovarian reserve, impaired oocyte quality, and obstructed ovulation.
   - Endometrial receptivity: Changes that hinder successful implantation.

   The management of endometriosis focuses on:
   - Reduction and removal of lesions
   - Pain relief and control
   - Fertility promotion
   - Recurrence prevention

   Current treatments include the following:
   - Pharmacological agents (e.g., hormonal therapies)
   - Surgical interventions (e.g., laparoscopic excision)
   - Interventional therapies
   - Assisted reproductive treatments (e.g., IVF)
6. Deep infiltrating endometriosis (DIE):
   DIE involves endometriotic lesions infiltrating ≥5 mm in depth.
   Common locations of DIE include the following:
   - Uterosacral ligament
   - Rectovaginal area and septum
   - Vaginal fornix
   - Bowel, bladder wall, and ureters [55] (see Fig. 7.69).

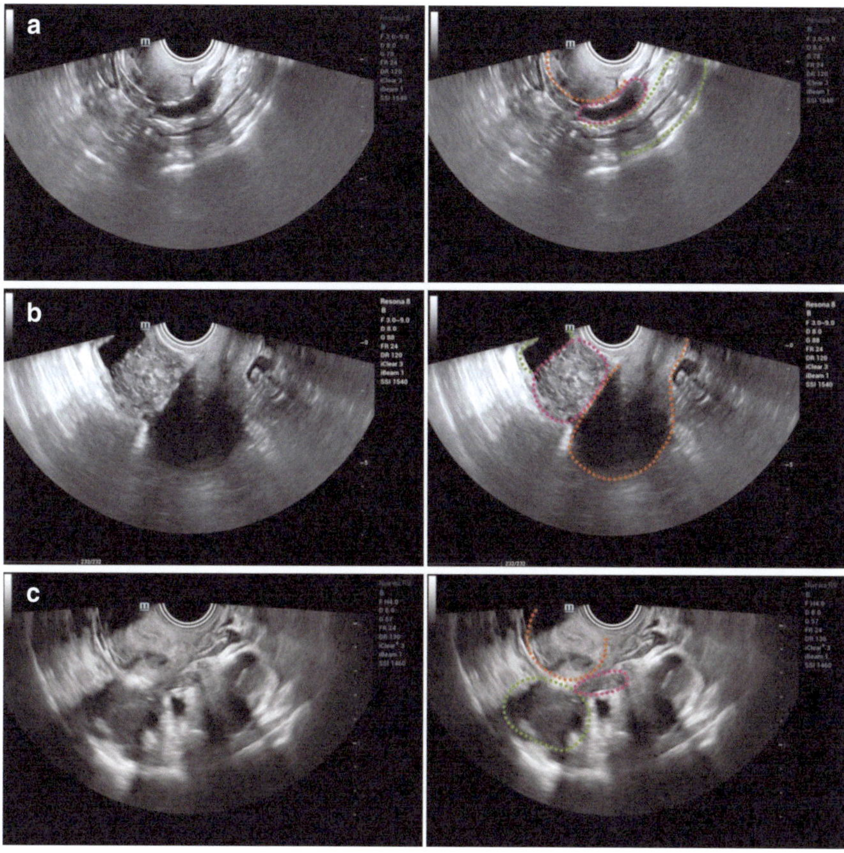

Fig. 7.69 (**a**) B-mode ultrasound shows a hypoechoic nodule with irregular morphology on the anterior wall of the rectum. The cervix is outlined in orange; the rectum is marked in green; the DIE is circled in pink. (**b**) B-mode ultrasound shows DIE in the bladder, characterized by a heterogeneous hypoechoic mass within the bladder, with many tiny cystic changes. The uterus is circled in orange; the bladder is marked in green; the DIE is circled in pink. (**c**) A hypoechoic nodule is visualized at the beginning of the left uterosacral ligament, which adheres to the right ovary. The cervix is circled in orange; the right ovary is circled in green; the DIE nodule is circled in pink

7.3.2 Polycystic Ovary Syndrome (PCOS)

1. Clinical overview:
   Polycystic ovary syndrome (PCOS), also known as Stein-Leventhal syndrome, is diagnosed based on the Rotterdam Criteria proposed by the European Society of Human Reproduction and Embryology (ESHRE) and the American Society for Reproductive Medicine (ASRM) in 2003. Diagnosis requires two of the following features, with other hyperandrogenic conditions excluded:
   (1) Oligo- or anovulation
   (2) Clinical and/or biochemical signs of hyperandrogenism
   (3) Polycystic ovaries observed on ultrasound: ≥12 follicles (2–9 mm in diameter) in one or both ovaries and/or ovarian volume ≥10 mL [56]
2. Clinical manifestations:
   Common clinical manifestations include the following:
   - Irregular periods: Scanty or absent menstruation, irregular uterine bleeding
   - Hyperandrogenism: Hirsutism, acne, and acanthosis nigricans
   - Infertility
   - Obesity
3. Ultrasonographic features:
   Ultrasound can identify polycystic ovarian morphology but does not provide a definitive diagnosis of PCOS. Assessments should exclude the presence of corpus luteum, cysts, or dominant follicles ≥10 mm in diameter. Key ultrasonographic features include the following:
   (1) Uniformly enlarged ovaries with clear borders, enhanced peripheral echogenicity, thickened medulla with increased echogenicity, and ≥12 follicles (2–9 mm) arranged in a "wheel-like" pattern around the ovary [57] (see Fig. 7.70).
   (2) Absence of dominant follicles during continuous ovulation monitoring.
   (3) Endometrial hyperplasia of varying degrees due to prolonged estrogen exposure.

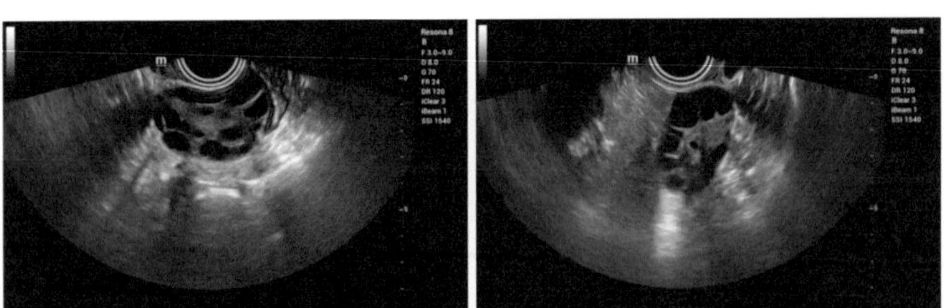

Fig. 7.70 These two ultrasound images show uniformly enlarged bilateral ovaries, each containing ≥12 follicles ranging from 2 to 9 mm in diameter

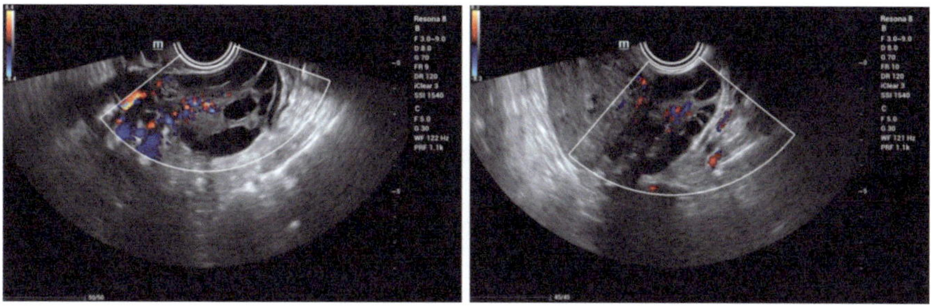

Fig. 7.71 Gray-scale ultrasound reveals polycystic changes in the ovary, while color Doppler ultrasound detects blood vessels running through the ovarian medulla

(4) Color Doppler findings: Moderate-resistance arterial spectra in the medullary ovarian artery may be detected (see Fig. 7.71).

4. Impact on fertility and treatment principles:

   PCOS impacts fertility by causing ovulation disorders, reducing endometrial receptivity, and lowering oocyte quality. Endocrine-metabolic abnormalities associated with PCOS can further impair conception. Additionally, PCOS is strongly linked to pregnancy complications. Fertility treatments include the following:

   - Pharmacological ovulation induction therapy
   - In vitro fertilization and embryo transfer (IVF-ET)
   - Laparoscopic ovarian perforation

7.3.3 Overview of Ovarian Tumors

1. Histologic classification:

   The most current World Health Organization (WHO) classification of ovarian oncology was developed in 2020, providing a standardized framework for diagnosing and managing ovarian tumors [58].

2. Staging of ovarian cancer:

   The International Federation of Gynecology and Obstetrics (FIGO) staging system, last revised in 2014, is widely used to assess the extent of cancer and guide treatment decisions [59].

3. Clinical manifestations:

   (1) Benign tumors:

   Large benign ovarian tumors may cause abdominal distension, masses, and compression symptoms such as frequent urination, dysuria, and constipation. On gynecological examination, the mass is typically cystic or solid, smooth-surfaced, and mobile.

(2) Malignant tumors:

Malignant ovarian tumors, often bilateral, manifest in advanced stages as abdominal pain, distension, cachexia, and pelvic effusion. Masses are mostly solid, with uneven surfaces and limited mobility.

4. Complications and ultrasonographic features:

(1) Torsion:

Ovarian torsion is a common gynecological emergency and typically presents with sudden severe lower abdominal pain, often triggered by a change in body position. The pain is frequently associated with nausea, vomiting, and, in severe cases, shock. Ultrasonographic features of torsion include the following:

(a) Mass identification:

A solid mass between the cyst and the uterus, often close to the uterus, irregular in shape with clear or unclear contours. The mass may show mixed medium-low echogenicity with thin low-echo strips (the "whirlpool sign"). On dynamic scanning, this mass may demonstrate spiral motion, indicating the twisted vascular pedicle. This is a characteristic sign of ovarian torsion.

(b) Cyst features:

Post-torsion, the cyst appears elevated and under tension (usually >5 cm), with anechoic interiors and multiple bright spots. Due to edema, the cyst wall may be thickened.

(c) Tenderness test:

Using the transducer to perform a tenderness test on the mass and its pedicle may yield positive results.

Color Doppler ultrasound can reveal the dilated blood vessels with meandering paths in the pedicle [60, 61] (see Figs. 7.72 and 7.73).

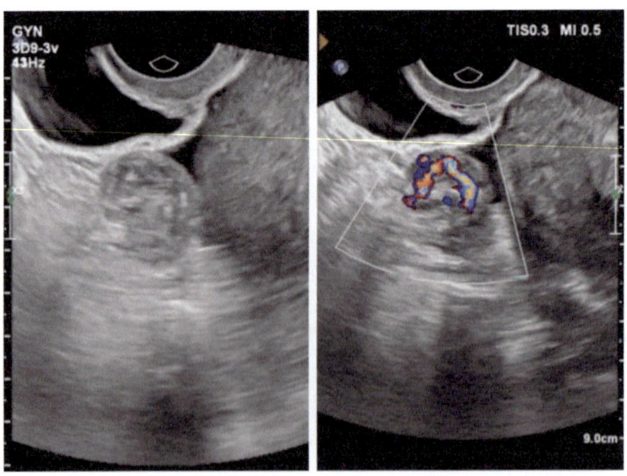

Fig. 7.72 Left: Gray-scale ultrasound reveals a mass with a "whirlpool sign". Right: Color Doppler ultrasound shows a spiral pattern of blood flow within the mass

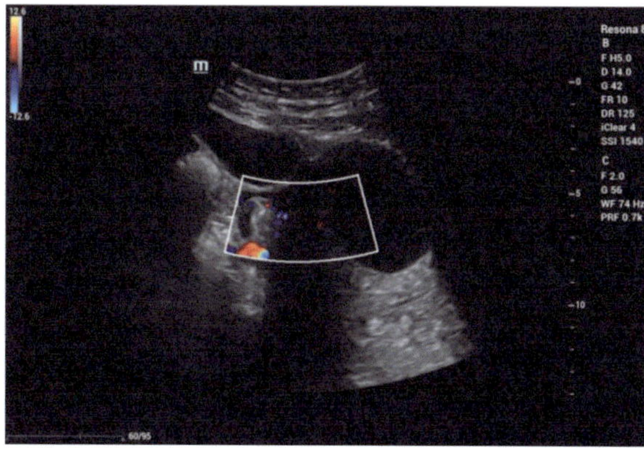

Fig. 7.73 The mass is located adjacent to the cyst, and color Doppler ultrasound shows a spiral pattern of blood flow within the mass

(2) Rupture:

Ovarian cyst rupture is a common gynecological emergency. Its ultrasonographic features include the following:

(a) Cyst size decrease or disappearance: The original cyst may shrink in size or even disappear following rupture.

(b) Hematoma formation: In cases of hematoma, a mixed echogenic mass can be detected in the ipsilateral adnexal area. This mass typically has an irregular morphology and is often associated with pelvic effusion.

These findings indicate an ovarian cyst rupture, and help guide further management [62] (see Figs. 7.74 and 7.75).

(3) Infection:

Though rare, infection is usually secondary to torsion or rupture. It presents with abdominal pain, fever, and peritoneal signs such as rebound tenderness and muscle tension. Initial treatment includes antibiotics, followed by surgical intervention.

(4) Malignant transformation:

Rapid growth of a tumor in a short period of time may suggest malignant transformation, requiring prompt surgical intervention.

Ultrasonographic features:

(a) Rapid enlargement: The mass increases in size quickly.

(b) Disorganized internal echoes: The internal echoes become irregular, with increased solid components.

(c) Enhanced blood flow: There is a significant increase in blood flow signals within the mass.

(d) Pelvic effusion: The development of pelvic effusion is often observed.

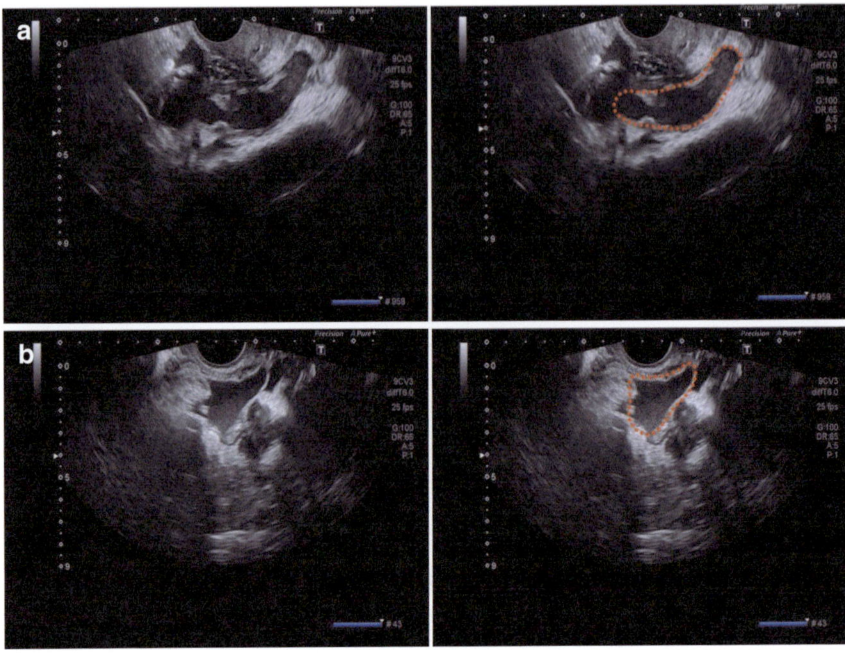

Fig. 7.74 (**a**) A crumpled chocolate cyst. The chocolate cyst is circled in orange. (**b**) Hypoechoic pelvic effusion developed after the rupture of a chocolate cyst. The pelvic fluid is circled in orange

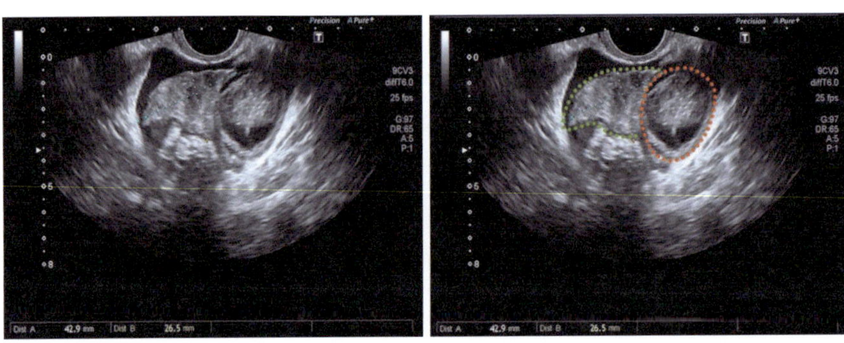

Fig. 7.75 Corpus luteum rupture with adjacent hematoma formation. The corpus luteum is circled in orange; the hematoma formed after rupture is outlined in green

5. Impact on fertility and treatment principles
   Large ovarian tumors can interfere with egg (oocyte) production and reduce ovarian reserve. Surgical treatment, especially if it involves the removal of the tumor, may further damage normal ovarian tissue and decrease ovarian reserve.
   For patients with reproductive needs, fertility-preserving surgery should be performed based on histological classification and staging of the tumor [63]. However, even fertility-preserving surgeries may have risks related to reduced ovarian reserve.

7.3.4 Ovarian Tumor-Like Conditions

Ovarian tumor-like conditions, also known as nonneoplastic ovarian cysts, are the most common group of ovarian disorders. These conditions include follicular cysts, corpus luteum cysts, theca lutein cysts, and ovarian hyperstimulation syndrome (OHSS). While these conditions are generally benign, they can present with symptoms similar to neoplastic tumors, requiring differentiation and appropriate management.

1. Follicular cyst
   (1) Clinical overview:
   Follicular cysts are typically single but can occasionally be multiple. These cysts appear as blister-like protrusions from the surface of the ovary. The wall of the cyst is thin, the inner surface is smooth, and the fluid within is clear and yellowish. Most follicular cysts are small, often measuring no more than 5 cm in diameter. The majority will either gradually resolve or rupture on their own within 4–6 weeks.
   (2) Ultrasonographic features:
   Follicular cysts typically appear as round or oval anechoic areas within the ovary, with clear borders and a thin, smooth cyst wall. These cysts are most often single and protrude from the ovary's surface. Their internal diameter ranges from 1 to 3 cm, rarely exceeding 5 cm. These cysts may resolve spontaneously upon follow-up ultrasound exams [64] (see Fig. 7.76).
   (3) Differential diagnosis:
   Follicular cysts need to be differentiated from ovarian cystadenomas and chocolate cysts. If the distinction is unclear during a single ultrasound scan, follow-up examinations can be used to observe the cyst's resolution, as follicular cysts typically resolve without intervention over time.
2. Corpus luteum cyst
   (1) Clinical overview:
   Following ovulation, the ruptured follicle transforms into the corpus luteum. When a significant amount of blood accumulates within the follicle or corpus luteum cavity, it can develop into a corpus luteum hematoma. This

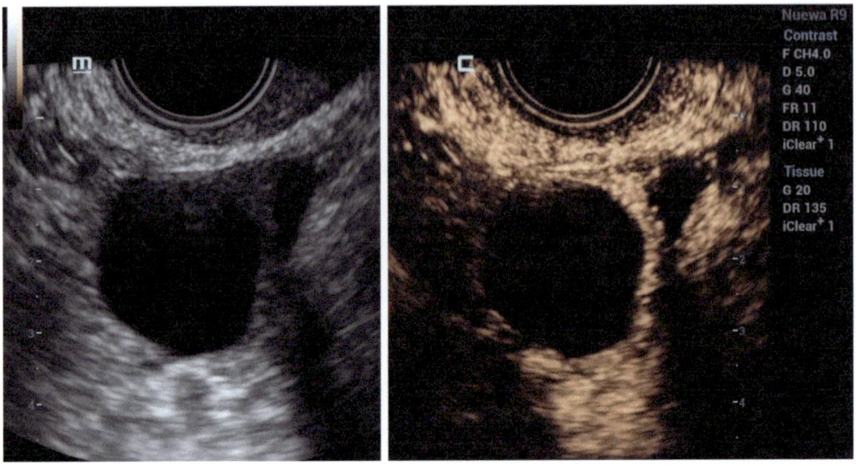

Fig. 7.76 The left panel shows a single oval anechoic area in the ovary with clear boundaries and thin, smooth cyst walls. The right panel demonstrates the absence of blood flow within the cyst, as shown in SonoVue contrast mode

hematoma may eventually liquefy, resulting in the formation of a corpus luteum cyst. Typically, these cysts are solitary, with an internal diameter usually not exceeding 5 cm, though they can occasionally reach up to 10 cm. The cystic fluid is often translucent or brownish in color. Corpus luteum cysts are most commonly encountered during the mid to late phases of the menstrual cycle or in early pregnancy.

(2) Ultrasonographic features:
Ultrasonographically, a corpus luteum cyst appears as a complex cystic mass characterized by a reticular pattern of internal echoes [65].

(a) Early stage:
The cyst appears as a subcircular, thick-walled structure with clear borders. The inner lining is rough, and the cyst may have a heterogeneous hypoechoic appearance resembling solid components (see Fig. 7.77).

(b) Intermediate stage:
As the blood begins to coagulate, the cyst wall becomes thinner and more regular. The inner wall remains smooth, and the intracystic echogenicity decreases, often showing a "spider-web" appearance (see Fig. 7.78).

(c) Late stage:
As blood is absorbed, the cyst shrinks and transforms into a white body (corpus albicans), which appears as a solid, slightly hyperechoic mass with poorly defined boundaries from the surrounding ovarian tissue (see Fig. 7.79).

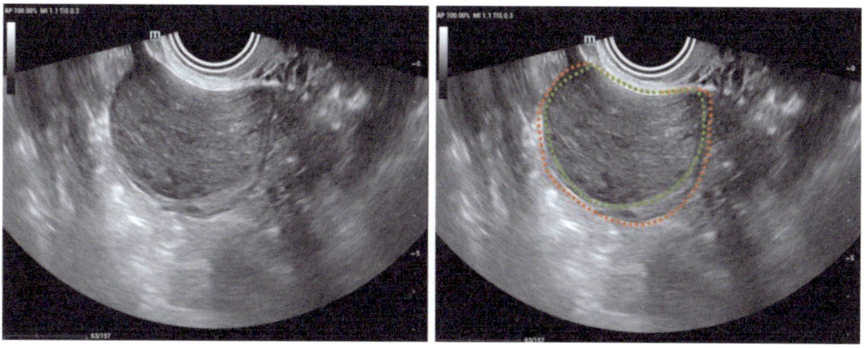

Fig. 7.77 An early-stage corpus luteum cyst, presenting as a subcircular cyst in the ovary with well-defined borders, solid components, and disorganized, heterogeneous hypoechoicity within the cyst. The ovary is circled in orange; the cyst is circled in green

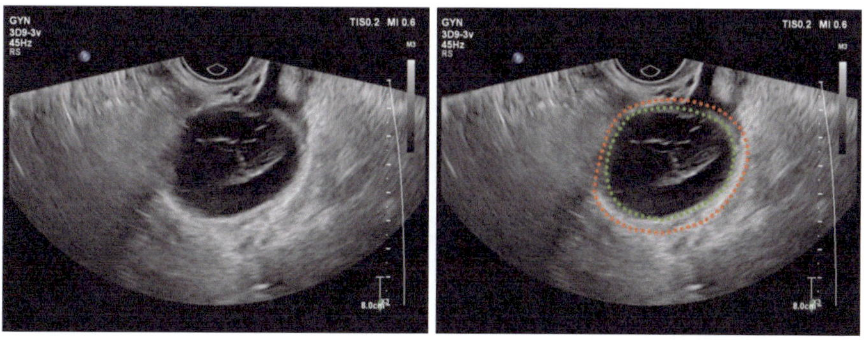

Fig. 7.78 An intermediate-stage corpus luteum cyst, characterized by the presence of fishnet-like structures of varying thickness within the cyst. The ovary is circled in orange; the cyst is circled in green

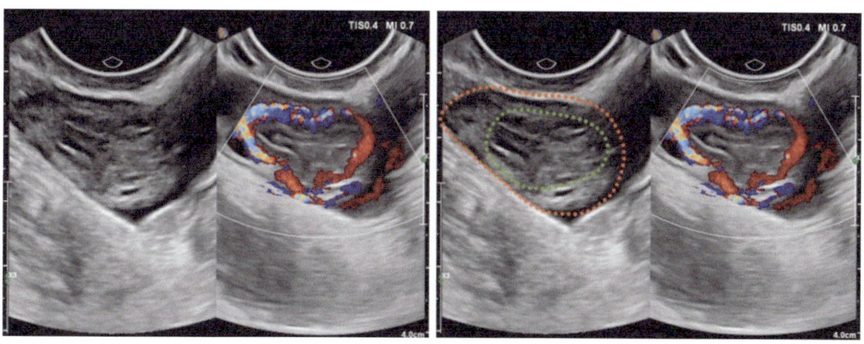

Fig. 7.79 Left: Gray-scale ultrasound shows a late-stage corpus luteum cyst, exhibiting internal solid, heterogeneous, and slightly hyperechoic patterns that are poorly demarcated from the surrounding ovarian tissue. Right: Color Doppler ultrasound shows peripheral circumferential blood flow signals in the cyst wall. The ovary is circled in orange; the late-stage corpus luteum cyst is circled in green

(3) Color Doppler and spectral Doppler ultrasound:
Abundant peripheral circumferential blood flow signals may be observed within the wall of the corpus luteum cyst. The blood flow often shows a high-velocity, low-resistance spectrum (see Fig. 7.79).

3. Theca lutein cyst
   (1) Clinical overview:
   Theca lutein cysts are often bilateral but can occasionally be unilateral.
   (2) Ultrasonographic features:
   Both ovaries are usually enlarged, presenting with a multicystic pattern. Multiple well-defined anechoic areas with thin, smooth walls are seen within the ovaries (see Fig. 7.80).
   (3) Differential diagnosis:
   On ultrasound, differentiating between OHSS and theca lutein cysts can be challenging [66]. However, OHSS typically develops after artificially induced ovulation, whereas theca lutein cysts are more commonly associated with trophoblastic disorders.

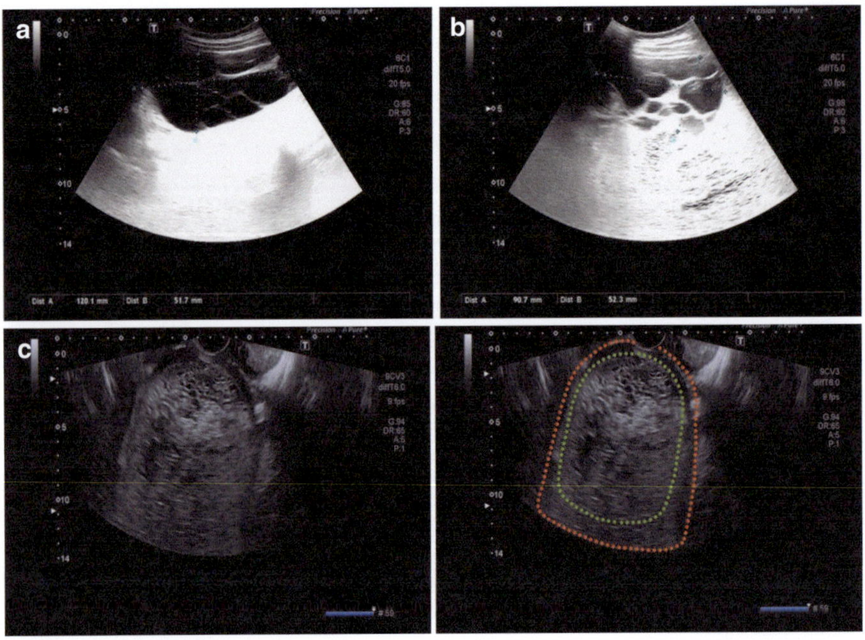

Fig. 7.80 (**a**) The right ovary is enlarged and multicystic. (**b**) The left ovary is enlarged and multicystic. (**c**) This patient has a concomitant intrauterine hydatidiform mole. The uterus is circled in orange; the hydatidiform mole is circled in green

7.3.5 Common Ovarian Tumors

1. Mature Cystic Teratomas
   (1) Clinical overview:
   Mature cystic teratomas, also known as dermoid cysts, are tumors composed of tissues derived from two or three germ layers. These tumors vary in size and are typically round with a smooth surface, well-encapsulated, and often unilocular and cystic. The cysts are filled with sebaceous material and hair and may occasionally feature a small nodule-like protrusion [67].
   (2) Ultrasonographic features:
   Mature cystic teratomas can present as cystic, mixed cystic-solid, or solid masses. Key ultrasonographic signs include the following:
   (a) Mural nodule(s):
   Single or multiple elevated, highly echogenic nodules may be seen on the inner wall of the cystic tumor, often with posterior acoustic shadowing. These strongly echogenic nodules are typically composed of dental or skeletal elements (see Fig. 7.81).
   (b) Fat–fluid level sign:
   A distinct horizontal demarcation line between the hyperechoic (lipid-rich) and anechoic (containing epithelial debris, hair, etc.) areas within the cystic tumor. The denser materials, such as hair and epithelial debris, sink to the bottom, forming this characteristic line (see Fig. 7.82).
   (c) Echogenic white ball (floating ball):
   Single or multiple round or oval hyperechoic masses with well-defined borders may be seen within the anechoic zone of the cyst. These masses, which float or settle to one side, are mostly composed of lipids and hair (see Fig. 7.83).

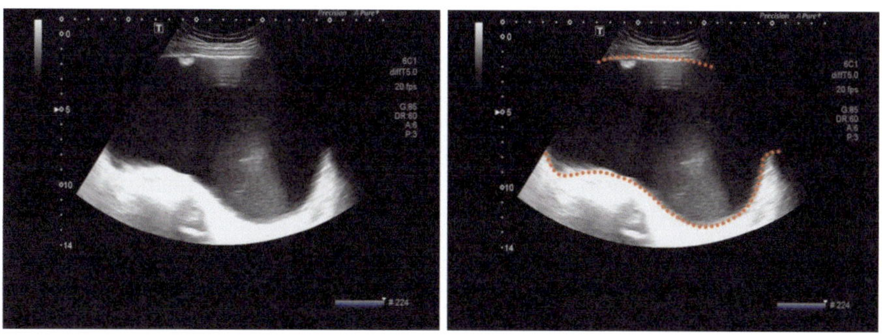

Fig. 7.81 A single strongly echogenic nodule on the inner wall of the cystic tumor. The cystic teratoma is circled in orange

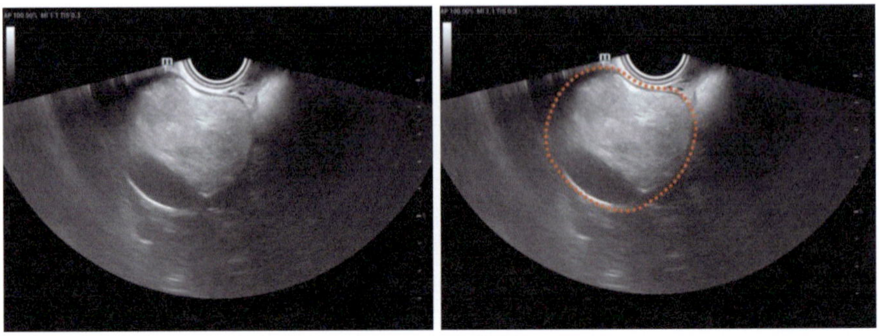

Fig. 7.82 Fat-fluid level sign in the cystic teratoma. The cystic teratoma is circled in orange

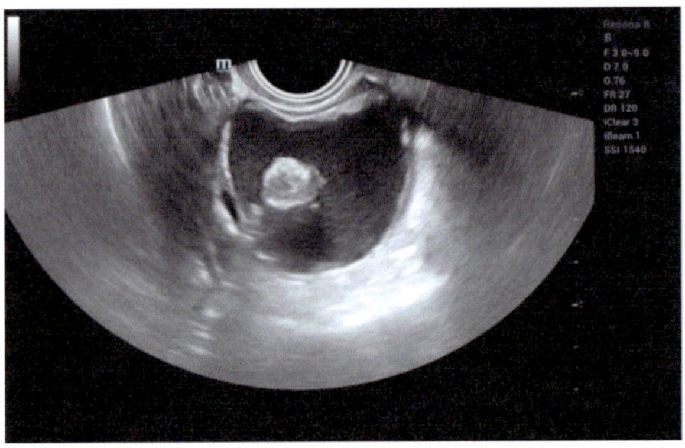

Fig. 7.83 Echogenic white ball sign: A floating hyperechoic mass is seen within the cystic teratoma

(d) Dots and/or lines:
Caused by hair within the cystic tumor, these strongly echogenic, short streaks appear within the anechoic region, typically arranged parallel to each other (see Fig. 7.84).

(e) Completely echogenic lesion:
Viscous lipids present as homogeneous, dense, echoic spots that float within the lesion area and move with pressure or manipulation (see Fig. 7.85).

(f) Polycystic sign:
Small sacs within the anechoic area of the cyst, creating the appearance of "a sac within a sac" (see Fig. 7.86).

(g) Sign of heterogeneous structures:
A mixture of the above-described echogenic features is observed, as the cyst contains components from multiple tissues (see Fig. 7.87).

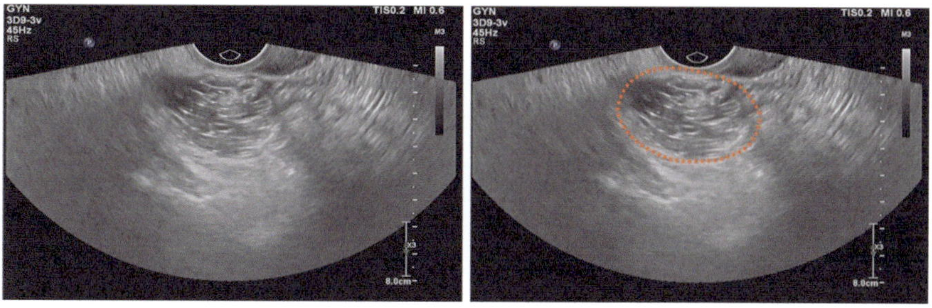

Fig. 7.84 "Streaks" within the cystic teratoma. The cystic teratoma is circled in orange

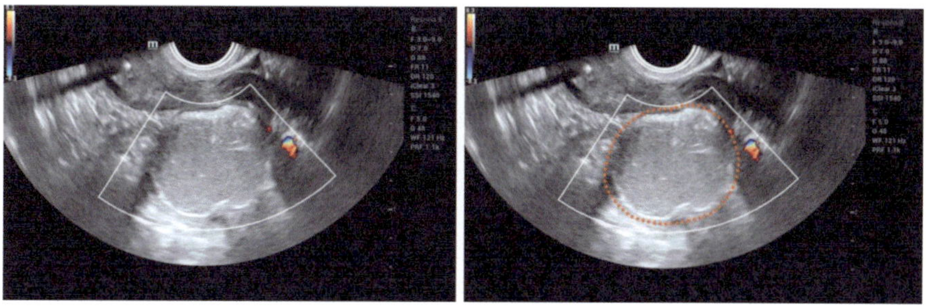

Fig. 7.85 Completely echogenic lesion. The cystic teratoma is circled in orange

Fig. 7.86 Polycystic sign

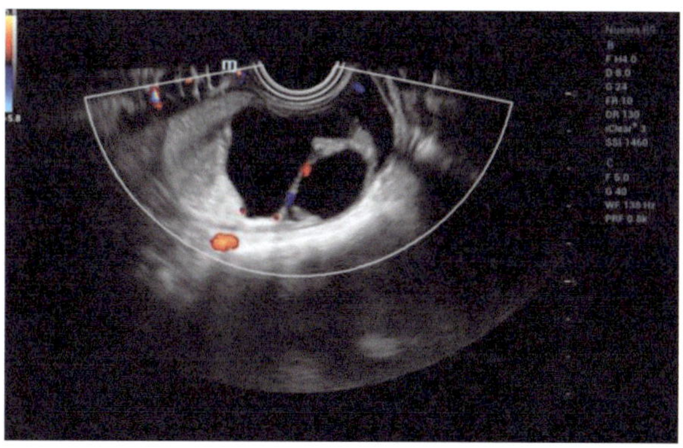

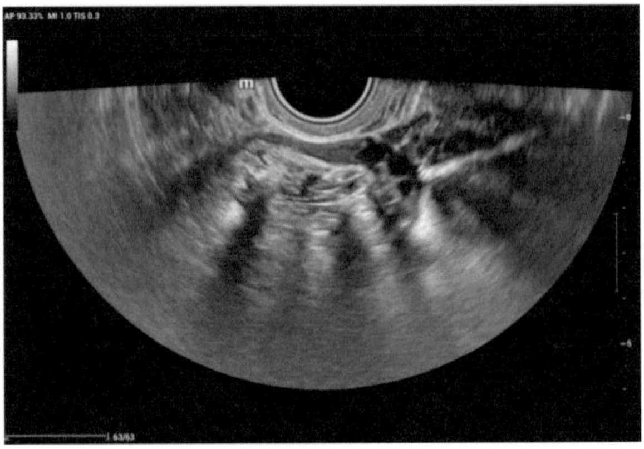

Fig. 7.87 Sign of heterogeneous structures

(3) Color Doppler ultrasound:
Most mature cystic teratomas exhibit little to no blood flow. However, in some cases, the tumor may contain specialized tissue components, such as nerve tissue or thyroid tissue, which may show detectable blood flow signals within the solid components (see Fig. 7.88).

(4) Differential diagnosis:
A teratoma may sometimes need to be differentiated from normal intestinal gas. Intestinal peristalsis can cause the position of the gas to change, in contrast to the fixed position of the teratoma. If differentiation remains difficult due to slow intestinal movement, the patient may be advised to repeat the examination after defecation.

2. Ovarian thecoma-fibroma group (OTFG)

(1) Clinical overview:
The ovarian thecoma-fibroma group (OTFG) comprises tumors classified based on the varying content of thecal cells and fibroblasts. The three subtypes include the following:
(a) Thecoma (or theca cell tumor): Composed entirely of thecal cells.
(b) Thecoma-fibroma: Contains both thecal cells and fibroblasts in varying proportions.
(c) Fibroma: Made up entirely of fibroblasts, with almost no thecal cells.

(2) Ultrasonographic features:
OTFG tumors consist of cells with characteristics of both thecal cells and fibroblasts. The greater the proportion of thecal cells, the more prominent the posterior echogenic enhancement, whereas the higher the content of fibroblasts, the more pronounced the posterior acoustic attenuation. The typical ultrasonographic presentation of OTFG is a unilateral adnexal mass that is either solid or predominantly solid, round, well-defined, and surrounded by peripheral membranes. The mass typically appears hypoechoic, with granular or striated hyperechoic patterns within, and shows posterior enhancement or attenuation of echoes.

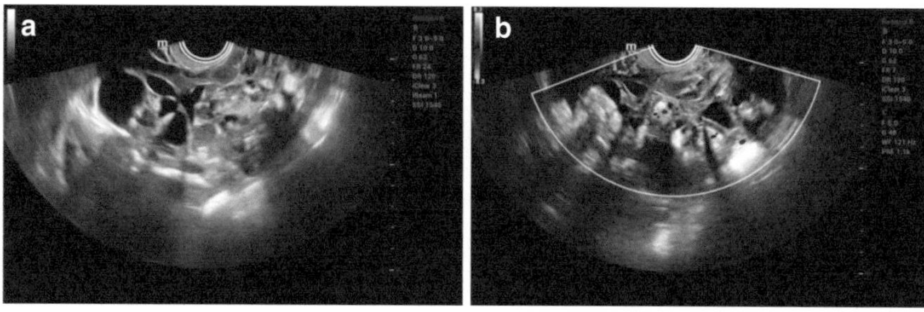

Fig. 7.88 (**a**) This image shows a teratoma with heterogeneous internal echogenicity, confirmed by histopathologic testing as a cystic-solid mature teratoma with abundant CNS content. (**b**) This image shows blood flow signals in the solid portion of the teratoma

Color Doppler ultrasound reveals a small to moderate amount of blood flow signals inside the mass [68]. A small number of patients may present with pleural effusion and/or ascites. In some cases, estrogen-producing tumors can lead to endometrial thickening (see Figs. 7.89 and 7.90).

3. Granulosa cell tumors (GCTs)
   (1) Clinical overview:
   Granulosa cell tumors (GCTs) are the most common type of sex cord-stromal tumor, typically presenting with low-grade malignancy.
   (2) Ultrasonographic features:
      (a) Mass characteristics: The tumor has clear boundaries, an intact envelope, and regular morphology.
      (b) Internal echogenicity: GCTs often appear as multilocular cystic or mixed cystic-solid masses. In mixed cystic-solid masses, the cystic portion typically contains multiple compartments, and the walls are thick with uneven thickness [69] (see Fig. 7.91).
      (c) Associated findings: GCTs are frequently associated with endometrial thickening, endometrial polyps, or even endometrial cancer.
      (d) Color Doppler and spectral Doppler ultrasound: Abundant blood flow signals are usually detected within the solid portion of the mass [70]. A low-resistance arterial spectrum is often observed (see Fig. 7.92).
4. Ovarian cystadenoma
   (1) Clinical overview:
   Ovarian cystadenomas are classified into serous and mucinous subtypes based on their pathological characteristics.

   Serous ovarian cystadenoma: This type accounts for approximately 25% of all benign ovarian tumors. These cystadenomas can vary in size, ranging from 5 to 10 cm in diameter, and typically have a smooth surface. The cysts are filled with yellowish, clear fluid. Serous cystadenomas are further divided into two subtypes:

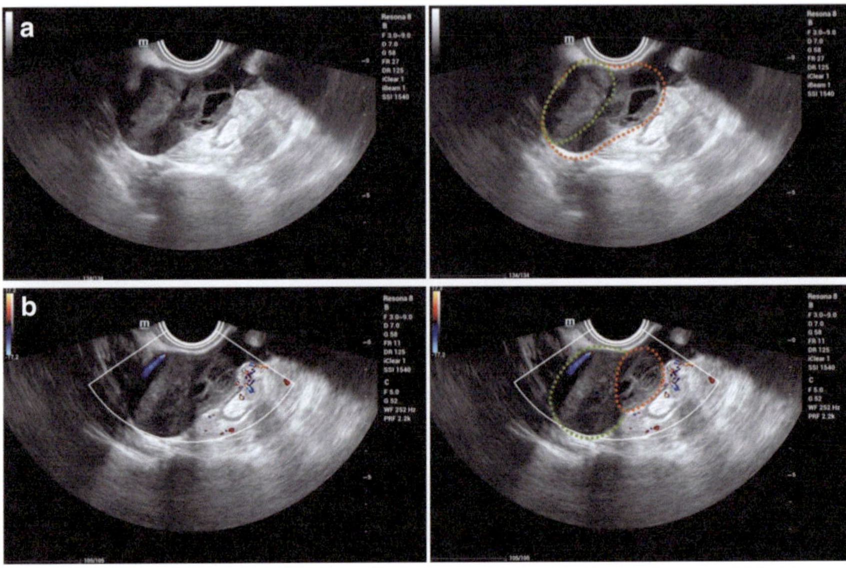

Fig. 7.89 (**a**) Ovarian tissue is observed surrounding the mass, which has clear boundaries, regular morphology, and is hypoechoic internally. The ovary is circled in orange; the mass is circled in green. (**b**) Color Doppler ultrasound reveals a small amount of blood flow signals within the mass (pathological testing confirmed the diagnosis as a theca cell tumor). The ovary is circled in orange; the mass is circled in green

- Simple Serous Cystadenomas: These are smooth-lined and generally unilocular.
- Papillary Serous Cystadenomas: These are often multilocular and feature internal papillary projections into the tumor. In some cases, calcifications can be observed microscopically, appearing as grit-like bodies growing outward from the tumor wall [71].

  Mucinous ovarian cystadenoma: Mucinous cystadenomas account for about 20% of all benign ovarian tumors and are typically unilateral. These tumors are large, often ranging from 10 to 30 cm in diameter, and can occupy the entire pelvic or abdominal cavity. The cysts are filled with mucinous or jelly-like fluid. Mucinous cystadenomas are predominantly multilocular with smooth surfaces, and in about 10% of cases, papillary projections are present on the tumor walls.

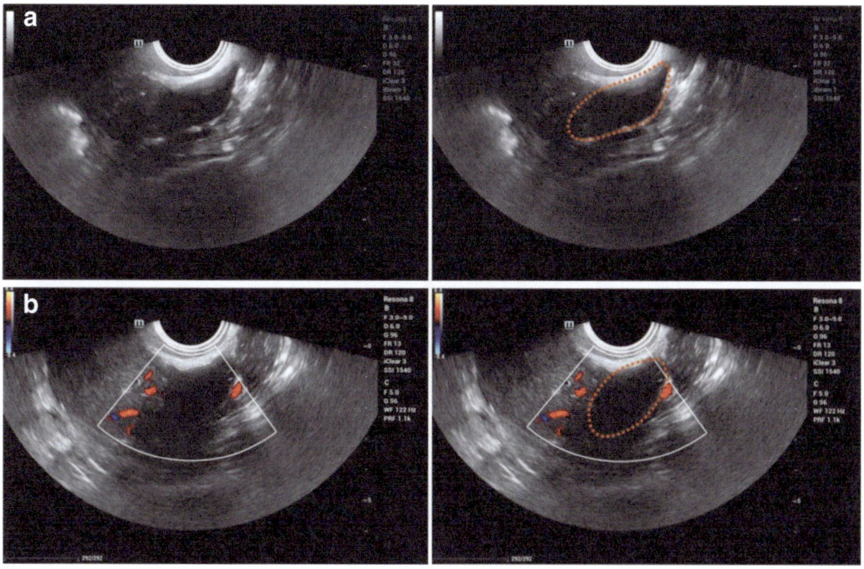

Fig. 7.90 (**a**) The ovary is completely occupied by a mass, which appears as a solid lesion in the adnexal region, with well-defined borders, regular morphology, internal hypoechoicity, and posterior echo attenuation. The tumor is circled in orange. (**b**) Color Doppler ultrasound shows no blood flow within the mass (pathological testing confirmed the diagnosis as a fibroma). The tumor is circled in orange

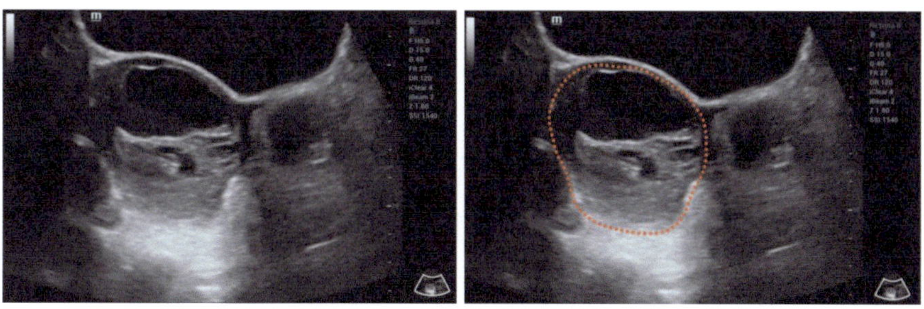

Fig. 7.91 B-mode ultrasound shows a mixed cystic-solid mass with well-defined borders, an intact envelope, and regular morphology. The tumor is circled in orange

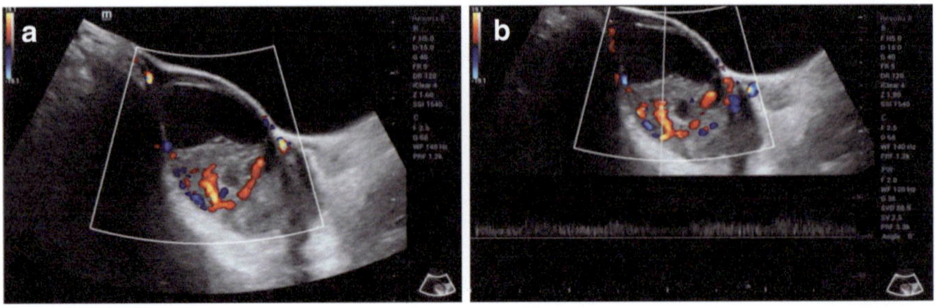

Fig. 7.92 (**a**) Rich blood flow signals detected within the mass. (**b**) Low-resistance arterial spectrum identified in the mass

(2) Ultrasonographic features:

Serous ovarian cystadenoma:

(a) Simple cystadenomas:

These are well-defined, round, or ovoid, predominantly unilocular, with a smooth inner wall.

(b) Papillary cystadenomas:

These are generally multilocular, with single or multiple medium-to-low echogenic papillary projections of varying sizes protruding into the tumor. Calcifications between the papillary projections may appear as strong echogenic spots. When the papillary projections are very small, only localized thickening of the tumor wall is observed. The larger and more extensive the papillary projections are, as well as the wider their base, the higher the potential malignancy of the tumor.

(c) Cystic composition:

The tumor is anechoic or shows sparse punctate echoes.

(d) Color Doppler and spectral Doppler ultrasound:

Color Doppler may reveal punctate flow signals within the tumor wall, septa, and papillary projections. A low-velocity, moderate-resistance flow spectrum is typically observed on spectral Doppler ultrasound.

If there is abundant blood flow within the tumor wall, septa, or papillary projections, malignancy should be considered [65] (see Figs. 7.93 and 7.94).

Mucinous ovarian cystadenoma:

(a) General features:

The tumor is well-defined, round, or ovoid, typically unilateral and multilocular (occasionally unilocular), large in size (diameter >10 cm), and has a uniformly thickened wall (>5 mm).

(b) Internal echoes:

The tumor shows poor intratumor sonolucency, with dense, fine, bright spot echoes within the anechoic area [72].

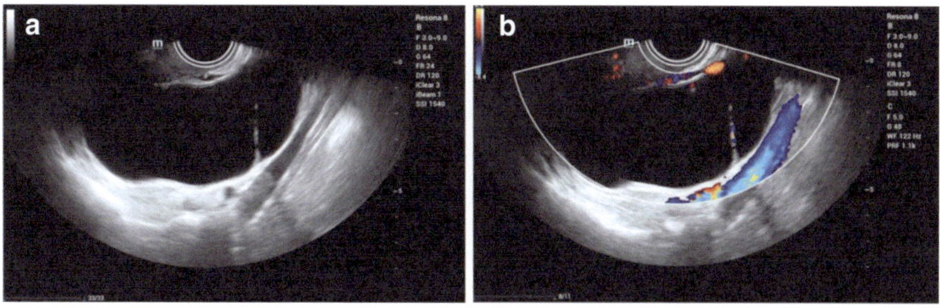

Fig. 7.93 (**a**) B-mode ultrasound reveals a simple serous ovarian cystadenoma characterized by a well-defined, ovoid shape, smooth inner walls, and a single septum. (**b**) Color Doppler ultrasound reveals blood flow signals in the cystic wall and septum

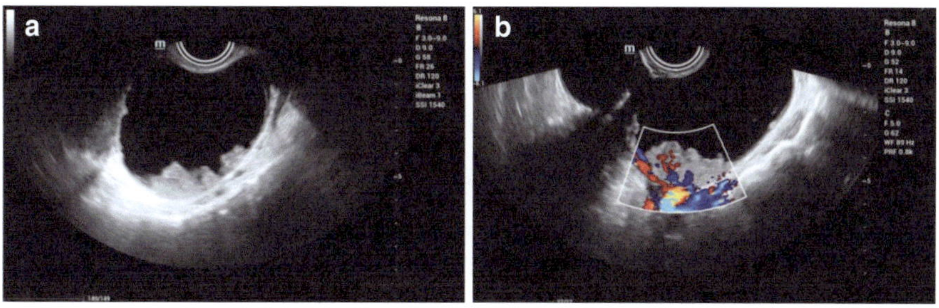

Fig. 7.94 (**a**) B-mode ultrasound shows a papillary serous ovarian cystadenoma featuring medium-low echogenic papillary projections of varying sizes on the tumor wall. (**b**) Color Doppler ultrasound demonstrates blood flow signals within the solid projections

(c) Solid components and borderline tumors:
If a tumor contains more than 10 subcapsular, honeycomb-like nodules or solid papillary projections, the possibility of a borderline tumor should be considered. Malignancy should be suspected for multilocular mixed cystic-solid tumors [73].

(d) Color Doppler and spectral Doppler ultrasound:
Punctate blood flow signals can be detected in tumor and septal walls. A low-velocity, medium-resistance arterial spectrum is typically observed. If abundant blood flow exists in the tumor wall, septal walls, or papillary projections, a borderline or malignant tumor should be considered (see Figs. 7.95, 7.96, and 7.97).

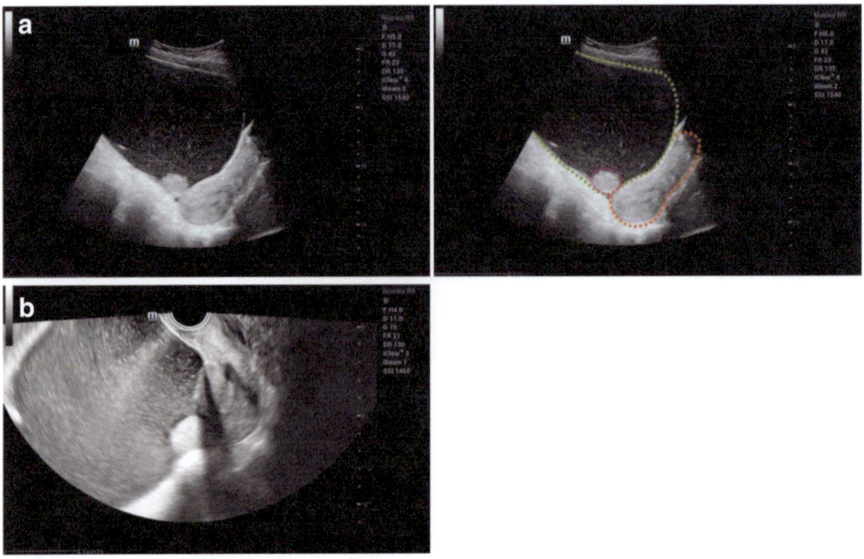

Fig. 7.95 (**a**) Transabdominal ultrasound image of a unilocular mucinous cystadenoma. The uterus is outlined in orange; the tumor is circled in green; the mucinous deposit is circled in pink. (**b**) Transvaginal ultrasound image of the same case

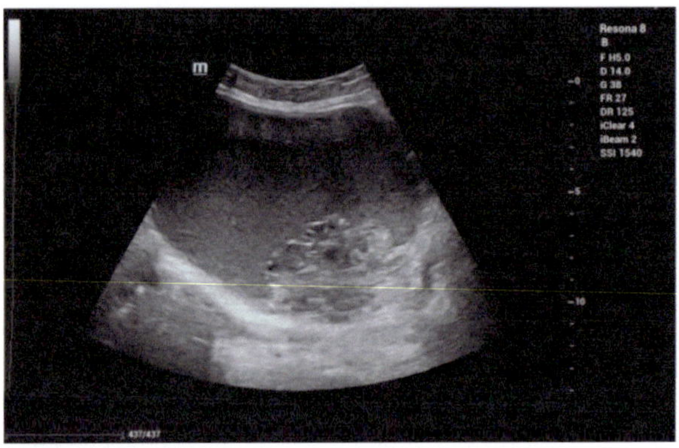

Fig. 7.96 Honeycomb-like nodule observed; pathological testing confirmed this case as a borderline mucinous cystadenoma

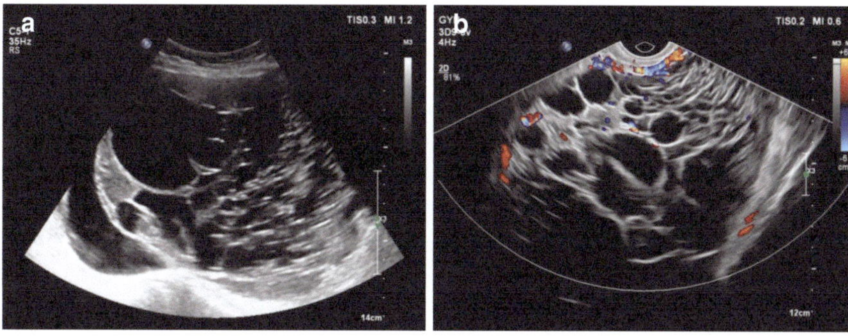

Fig. 7.97 (**a**) Mucinous cystadenoma showing a large multilocular tumor with poor internal sonolucency. (**b**) Color Doppler ultrasound shows blood flow within septa

(3) Differential diagnosis:

Distinguishing a simple ovarian cyst from a simple serous cystadenoma can be challenging on an initial ultrasound examination. Follow-up imaging to monitor changes in cyst size may help make an accurate differentiation.

5. Epithelial ovarian cancer

(1) Clinical overview:

Epithelial ovarian cancer accounts for approximately 90% of all ovarian cancers and includes several histological subtypes [74]. According to the WHO classification, the five primary subtypes are high-grade serous carcinoma (HGSOC), low-grade serous carcinoma (LGSC), endometrioid carcinoma (EC), clear cell carcinoma (CCC), and mucinous carcinoma (MC) [75].

HGSOC exhibits a heterogeneous growth pattern characterized by large papillae, glandular and solid structures, occasional micropapillary formations, and frequent necrosis [76]. Based on their epithelial composition, mucinous carcinomas are subdivided into gastrointestinal (GI)-type and endocervical-type. GI-type mucinous carcinomas are typically larger and multilocular, whereas endocervical-type mucinous carcinomas are smaller with fewer locules [73].

(2) Ultrasonographic features:

Epithelial ovarian cancers exhibit a range of appearances, including predominantly cystic, mixed cystic-solid, or predominantly solid masses:

(a) Predominantly cystic tumors:

These tumors often display irregular thickening of the tumor wall, thick and uneven septations, and anechoic fluid within the cystic cavity, sometimes accompanied by fine, bright spot echoes.

(b) Predominantly solid tumors:

These masses typically have irregular shapes, are heterogeneous and hypoechoic, and may include irregular fluid-filled areas due to hemorrhagic necrosis.

(c) Advanced disease features:

Ovarian cancer frequently presents with ascites. In advanced stages, there may be carcinomatous infiltration of the uterus and intestines or extensive peritoneal metastases.

(d) Color Doppler and spectral Doppler ultrasound:

Color Doppler often reveals abundant blood flow signals within the tumor wall, septa, and solid components. A high-velocity, low-resistance arterial spectrum is a common finding on spectral Doppler ultrasound (see Figs. 7.98 and 7.99).

(3) Differential diagnosis:

Ovarian cystadenocarcinoma must be distinguished from benign ovarian tumors. Key differences are summarized in Table 7.5.

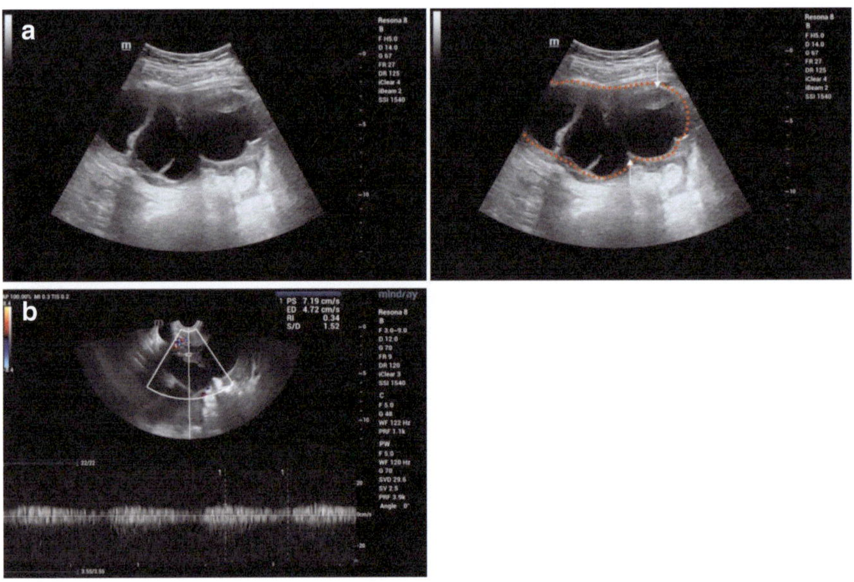

Fig. 7.98 (**a**) B-mode ultrasound reveals a predominantly cystic tumor with irregular thickening of the tumor wall and thick, uneven septations. The tumor is circled in orange; the upper arrow points to a thick segment of the tumor wall, and the lower arrow points to a thin segment. (**b**) Spectral Doppler ultrasound shows a low-resistance arterial spectrum

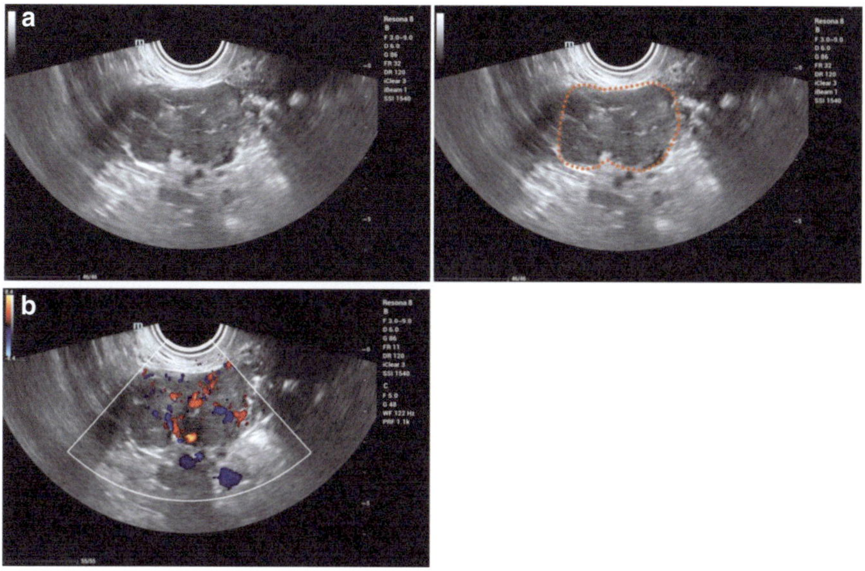

Fig. 7.99 (**a**) Ultrasound shows a solid, internally hypoechoic mass with unclear borders and irregular morphology. The tumor is circled in orange. (**b**) Color Doppler ultrasound shows abundant blood flow signals within the tumor

Table 7.5 Differential features of epithelial ovarian cancer and benign ovarian tumors

		Benign ovarian tumors	Epithelial ovarian cancer
Symptoms and signs	Duration of disease	Long, slow progression	Short, rapid progression
	Signs	Unilateral, with a smooth surface, mostly cystic or regular and solid, exhibiting good mobility and without ascites	Primarily bilateral, with a nodular surface, solid or cystic-solid, accompanied by hemorrhagic ascites
	General condition	Good	Gradual development of cachexia
Ultrasonographic features	Internal echogenicity	Predominantly cystic or uniformly solid	Predominantly solid or mixed cystic-solid, with chaotic echoes in the solid portion, poor sonolucency in the cystic area, and tiny bright spots
	Morphology and margins	Regular, smooth	Irregular, nodular
	Cyst wall and septa	Thin and uniform wall, smooth inner wall	Thick-walled, uneven inner wall
	Papillary structures	Small, few, regular	Large, numerous, irregular
	Color Doppler ultrasound	No or little blood flow	Solid portion with abundant blood flow
	Arterial spectrum on spectral Doppler	Low-velocity, high-resistance (>0.5)	High-velocity, low-resistance (≤0.5)
	Peritoneal effusion (ascites)	Mostly absent, but OTFG may be accompanied by effusion	Present and typically hemorrhagic
	Distant metastasis	No	Yes

7.4 Tubal-Related Diseases

7.4.1 Infectious Diseases of the Fallopian Tubes

1. Hydrosalpinx
   (1) Clinical overview:
   Hydrosalpinx results from tubal infection or other factors that cause adhesions between the fallopian tube and surrounding tissues, leading to tubal atresia. The subsequent accumulation of serous exudate or resorption of tubal pus transforms the condition into chronic tubal infection [77]. It is most frequently observed in sexually active women.

(2) Clinical manifestations:
Patients commonly present with the following:
- Lower abdominal pain
- Irregular menstruation
- Increased leucorrhea
- Infertility

During gynecological examination, unilateral or bilateral thickening of the fallopian tube with tenderness may be palpated.

(3) Ultrasonographic features:
Visualization of hydrosalpinx on ultrasound depends on the volume of fluid in the fallopian tube. In cases with minimal fluid, it may appear only as a simple tube thickening. When a substantial amount of fluid is present, it manifests as unilateral or bilateral cystic masses adjacent to the uterus. These masses are tortuous and tubular or sausage-like in shape, with clear borders and thick walls. The internal sonolucency ranges from anechoic to low-level echoes, and the ovaries remain unaffected. Color Doppler ultrasound may reveal a few streaks of blood flow signals within the sac walls.

Three characteristic ultrasonographic signs of hydrosalpinx are described in the literature [78–80]:

(a) Waist sign:
A tubular cystic structure with indentations along the walls, resembling a human waist. This feature is observed on the sagittal section of a specific fallopian tube segment and arises from the diameter transition between the wider ampulla and the narrower isthmus of the fallopian tube (see Fig. 7.100).

(b) Cogwheel sign:
In transverse sections of tubular cystic structures in the adnexal region, small bulging echoes (<3 mm) are seen along the inner wall, resembling a cogwheel. This appearance is due to folds in the tubal mucosa and is sometimes referred to as the "beads-on-a-string" sign (see Fig. 7.101).

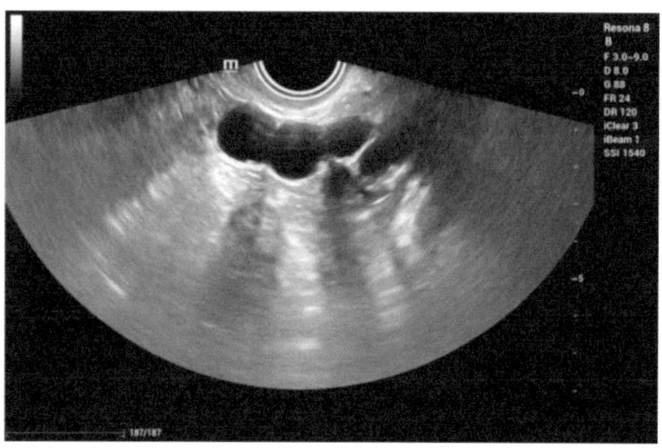

Fig. 7.100 Waist sign

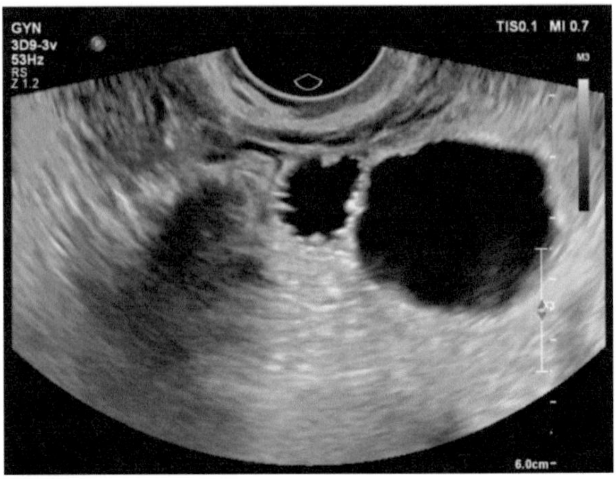

Fig. 7.101 Cogwheel sign

(c) Incomplete septation sign:
This sign features a septal band originating from one side of the inner wall of a tubular cystic mass, extending toward but not connecting to the opposite wall. This incomplete septation is formed by the folding of two layers of tubal walls along the curvature of the dilated tube (see Fig. 7.102).

(4) Differential diagnosis:
Hydrosalpinx must be differentiated from pelvic encapsulated effusion, which presents as an irregularly shaped fluid collection encircling the uterus or adnexa. This fluid may contain septations; in some cases, the bilateral fallopian tubes are distinctly visualized against the background of the effusion (see Fig. 7.103).

(5) Impact on fertility and treatment principles:
Hydrosalpinx reduces the likelihood of spontaneous pregnancy and can significantly impair the success rates of IVF-ET.

Surgical options: For younger patients with minimal effusion, mild adhesions (not visible on ultrasound), a short duration of infertility, and a strong desire for natural conception, salpingoplasty or salpingostomy may be considered.

IVF-ET recommendation: In cases of severe hydrosalpinx visible on ultrasound, particularly in older patients, IVF-ET is recommended after surgical or medical treatment to address the hydrosalpinx, improving the likelihood of successful implantation and pregnancy.

2. Pyosalpinx (tubal abscess) and tubo-ovarian abscess (TOA)

(1) Clinical overview:
Pelvic abscesses encompass a range of conditions, including tubal abscess, ovarian abscess, tubo-ovarian abscess, and abscesses arising from acute inflammation of pelvic connective tissues.

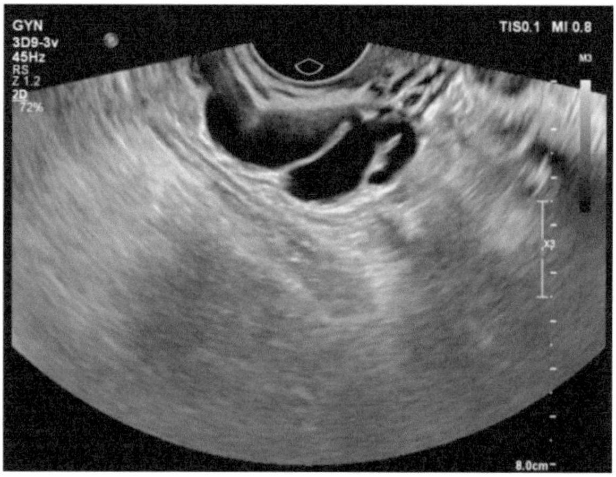

Fig. 7.102 Incomplete septation sign

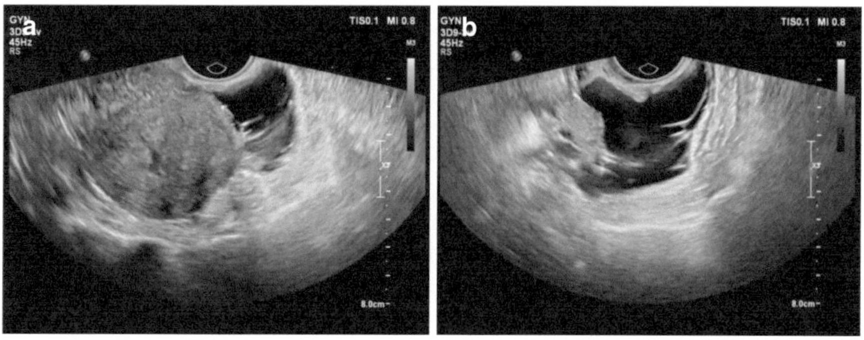

Fig. 7.103 (**a**) Pelvic encapsulated effusion with irregular morphology, multiple segregations within the effusion, and the effusion encircling the uterus. (**b**) Pelvic encapsulated effusion in a different section of the same patient, showing irregular morphology, multiple segregations, and the effusion encircling the ovaries

(2) Clinical manifestations:

Patients may present with acute lower abdominal pain or distension, often accompanied by systemic symptoms such as high fever, chills, nausea, and vomiting. Additional symptoms include the following:

- Vaginal discharge: Profuse, purulent discharge, sometimes with a foul odor.
- Urinary symptoms: Frequent urination, urgency, or urinary retention due to the bladder being compressed by the abscess.
- Gastrointestinal symptoms: Diarrhea, rectal tenesmus, or altered bowel habits if the abscess involves or compresses the rectum [81, 82].

Gynecological examination usually reveals

- Discharge: Purulent vaginal discharge is typically observed.

- Cervical motion tenderness: A hallmark finding suggestive of pelvic infection.
- Mass in the posterior fornix: A tender, palpable mass may be detected, particularly when the abscess is located in a low position within the pelvis.

(3) Ultrasonographic features:
The progression of infection typically follows a sequence: initial thickening of the fallopian tube, formation of a tubal abscess, and eventually, a tubo-ovarian abscess. Pelvic effusion is often present, and probe-induced tenderness is a notable finding during ultrasonography.

(a) Pyosalpinx/tubal abscess:
General appearance: A tortuous, tubular cystic mass with well-defined boundaries located in the adnexal region.

Cystic characteristics: The mass may display incomplete septations with thickened, coarse walls.

Internal echoes: Due to floating pus or debris, the mass often exhibits poor sonolucency [83], along with dense, fine, bright spot echoes or flocculent echoes. These echoes may shift when the probe applies pressure, or the patient changes position.

Signs of gas formation: In cases of infection with gas-producing bacteria, strong echogenic spots, formed by tiny air bubbles, may be visible within the mass.

Adhesions: Ipsilateral ovarian tissue adherent to the mass is commonly seen.

Ovary appearance: In mild ovarian inflammation, the ovary may appear enlarged, with uneven internal echogenicity and a blurred follicular structure, though an abscess may not yet be present.

Color Doppler findings: Stellate blood flow signals may be detected in the cystic wall and septal walls, with more abundant blood flow observed in the ipsilateral ovary (see Fig. 7.104).

(b) Tubo-Ovarian Abscess (TOA):
Along with the findings described for pyosalpinx/tubal abscess, a cystic mass within the ipsilateral ovary is also noted.

Cystic mass characteristics: This mass is typically round or oval with a thick wall, a rough inner lining, and poor sonolucency. Dense, dotted, bright, or flocculent echoes are often visible floating within the mass.

Fusion: Distinction between ovarian and tubal abscesses is challenging as they often merge into a mixed echogenic mass [82].

Color Doppler findings: A few streaks of blood flow signals can be detected within the wall of the mass, septations, and solid areas of the mass (see Fig. 7.105).

(4) Impact on reproductive function and treatment principles:
Both pyosalpinx and TOA may lead to infertility or ectopic pregnancy. The likelihood of infertility rises significantly with the duration of the condition, highlighting the importance of early intervention. For mild cases with minimal pelvic mass, antibiotics may be sufficient. However, in cases

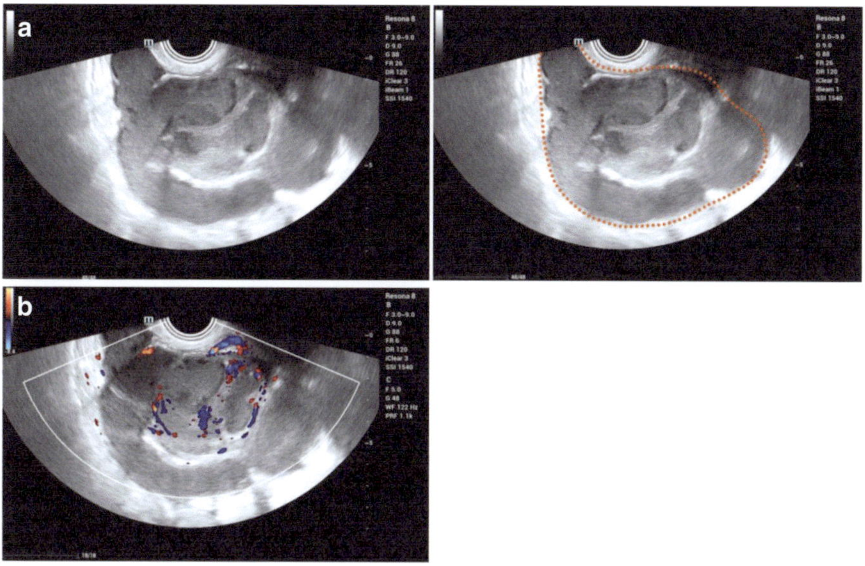

Fig. 7.104 (**a**) Tubal abscess on B-mode ultrasound showing a tortuous tubular cystic mass with well-defined borders, incomplete septation, poor sonolucency, and dense, fine, punctate echoes. The tubal abscess is circled in orange. (**b**) Color Doppler ultrasound shows abundant blood flow signals in the incomplete septations

involving large abscesses, drainage or surgical intervention is typically required to prevent further complications and preserve reproductive function.

3. Female genital tuberculosis (FGTB)
   (1) Clinical overview:
   Female genital tuberculosis (FGTB) typically results from primary pulmonary tuberculosis and is most commonly associated with tubal involvement. Tubal tuberculosis is the most prevalent form of FGTB and often presents bilaterally [84].
   (2) Clinical manifestations:
   FGTB primarily affects women of childbearing age. Due to its chronic nature and the nonspecificity of its symptoms, the condition often presents with the following:
   - Abdominal pain
   - Distension

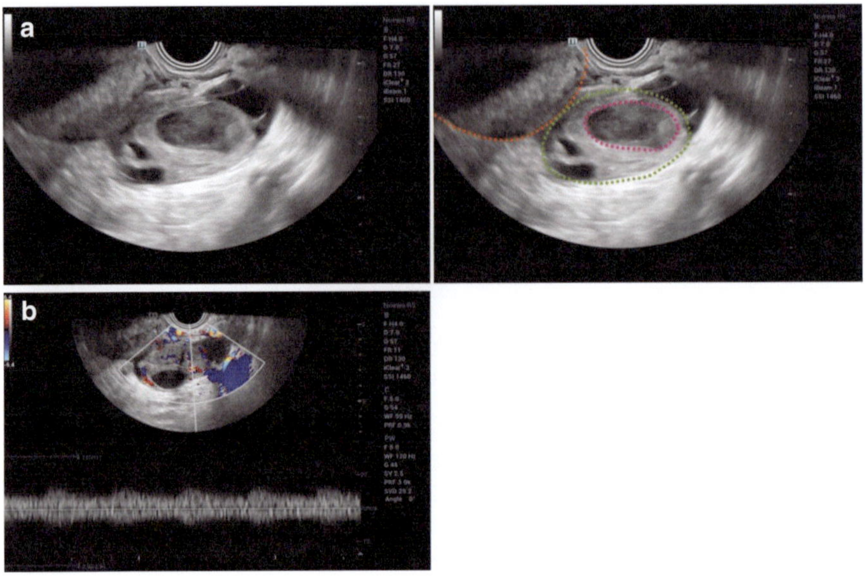

Fig. 7.105 (**a**) Ovarian abscess on B-mode ultrasound showing a thick-walled cystic mass with poor sonolucency and dense, fine, punctate echoes within the mass. The uterus is outlined in orange; the ovary is circled in green; the ovarian abscess is circled in pink. (**b**) Doppler ultrasound reveals an arterial spectrum in the wall of the mass

- Palpable masses
- Infertility
- Menstrual irregularities

However, systemic tuberculosis symptoms, such as afternoon fever and night sweats, are generally absent.

(3) Ultrasonographic features:

The pathologic changes in tuberculous lesions often overlap, and the involvement of multiple organs leads to complex and varied ultrasound presentations.

(a) Fluid accumulation type:

An irregularly shaped dark fluid collection may be seen in the pelvis, often with incomplete septations and lattice-like ascites (fibrous bands within the ascitic fluid) or loculated ascites [85]. Color Doppler ultrasound may reveal blood flow signals within the septations (see Fig. 7.106).

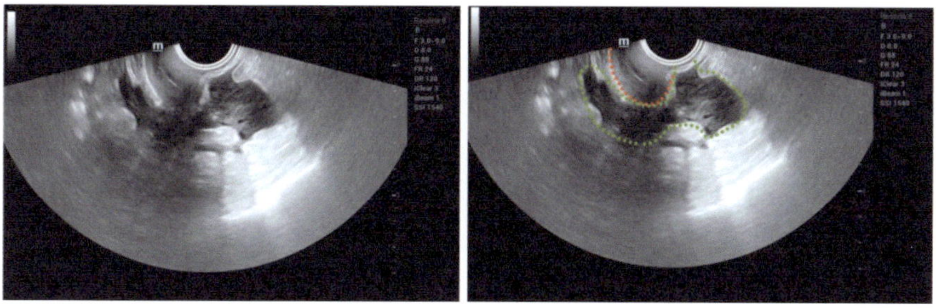

Fig. 7.106 Pelvic fluid with grid-like separations and fine dot-like echoes. The cervix is marked with an orange dotted line, and the fluid accumulated in the pelvis is circled in green

(b) Mass type:
The mass can be classified based on its internal echogenicity into cystic, solid, or mixed cystic-solid. It typically appears as an irregular mass surrounding the uterus, with poorly defined borders and clear adhesions to the surrounding tissues. A solid mass often shows heterogeneous medium-to-high echogenicity, potentially with bright, highly echogenic spots or clusters. A cystic mass is usually characterized by thick walls and small bright echoes within. Color Doppler ultrasound may detect blood flow signals within the solid portion or the cystic wall (see Fig. 7.107).

(c) Mixed type:
This is the most common presentation and involves the coexistence of fluid and mass characteristics. In simple tubal tuberculosis, the affected fallopian tube may appear enlarged, with wall thickening and luminal dilation. The lumen may become hypoechoic, resembling a solid mass due to the filling with caseous matter, although no blood flow signal is typically detected [86]. In cases with tuberculous peritonitis, thickening of the peritoneum and omentum may be observed, sometimes with small nodules (see Fig. 7.108). If endometrial tuberculosis is present, the endometrium may appear thinned with uneven echogenicity, exhibiting multiple strong echogenic spots or patches and/or adhesions within the uterine cavity.

(4) Differential diagnosis:
Tuberculosis of the fallopian tube must be distinguished from ovarian malignancies based on several key differences:

(a) Patient age: Ovarian malignancies typically occur in middle-aged and elderly women, while tuberculosis predominantly affects women of childbearing age.

(b) Mass characteristics: Ovarian malignancies often present as larger masses, with abundant blood flow signals detectable by color Doppler

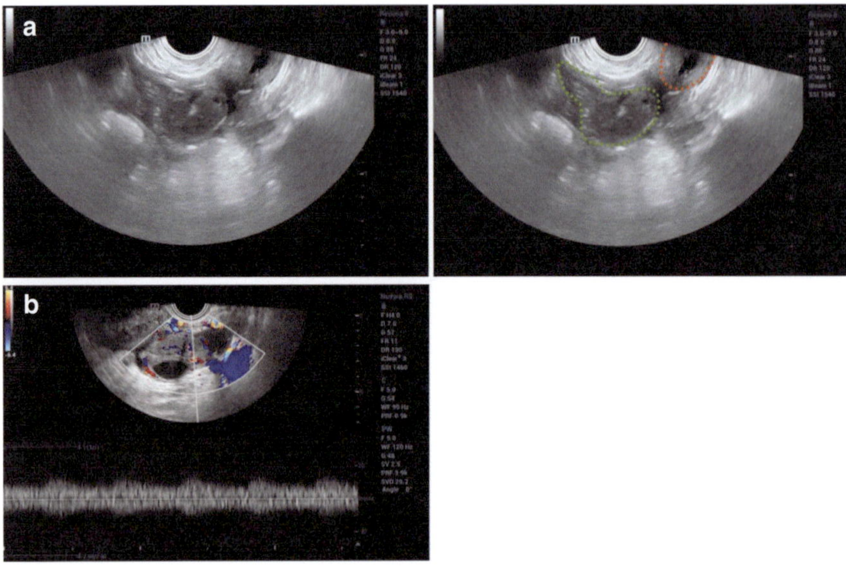

Fig. 7.107 (**a**) Ultrasound image showing a mass adjacent to the uterus with irregular alignment and a hypoechoic interior, surrounded by multiple hyperechogenic spots. The mass is circled in green; the uterus is outlined in orange. (**b**) Color Doppler ultrasound shows rich blood flow signals within the mass

ultrasound. In contrast, tuberculosis-related masses are generally smaller, with more severe adhesions to surrounding pelvic organs.

(c) Other ultrasound features: In cases of ovarian tuberculosis, there are more distinct septations and a higher frequency of hyperechogenic spots or clusters within the effusion, as compared to ovarian malignancies.

(5) Impact on fertility and treatment principles:

FGTB can cause irreversible damage to the fallopian tubes, endometrium, ovaries, and other reproductive organs. This, combined with immune dysfunction, can result in complications such as infertility, ectopic pregnancy, miscarriage, and ovarian hypofunction [87]. Early-stage FGTB can often be fully treated with anti-tuberculosis medications, while advanced cases may require a combination of anti-tuberculosis therapy and surgical intervention.

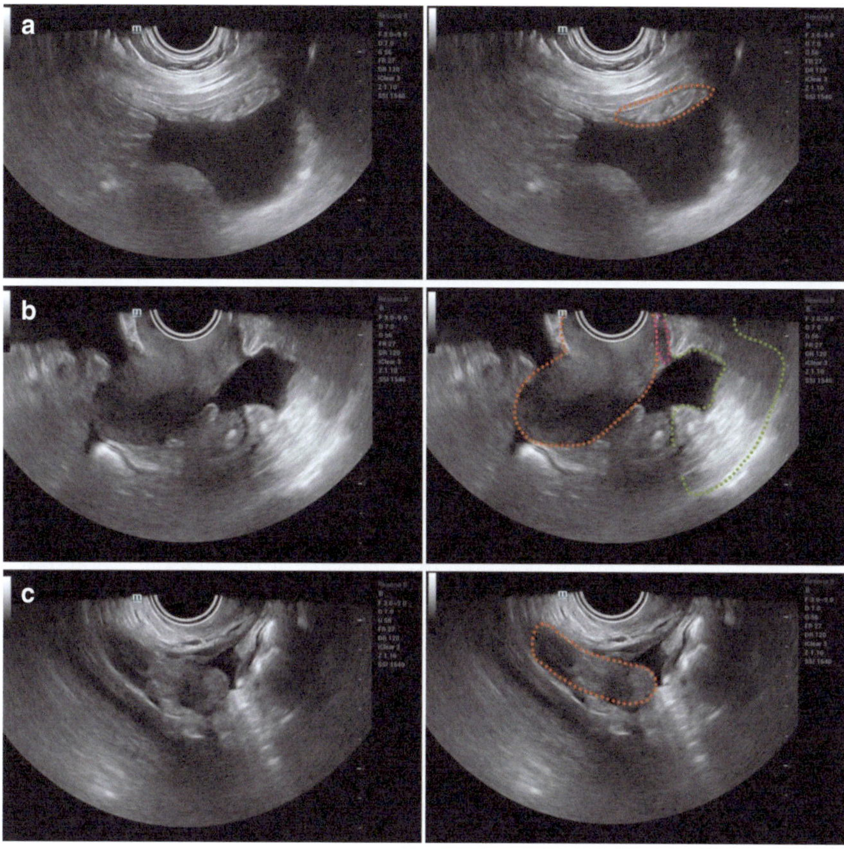

Fig. 7.108 (**a**) Pelvic tuberculosis with tuberculous peritonitis showing nodular thickening of the peritoneum. The peritoneum is circled in orange. (**b**) Pelvic tuberculosis with tuberculous peritonitis showing adhesion of the uterus to the posterior rectum. The uterus is outlined in orange; the rectum is outlined in green; the adhesions is circled in pink. (**c**) Pelvic tuberculosis with tuberculous peritonitis showing a thickened fallopian tube. The thickened fallopian tube is circled in orange

7.4.2 Primary Fallopian Tube Carcinoma (PFTC)

1. Clinical overview:
   Primary fallopian tube carcinoma (PFTC) originates in the lumen of the fallopian tube. It typically begins as a nodule, gradually leading to thickening of the fallopian tube wall, and may further progress into a cauliflower-like tumor that fills the fallopian tube lumen [88].
2. Clinical manifestations:
   The characteristic clinical presentation of PFTC is the "triad" of vaginal discharge or bleeding, abdominal pain, and an abdominal mass, with vaginal discharge being the most common symptom.
3. Ultrasonographic features:
   (1) Based on internal echogenicity, PFTC can be classified into three types:
      (a) Cystic: The mass occludes the infundibulum of the fallopian tube, causing dilation due to the accumulation of fluid or blood. Hydrosalpinx may present with an unevenly thickened wall, with papillary projections visible on the inner surface.
      (b) Solid: A solid, hypoechoic mass appears in the adnexal region, often sausage-shaped or irregular, with an irregular contour and heterogeneous echogenicity [89] (see Fig. 7.109).
      (c) Mixed cystic-solid: A mixed cystic-solid mass is seen in the adnexal area, typically sausage-shaped or irregular. The solid component appears cauliflower-shaped and exhibits heterogeneous echogenicity (see Fig. 7.110).
   (2) If the ipsilateral ovary is not involved, it may appear normal on ultrasound.
   (3) The presence of intrauterine fluid is common, and tiny bright spots may be visible within the anechoic area of fluid in the uterine cavity.
   (4) Color Doppler ultrasound may reveal abundant blood flow signals within the mass's solid component, along the cystic wall, and within the septations.

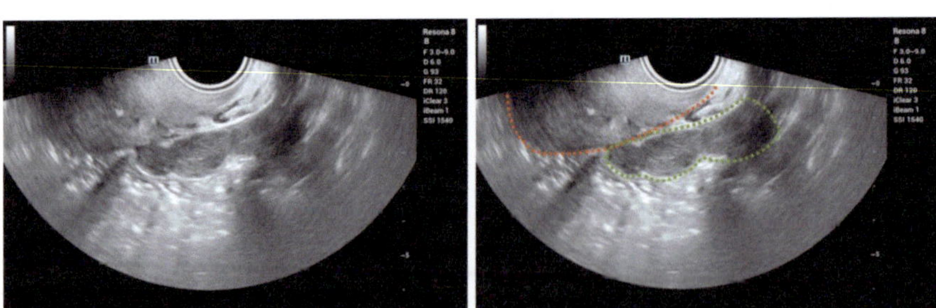

Fig. 7.109 B-mode ultrasound shows a solid hypoechoic mass in the adnexal area with a sausage-like shape and irregular contours. The uterus is outlined in orange; the solid hypoechoic tumor circled in green

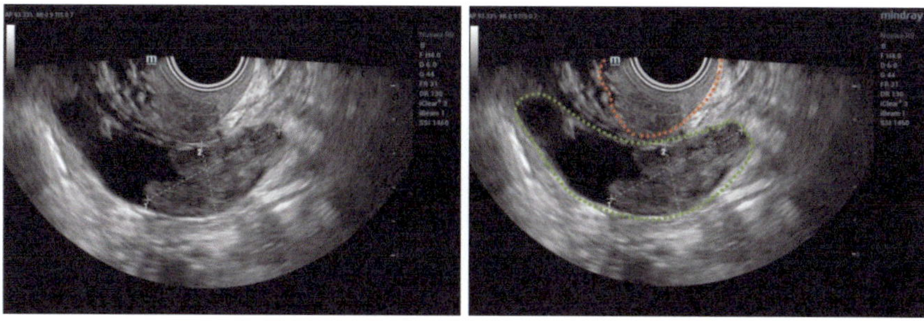

Fig. 7.110 Mixed cystic-solid PFTC. The cervix is marked in orange; the mixed cystic-solid PFTC is circled in green

Spectral Doppler ultrasound often shows a low-resistance arterial flow spectrum.

4. Impact on fertility and treatment principles:
   Unilateral adnexectomy, a conservative surgical option, is considered only for carefully selected patients with unilateral PFTC in situ who wish to preserve fertility. Conservative surgery is not recommended in cases of invasive carcinoma or when both fallopian tubes are likely to be affected.

7.4.3 Paraovarian Cyst

1. Clinical overview:
   A paraovarian cyst originates in the broad ligament between the two lobes, with its lumen not communicating with either the fallopian tube or the ovary [90].
2. Clinical manifestations:
   When the cyst becomes large, it may cause abdominal distension, pain, and pressure symptoms on adjacent organs. In some cases, torsion or rupture of the cyst can lead to acute abdominal symptoms.
3. Ultrasonographic features:
   Paraovarian cysts can be classified as simple or complex based on their echogenicity.
   (1) Simple cysts:
   These are more common and appear as single or multiple, round, thin- and smooth-walled anechoic areas in the adnexal region. The ipsilateral ovary is typically visible and can be clearly separated from the cyst (see Fig. 7.111).
   (2) Complex cysts:
   Less common, complex cysts appear with septations or fine punctate echoes within the cyst, along with single or multiple papillary projections on the inner wall. Color Doppler ultrasound may reveal blood flow signals within these projections. The ipsilateral ovary can usually be visualized and distinguished from the cyst.

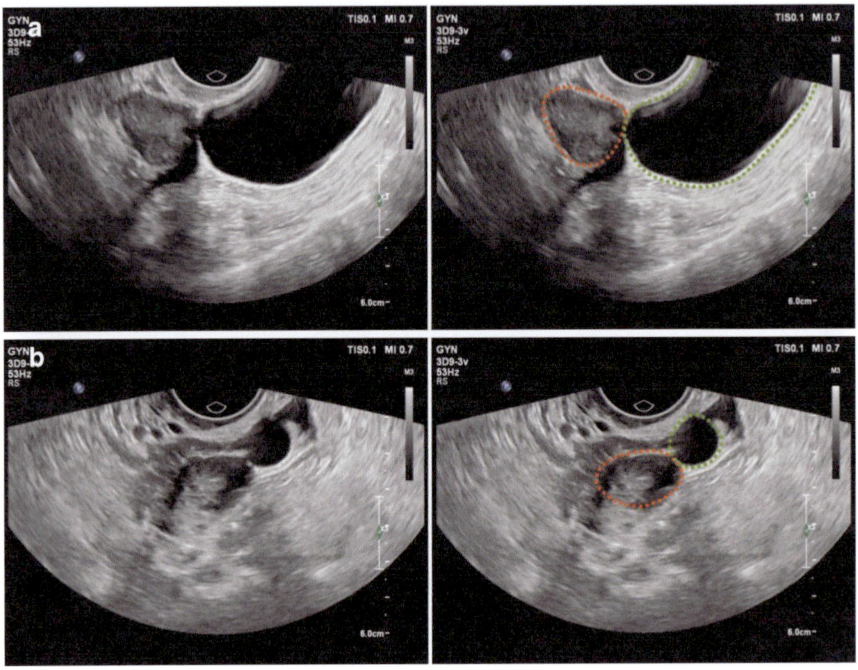

Fig. 7.111 (**a**) Paraovarian cyst seen as a fluid area adjacent to the ovary. The ovary is circled in orange; the paraovarian cyst is outlined in green. (**b**) Paraovarian cyst located adjacent to the ovary with the infundibulum of the fallopian tube visible at the periphery. The ovary is circled in orange; the paraovarian cyst is circled in green; the infundibulum of the fallopian tube is circled in pink

4. Differential diagnosis:

   In the case of an adnexal cyst, if the ipsilateral ovary cannot be visualized, an ovarian cyst should be the first consideration. A paraovarian cyst should only be suspected when the ipsilateral ovary is visible and not associated with the cyst.
5. Impact on fertility and treatment principles:

   Surgery may be considered in cases where the cyst is located near the infundibulum of the fallopian tube and is affecting the tube's normal function, or in situations where the cyst is large, experiencing torsion of the pedicle, rupturing, or causing compression symptoms.

References

1. Chan YY, Jayaprakasan K, Zamora J, et al. The prevalence of congenital uterine anomalies in unselected and high-risk populations: a systematic review. Hum Reprod Update. 2011;17(6):761–71.
2. Prior M, Richardson A, Asif S, et al. Outcome of assisted reproduction in women with congenital uterine anomalies: a prospective observational study. Ultrasound Obstet Gynecol. 2018;51(1):110–7.
3. Habiba M, Heyn R, Bianchi P, et al. The development of the human uterus: morphogenesis to menarche. Hum Reprod Update. 2021;27(1):1–26.
4. Herlin MK. Genetics of Mayer-Rokitansky-Küster-Hauser (MRKH) syndrome: advancements and implications. Front Endocrinol (Lausanne). 2024;15:1368990.
5. Ludwin A, Lindheim SR. Unicornuate uterus and the non-communicating functional horn: continued debate on the diagnosis, classification, and treatment. Fertil Steril. 2020;113(4):772–3.
6. Tellum T, Bracco B, De Braud LV, et al. Reproductive outcome in 326 women with unicornuate uterus. Ultrasound Obstet Gynecol. 2023;61(1):99–108.
7. Bhagavath B, Ludwin A, Lindheim SR. Reunification of the unicornuate uterus and the remnant horn- proceed with caution! Fertil Steril. 2020;114(5):981–2.
8. Latif NFBA, Guan Z, Asare S, et al. Robotic-assisted single-site abdominal cerclage in the bicornuate uterus patient with cervical insufficiency. Fertil Steril. 2024;121(5):887–9.
9. Fox NS, Connolly CT, Hill MB, et al. Pregnancy outcomes in viable pregnancies with a septate uterus compared with viable pregnancies after hysteroscopic uterine septum resection. Am J Obstet Gynecol MFM. 2019;1(2):136–43.
10. Grimbizis GF, Camus M, Tarlatzis BC, et al. Clinical implications of uterine malformations and hysteroscopic treatment results. Hum Reprod Update. 2001;7(2):161–74.
11. Wilson D, Bordoni B. Embryology, Mullerian ducts (paramesonephric ducts). In: StatPearls [Internet]. StatPearls Publishing; 2023.
12. Chan YY, Jayaprakasan K, Tan A, et al. Reproductive outcomes in women with congenital uterine anomalies: a systematic review. Ultrasound Obstet Gynecol. 2011;38(4):371–82.
13. Grimbizis GF, Gordts S, Di Spiezio SA, et al. The ESHRE/ESGE consensus on the classification of female genital tract congenital anomalies. Hum Reprod. 2013;28(8):2032–44.
14. Ludwin A, Coelho Neto MA, Ludwin I, et al. Congenital Uterine Malformation by Experts (CUME): diagnostic criteria for T-shaped uterus. Ultrasound Obstet Gynecol. 2020;55(6):815–29.
15. Drakonaki EE, Tritou I, Pitsoulis G, et al. Hematocolpometra due to an imperforate hymen presenting with back pain: sonographic diagnosis. J Ultrasound Med. 2010;29(2):321–2.
16. Anselm OO, Ezegwui UH. Imperforate hymen presenting as acute urinary retention in a 14-year-old Nigerian girl. J Surg Tech Case Rep. 2010;2(2):84–6.
17. Lee KH, Hong JS, Jung HJ, et al. Imperforate hymen: a comprehensive systematic review. J Clin Med. 2019;8(1):56.
18. Grant A, Carpenter CP, Li B, et al. Hydrometrocolpos: a contemporary review of the last 5 years. Curr Urol Rep. 2023;24(12):601–10.
19. Ruggeri G, Gargano T, Antonellini C, et al. Vaginal malformations: a proposed classification based on embryological, anatomical and clinical criteria and their surgical management (an analysis of 167 cases). Pediatr Surg Int. 2012;28(8):797–803.
20. Cunha GR, Robboy SJ, Kurita T, et al. Development of the human female reproductive tract. Differentiation. 2018;103:46–65.
21. Kang J, Zhou Q, Chen N, et al. Clinical and genetic characteristics of a cohort with distal vaginal atresia. Int J Mol Sci. 2022;23(21):12853.
22. Tanitame K, Tanitame N, Urayama S, et al. Congenital anomalies causing hemato/hydrocolpos: imaging findings, treatments, and outcomes. Jpn J Radiol. 2021;39(8):733–40.
23. Heinonen PK. Longitudinal vaginal septum. Eur J Obstet Gynecol Reprod Biol. 1982;13(4):253–8.

24. Heinonen PK. Complete septate uterus with longitudinal vaginal septum. Fertil Steril. 2006;85(3):700–5.
25. Zhang Y, Liu Q. Diagnosis and treatment of 46 patients with oblique vaginal septum syndrome. J Obstet Gynaecol. 2022;42(8):3731–6.
26. Sanderson PA, Critchley HO, Williams AR, et al. New concepts for an old problem: the diagnosis of endometrial hyperplasia. Hum Reprod Update. 2017;23(2):232–54.
27. Chandra V, Kim JJ, Benbrook DM, et al. Therapeutic options for management of endometrial hyperplasia. J Gynecol Oncol. 2016;27(1):e8.
28. Berceanu C, Cernea N, Căpitănescu RG, et al. Endometrial polyps. Romanian J Morphol Embryol. 2022;63(2):323–34.
29. Di Spiezio SA, Calagna G, Guida M, et al. Hysteroscopy and treatment of uterine polyps. Best Pract Res Clin Obstet Gynaecol. 2015;29(7):908–19.
30. Vitale SG, Haimovich S, Laganà AS, et al. Endometrial polyps. An evidence-based diagnosis and management guide. Eur J Obstet Gynecol Reprod Biol. 2021;260:70–7.
31. Pecorelli S. Revised FIGO staging for carcinoma of the vulva, cervix, and endometrium. Int J Gynecol Obstet. 2009;105(2):103–4.
32. Rodolakis A, Biliatis L, Morice P, et al. European Society of Gynecological Oncology Task Force for Fertility Preservation: clinical recommendations for fertility-sparing management in young endometrial cancer patients. Int J Gynecol Cancer. 2015;25(7):1258–65.
33. Chen L, Zhang H, Wang Q, et al. Reproductive outcomes in patients with intrauterine adhesions following hysteroscopic adhesiolysis: experience from the largest women's hospital in China. J Minim Invasive Gynecol. 2017;24(2):299–304.
34. Stewart EA, Laughlin-Tommaso SK, Catherino WH, et al. Uterine fibroids. Nat Rev Dis Primers. 2016;2:16043.
35. De La Cruz MS, Buchanan EM. Uterine fibroids: diagnosis and treatment. Am Fam Physician. 2017;95(2):100–7.
36. Ferrari F, Forte S, Valenti G, et al. Current treatment options for cervical leiomyomas: a systematic review of literature. Medicina (Kaunas). 2021;57(2):92.
37. Munro MG, Critchley HO, Broder MS, et al. The FIGO classification system (PALM-COEIN) for causes of abnormal uterine bleeding in nongravid women of reproductive age. Int J Gynaecol Obstet. 2011;113(1):3–13.
38. Awiwi MO, Badawy M, Shaaban AM, et al. Review of uterine fibroids: imaging of typical and atypical features, variants, and mimics with emphasis on workup and FIGO classification. Abdom Radiol (NY). 2022;47(7):2468–85.
39. McLucas B. Diagnosis, imaging and anatomical classification of uterine fibroids. Best Pract Res Clin Obstet Gynaecol. 2008;22(4):627–42.
40. Murase E, Siegelman ES, Outwater EK, et al. Uterine leiomyomas: histopathologic features, MR imaging findings, differential diagnosis, and treatment. Radiographics. 1999;19(5):1179–97.
41. Carranza-Mamane B, Havelock J, Hemmings R, et al. The management of uterine fibroids in women with otherwise unexplained infertility. J Obstet Gynaecol Can. 2015;37(3):277–88.
42. Munro MG. Uterine polyps, adenomyosis, leiomyomas, and endometrial receptivity. Fertil Steril. 2019;111(4):629–40.
43. Van den Bosch T, de Bruijn AM, de Leeuw RA, et al. Sonographic classification and reporting system for diagnosing adenomyosis. Ultrasound Obstet Gynecol. 2019;53(5):576–82.
44. Harmsen MJ, Van den Bosch T, de Leeuw RA, et al. Consensus on revised definitions of Morphological Uterus Sonographic Assessment (MUSA) features of adenomyosis: results of modified Delphi procedure. Ultrasound Obstet Gynecol. 2022;60(1):118–31.
45. Di Donato N, Seracchioli R. How to evaluate adenomyosis in patients affected by endometriosis? Minim Invasive Surg. 2014;2014:507230.
46. Tanos V, Berry KE, Seikkula J, et al. The management of polyps in female reproductive organs. Int J Surg. 2017;43:7–16.
47. Wu Z, Zou B, Zhang X, et al. A large nabothian cyst causing chronic urinary retention: a case report. Medicine (Baltimore). 2020;99(6):e19035.

48. Bhatla N, Aoki D, Sharma DN, et al. Cancer of the cervix uteri. Int J Gynaecol Obstet. 2018;143(2):22–36.
49. Huang WC, Yang JM, Yang YC, et al. Ultrasonographic characteristics and cystoscopic correlates of bladder wall invasion by endophytic cervical cancer. Ultrasound Obstet Gynecol. 2006;27(6):680–6.
50. Scioscia M, Scardapane A, Virgilio BA, et al. Ultrasound of the uterosacral ligament, parametrium, and paracervix: disagreement in terminology between imaging anatomy and modern gynecologic surgery. J Clin Med. 2021;10(3):437.
51. Testa AC, Di Legge A, De Blasis I, et al. Imaging techniques for the evaluation of cervical cancer. Best Pract Res Clin Obstet Gynaecol. 2014;28(5):741–68.
52. Jain S, Dalton ME. Chocolate cysts from ovarian follicles. Fertil Steril. 1999;72(5):852–6.
53. Van den Bosch T, Van Schoubroeck D. Ultrasound diagnosis of endometriosis and adenomyosis: state of the art. Best Pract Res Clin Obstet Gynaecol. 2018;51:16–24.
54. Collins BG, Ankola A, Gola S, et al. Transvaginal US of endometriosis: looking beyond the endometrioma with a dedicated protocol. Radiographics. 2019;39(5):1549–68.
55. Guerriero S, Saba L, Pascual MA, et al. Transvaginal ultrasound vs magnetic resonance imaging for diagnosing deep infiltrating endometriosis: systematic review and meta-analysis. Ultrasound Obstet Gynecol. 2018;51(5):586–95.
56. Rotterdam ESHRE/ASRM-Sponsored PCOS Consensus Workshop Group. Revised 2003 consensus on diagnostic criteria and long-term health risks related to polycystic ovary syndrome. Fertil Steril. 2004;81(1):19–25.
57. Adams J, Franks S, Polson DW, et al. Multifollicular ovaries: clinical and endocrine features and response to pulsatile gonadotropin releasing hormone. Lancet. 1985;2(8469–70):1375–9.
58. WHO Classification of Tumors Editorial Board. Female genital tumors. WHO classification of tumors series. 5th ed. Lyon: International Agency for Research on Cancer; 2020.
59. Mutch DG, Prat J. 2014 FIGO staging for ovarian, fallopian tube and peritoneal cancer. Gynecol Oncol. 2014;133(3):401–4.
60. Moro F, Bolomini G, Sibal M, et al. Imaging in gynecological disease (20): clinical and ultrasound characteristics of adnexal torsion. Ultrasound Obstet Gynecol. 2020;56(6):934–43.
61. Garde I, Paredes C, Ventura L, et al. Diagnostic accuracy of ultrasound signs for detecting adnexal torsion: systematic review and meta-analysis. Gynecol Oncol. 2020;157(1):89–93.
62. Pulappadi VP, Manchanda S, Sk P, et al. Identifying corpus luteum rupture as the culprit for haemoperitoneum. Br J Radiol 2021;94(1117):20200383.
63. Sathoh T, Hatae M, Watanabe Y, et al. Outcomes of fertility-sparing surgery for stage I epithelial ovarian cancer: a proposal for patient selection. J Clin Oncol. 2010;28(10):1727–32.
64. Sayasneh A, Ekechi C, Ferrara L, et al. The characteristic ultrasound features of specific types of ovarian pathology (review). Int J Oncol. 2015;46(2):445–58.
65. Levine D, Brown DL, Andreotti RF, et al. Management of asymptomatic ovarian and other adnexal cysts imaged at US: Society of Radiologists in Ultrasound Consensus Conference Statement. Radiology. 2010;256(3):943–54.
66. Kurakula S, Muralidharan V, Chengappa Appaneravanda L, et al. Rupture of bilateral theca lutein cysts during pregnancy: a case report. Cureus. 2022;14(9):e29758.
67. Heremans R, Valentin L, Sladkevicius P, et al. Imaging in gynecological disease (24): clinical and ultrasound characteristics of ovarian mature cystic teratomas. Ultrasound Obstet Gynecol. 2022;60(4):549–58.
68. Chen H, Liu Y, Shen LF, et al. Ovarian thecoma-fibroma groups: clinical and sonographic features with pathological comparison. J Ovarian Res. 2016;9(1):81.
69. Pectasides D, Pectasides E, Psyrri A. Granulosa cell tumor of the ovary. Cancer Treat Rev. 2008;34(1):1–12.
70. Petrone M, Bergamini A, Tateo S, et al. Transvaginal ultrasound in evaluation and follow-up of ovarian granulosa cell tumors. Int J Gynecol Cancer. 2020;30(9):1384–9.
71. Okada S, Ohaki Y, Inoue K, et al. Calcifications in mucinous and serous cystic ovarian tumors. J Nippon Med Sch. 2005;72(1):29–33.

72. Marko J, Marko KI, Pachigolla SL, et al. Mucinous neoplasms of the ovary: radiologic-pathologic correlation. Radiographics. 2019;39(4):982–97.
73. Moro F, Zannoni GF, Arciuolo D, et al. Imaging in gynecological disease (11): clinical and ultrasound features of mucinous ovarian tumors. Ultrasound Obstet Gynecol. 2017;50(2):261–70.
74. Maturen KE, Shampain KL, Roseland ME, et al. Malignant epithelial tumors of the ovary: pathogenesis and imaging. Radiol Clin North Am. 2023;61(4):563–77.
75. Sambasivan S. Epithelial ovarian cancer: review article. Cancer Treat Res Commun. 2022;33:100629.
76. Lheureux S, Gourley C, Vergote I, et al. Epithelial ovarian cancer. Lancet. 2019;393(10177):1240–53.
77. Ng KYB, Cheong Y. Hydrosalpinx – salpingostomy, salpingectomy or tubal occlusion. Best Pract Res Clin Obstet Gynaecol. 2019;59:41–7.
78. Chen F, Jain MK, Bhatt S. The "waist sign" of a dilated fallopian tube. Abdom Radiol (NY). 2021;46(6):2985–6.
79. Della Grotta LM, Dyer RB, Holbert BL. The "cogwheel" sign of hydrosalpinx. Abdom Radiol (NY). 2019;44(10):3486–7.
80. Timor-Tritsch IE, Lerner JP, Monteagudo A, et al. Transvaginal sonographic markers of tubal inflammatory disease. Ultrasound Obstet Gynecol. 1998;12(1):56–66.
81. Greydanus DE, Cabral MD, Patel DR. Pelvic inflammatory disease in the adolescent and young adult: an update. Dis Mon. 2022;68(3):101287.
82. Lareau SM, Beigi RH. Pelvic inflammatory disease and tubo-ovarian abscess. Infect Dis Clin N Am. 2008;22(4):693–708.
83. Revzin MV, Moshiri M, Katz DS, et al. Imaging evaluation of fallopian tubes and related disease: a primer for radiologists. Radiographics. 2020;40(5):1473–501.
84. Tjahyadi D, Ropii B, Tjandraprawira KD, Parwati I, et al. Female genital tuberculosis: clinical presentation, current diagnosis, and treatment. Infect Dis Obstet Gynecol. 2022;2022:3548190.
85. Sharma JB, Khurana A, Hari S, et al. Evaluation of role of transabdominal and transvaginal ultrasound in diagnosis of female genital tuberculosis. J Hum Reprod Sci. 2021;14(3):250–9.
86. Yapar EG, Ekici E, Karasahin E,et al. Sonographic features of tuberculous peritonitis with female genital tract tuberculosis. Ultrasound Obstet Gynecol 1995;6(2):121–125.
87. Dahiya B, Kamra E, Alam D,et al. Insight into diagnosis of female genital tuberculosis. Expert Rev Mol Diagn 2022;22(6):625–642.
88. Ajithkumar TV, Minimole AL, John MM, et al. Primary fallopian tube carcinoma. Obstet Gynecol Surv. 2005;60(4):247–52.
89. Shaaban AM, Rezvani M. Imaging of primary fallopian tube carcinoma. Abdom Imaging. 2013;38(3):608–18.
90. Durairaj A, Gandhiraman K. Complications and management of paraovarian cyst: a retrospective analysis. J Obstet Gynaecol India. 2019;69(2):180–4.

8 Ultrasound Assessment of First-Trimester Pregnancy and Complications

Da Li and Xinlu Wang

The most commonly used indicators for assessing the outcomes of assisted reproductive treatments (ART) include the implantation rate, clinical pregnancy rate, early miscarriage rate, multiple pregnancy rate, ongoing pregnancy rate, and live birth rate. The clinical pregnancy rate is considered the most significant.

This chapter examines the ultrasound manifestations of normal first-trimester pregnancies, miscarriages, ectopic pregnancies, and multiple pregnancies, with a particular focus on early pregnancy outcomes in ART patients.

8.1 Ultrasound Evaluation of Normal Early Pregnancy

An early pregnancy refers to the period up to the end of the 12th week of gestation. Clinical manifestations of early pregnancy include the cessation of menstruation, symptoms such as nausea and vomiting, and a positive urine pregnancy test.

8.1.1 Ultrasonography

In normal cases, the gestational sac is located in the upper-middle part of the uterine cavity. It is surrounded by a complete, uniformly thick, hyperechoic ring measuring no less than 2 mm in thickness. This hyperechoic ring represents the decidua.

The "intradecidua sign" refers to an intrauterine round or oval fluid collection lying within the echogenic decidua. As the gestational sac enlarges, the

D. Li (✉) · X. Wang
Shengjing Hospital of China Medical University, Shenyang, China
e-mail: wangxl1@sj-hospital.org

D. Li et al. (eds.), *Ultrasonography of the Female Reproductive System*,
https://doi.org/10.1007/978-981-95-1373-4_8

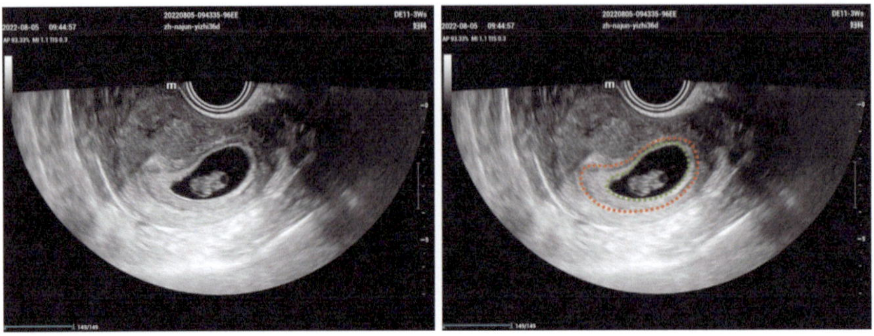

Fig. 8.1 The "double sac sign" of the gestational sac. The inner ring is circled in green; the outer ring is circled in orange

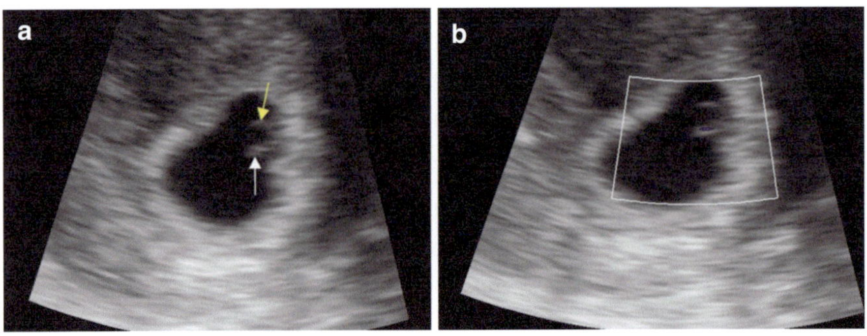

Fig. 8.2 (**a**) Sonogram of a yolk sac: The yellow arrow indicates the yolk sac within the gestational sac, and the white arrow points to the embryo. (**b**) Sonogram of a yolk sac with fetal heartbeat blood flow signals visualized on CDFI

characteristic "double-sac sign" becomes apparent, showing an intra-endometrial fluid collection surrounded by two concentric echogenic rings [1] (see Fig. 8.1).

The yolk sac is the first anatomical structure detectable by ultrasound within the gestational sac. The yolk sac is typically visualized on transvaginal ultrasound around the 5th week of gestation. On transabdominal ultrasound, it is generally visualized later than on transvaginal ultrasound.

In a normal pregnancy, the yolk sac appears as a spherical structure with a thin, thread-like wall and an anechoic center (see Fig. 8.2). Its diameter ranges from 3 to 8 mm, with an average of 5 mm. It usually disappears by the 12th week of gestation [2].

By 6 weeks of gestation, transvaginal ultrasound reveals an embryo measuring 2–3 mm in length, typically located adjacent to the yolk sac [3]. Between 6 and 6.5 weeks, fetal heartbeats can be detected using transvaginal ultrasound. Fetal skull osteogenesis begins at 8 weeks of gestation, with ossification becoming visible by the end of the 11th week [4]. By 10 weeks, the fetus begins to move its limbs.

8.1.2 Standardized Measurements in Early Pregnancy

The internal diameter of the gestational sac (excluding the hyperechoic ring) is measured in the largest longitudinal and transverse sections of the gestational sac, not the uterus. The average internal diameter is calculated as the sum of the maximum anterior-posterior, left-right, and top-bottom diameters, divided by three.

The crown-rump length (CRL) should be measured in the maximum longitudinal section of the embryo or in the fetal median sagittal plane. This measurement must be taken when the fetus is in a natural straight position, avoiding hyperextension or hyperflexion.

8.1.3 Weeks of Pregnancy (Gestational Age)

1. Estimation of gestational age in normal early pregnancy
   Blood HCG can be tested to confirm pregnancy from the 30th day of pregnancy. The gestational sac is typically identifiable on transvaginal ultrasound at approximately 5 weeks of gestation, and the embryo becomes visible on transvaginal ultrasound around 6 weeks of gestation [5].
   Before 7 weeks of gestation, particularly when the embryonic structure is not yet visible, the average internal diameter of the gestational sac is commonly used to estimate gestational age. The formula for calculating the average internal diameter is: Average internal diameter (mm) = (maximal longitudinal diameter + transverse diameter + anterior-posterior diameter)/3. The gestational age (in days) can then be estimated using the formula: Gestational age (days) = average internal diameter (mm) + 30 (see Fig. 8.3).
   Once the embryo or fetus is visible, measuring the CRL is the most accurate method for estimating gestational age during the first trimester [4]. While vari-

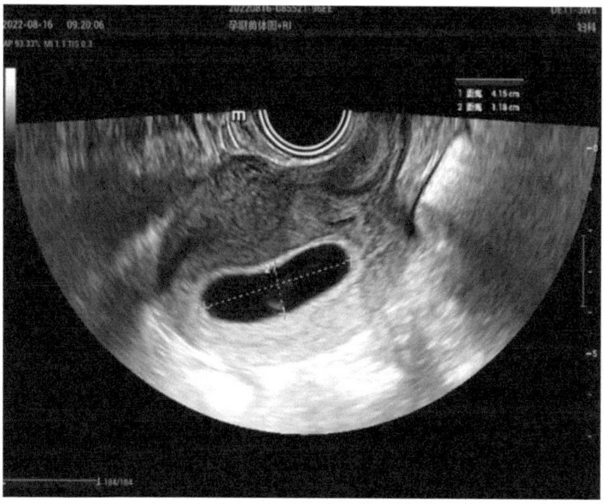

Fig. 8.3 Measurement of the average internal diameter of the gestational sac: Maximum transverse and anterior-posterior diameters are measured

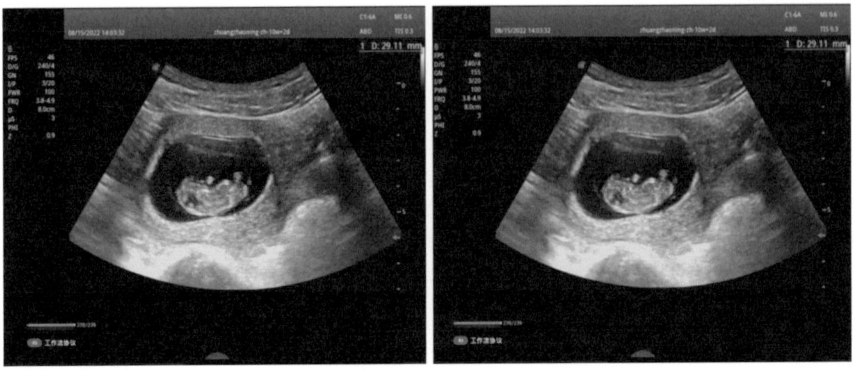

Fig. 8.4 The fetus in a neutral position. Measurement of the CRL, indicated by the dotted orange line

ous CRL equations have been proposed since 1975, there is no consensus on the most appropriate formula for pregnancy dating [6]. Alternatively, a standardized table of CRL in relation to gestational age can be used to determine the corresponding gestational week (see Fig. 8.4).

2. Estimation of gestational age in early pregnancy for patients conceived with ART
   (1) Patients conceived via intrauterine insemination (IUI)
   For patients conceived through intrauterine insemination (IUI), the date of ovulation is used to calculate the last menstrual period (LMP).
      - Patients with regular menstrual cycles: Gestational age can be calculated using the actual LMP.
      - Patients with polycystic ovary syndrome (PCOS) undergoing ovulation induction: These patients often experience variability in the length of the follicular phase, with the ovulation induction phase lasting a month or longer. In such cases, calculating gestational age based on the actual LMP can lead to overestimation. Instead, the date of ovulation should be used to determine the LMP, which is typically 14–15 days before ovulation.

   (2) Patients undergoing in vitro fertilization and embryo transfer (IVF-ET)
   For IVF-ET patients, menstrual cycles are often manipulated with artificial interventions, such as adjustments to the follicular phase or endometrial proliferation phase. Consequently, gestational age is calculated based on the date of embryo implantation, not the patient's actual LMP.
      - Cleavage-stage embryo implantation: The LMP is estimated as 17 days before the date of implantation.
      - Blastocyst implantation: The LMP is estimated as 19 days before the date of implantation.

   Follow-up timeline for IVF-ET patients:
      - Day 14 after implantation: A pregnancy test is performed (equivalent to 31 days of gestation for cleavage-stage embryos and 33 days for blastocysts).

- Day 20 after implantation: Ultrasound is performed to detect the presence of a gestational sac in the uterus (equivalent to 37 days for cleavage-stage embryos and 39 days for blastocysts).
- Days 30–35 after implantation: Ultrasound is conducted to detect fetal heartbeats (equivalent to 47–52 days for cleavage-stage embryos and 49–54 days for blastocysts).

8.1.4 Differential Diagnosis

An intrauterine gestational sac must be differentiated from intrauterine fluid accumulation.

Intrauterine fluid accumulation: Unlike a gestational sac, intrauterine fluid does not exhibit the double-ring sign nor contain an embryonic bud or yolk sac. On ultrasound, intrauterine fluid may appear with a few punctate echoes, accompanied by strong peripheral echoes from detached endometrial fragments.

In cases where intrauterine fluid accumulation is observed without a gestational sac, the possibility of ectopic pregnancy should be carefully considered. A thorough examination of both adnexa is essential to rule out this condition.

8.2 Miscarriage

Miscarriage rates are notably high in pregnancies achieved through ART, primarily involving biochemical pregnancies and miscarriages. Miscarriage is broadly defined as the loss of a pregnancy before viability [7].

Definitions:

- The intentional termination of a pregnancy before 28 weeks of gestation or of a fetus weighing less than 1000 g is referred to as an abortion.
- A spontaneous pregnancy loss is termed a miscarriage.
- Early miscarriage: The termination of a pregnancy before the 12th gestational week.
- Late miscarriage: The termination of a pregnancy between the 12th and 28th weeks of gestation.

In this section, we will discuss the main clinical manifestations, typical ultrasound findings, and key diagnostic features of various types of miscarriage.

Clinical manifestations:

The primary symptoms of miscarriage include the following:

- Cessation of menstruation
- Positive pregnancy test
- Vaginal bleeding
- Lower back pain, abdominal cramps, and pain [8]

The presentation of symptoms varies based on the timing of the miscarriage:

- Early miscarriages typically begin with vaginal bleeding, followed by abdominal pain.
- Late miscarriages often present with abdominal pain first, followed by vaginal bleeding.

Classification of miscarriages:

Miscarriages are categorized based on the stage of development and clinical symptoms into the following:

- Threatened miscarriage
- Inevitable miscarriage
- Incomplete miscarriage
- Missed miscarriage
- Complete miscarriage

8.2.1 Threatened Miscarriage

1. Clinical overview

   A threatened miscarriage represents the initial stage of potential pregnancy loss. Patients commonly present with symptoms such as light vaginal bleeding (or bloody discharge) and mild lower abdominal pain.

   Key clinical features include the following:

   - Cervix: Remains closed
   - Amniotic sac: Intact
   - Embryo and fetal heartbeats: Normal

   Threatened miscarriages are often associated with luteal insufficiency or increased uterine sensitivity. With appropriate treatment, the pregnancy may continue. However, worsening symptoms, such as increased vaginal bleeding and intensified abdominal pain, indicate a higher risk of progression to an inevitable miscarriage.

2. Typical ultrasonic features

   In cases of threatened miscarriage, ultrasound findings are generally unremarkable, with the following observations:

   - The uterus, gestational sac, and embryo or fetus size are consistent with the gestational age.
   - Fetal heartbeats are typically detectable.
   - The internal cervical os remains closed.

   In some cases, additional findings may include a limited crescent-shaped anechoic area or a cloud-like hypoechoic area adjacent to the gestational sac caused by the detachment of chorionic villi from the uterine wall and localized blood accumulation (see Fig. 8.5).

   Color Doppler flow imaging (CDFI):

   - Around the gestational sac: High-speed, low-resistance blood flow signals can be observed.

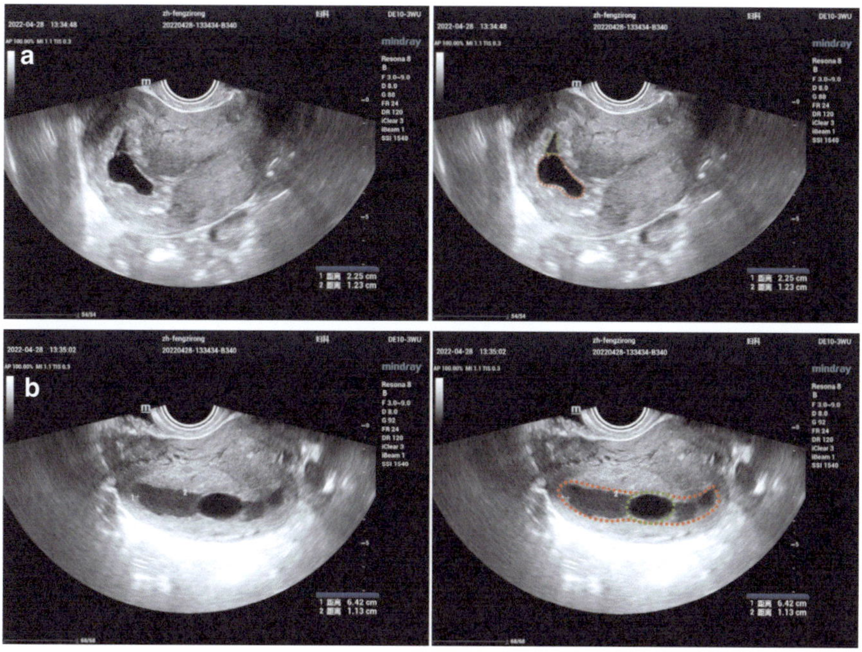

Fig. 8.5 (**a**) A case of threatened miscarriage (with intrauterine fluid): Sagittal view of the uterus showing an intrauterine gestational sac with an angular anechoic area anterior to it. The gestational sac is circled in orange; the angular anechoic area is circled in green. (**b**) A case of threatened miscarriage (with intrauterine fluid): Transverse view showing a large fluid area with punctate echoes adjacent to the gestational sac. The gestational sac is circled in orange; the fluid area is circled in green

- Embryo or fetus: Heartbeat blood flow signals are detected.
- Hypoechoic or anechoic area: No significant blood flow signals are observed.

Fetal heart rate:

- Before 6.5 weeks of gestation: less than 100 bpm.
- At 9 weeks of gestation: up to 180 bpm.
- At 14 weeks of gestation: around 140 bpm.
- A fetal heart rate of ≤110 bpm has shown higher diagnostic accuracy in predicting miscarriage [9].

3. Differential diagnosis
   (1) Threatened miscarriage vs. inevitable or incomplete miscarriage (early pregnancy):

   In early pregnancy, before the appearance of an embryonic bud, a threatened miscarriage must be distinguished from an inevitable or incomplete miscarriage.

   Clinical tip: In cases of mild vaginal bleeding, a follow-up ultrasound after 1 week is recommended to confirm the diagnosis.

(2) Threatened miscarriage with intrauterine hemorrhage vs. twin pregnancy: When intrauterine hemorrhage is detected, it should be differentiated from twin pregnancy:
- A dichorionic twin pregnancy on ultrasound reveals two gestational sacs.
- Each gestational sac is surrounded by a hyperechoic ring with a regular shape.
- A yolk sac and embryonic structure are identifiable within each gestational sac.

8.2.2 Early Embryonic (Fetal) Demise

1. Clinical overview

   Early embryonic demise, also referred to as a missed miscarriage or blighted ovum, represents an early stage in the natural course of miscarriage [10].

   Key clinical features include the following:

   History: Many patients have prior symptoms of a threatened miscarriage.

   Symptoms:
   - Cessation of menstruation and early pregnancy symptoms
   - The gradual disappearance of pregnancy symptoms as the condition progresses

   Uterine size:
   - No further uterine enlargement.
   - Uterus size may be smaller than expected for the gestational age.

   Pregnancy test: May turn negative at the time of diagnosis.
2. Typical ultrasonic features

   On ultrasound, early embryonic demise is characterized by the following:

   Gestational sac:
   - An intact sac is visible within the uterine cavity.
   - It may lack an embryo, or the embryo is present but shows no cardiac activity [10].

   Diagnostic thresholds:
   - Fetal demise is suspected when
   - CRL >6 mm without detectable cardiac activity.
   - Gestational sac >20 mm without a visible embryo or yolk sac.

   Confirmation:

   To minimize diagnostic errors, the diagnosis should be confirmed with a follow-up ultrasound 7–14 days later [11]. (Refer to Figs. 8.6, 8.7, 8.8, 8.9, and 8.10 for examples.)

8.2.3 Incomplete Miscarriage

1. Clinical overview

   An incomplete miscarriage refers to the partial expulsion of products of conception, with no intact gestational sac remaining [12].

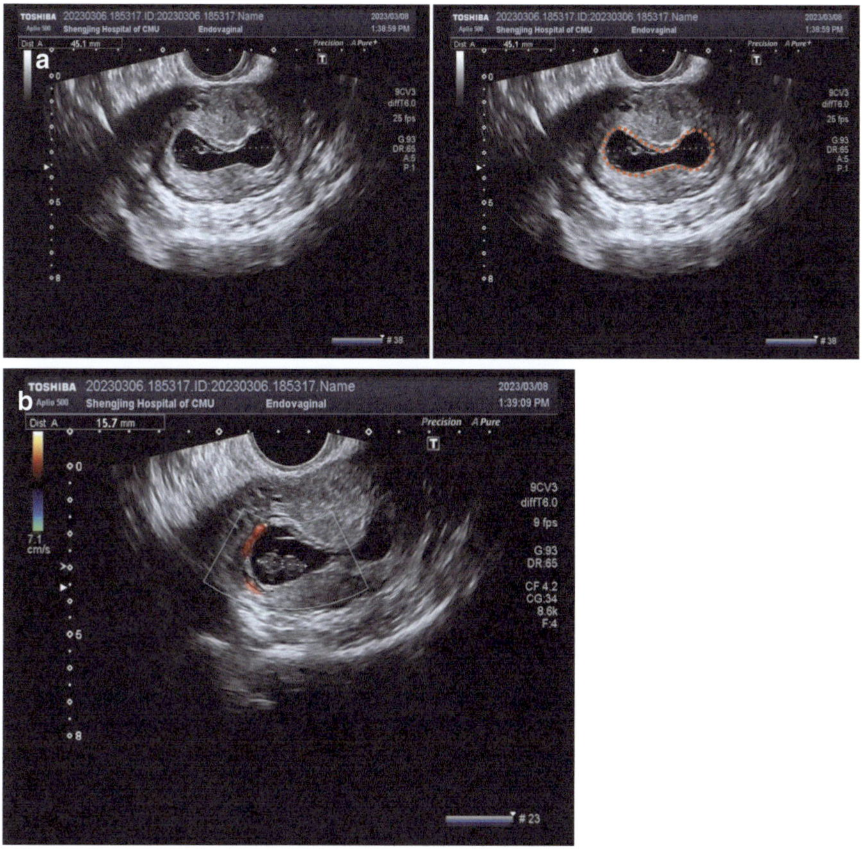

Fig. 8.6 (**a**) Early fetal demise: An irregularly shaped gestational sac visualized in the uterus. The irregularly shaped gestational sac is circled in orange. (**b**) Early fetal demise: CDFI showing no significant blood flow in the embryo

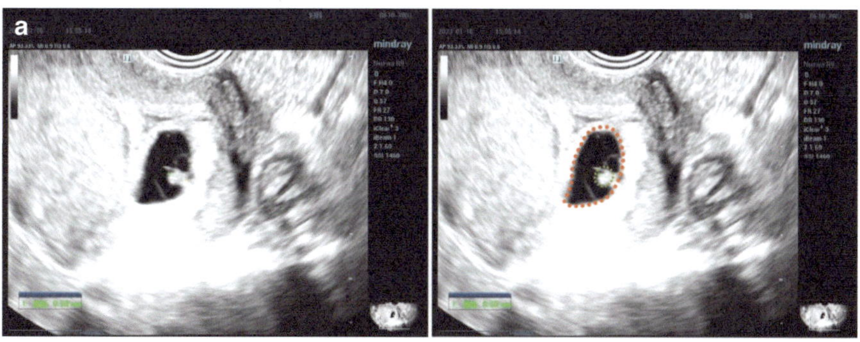

Fig. 8.7 (**a**) A case of early embryonic demise: The gestational sac visualized inside the uterine cavity with an embryonic structure. The gestational sac is circled in orange; the embryonic structure is circled in green. (**b**) No heartbeat in the embryonic structure. The gestational sac is circled in orange; the embryonic bud is circled in green

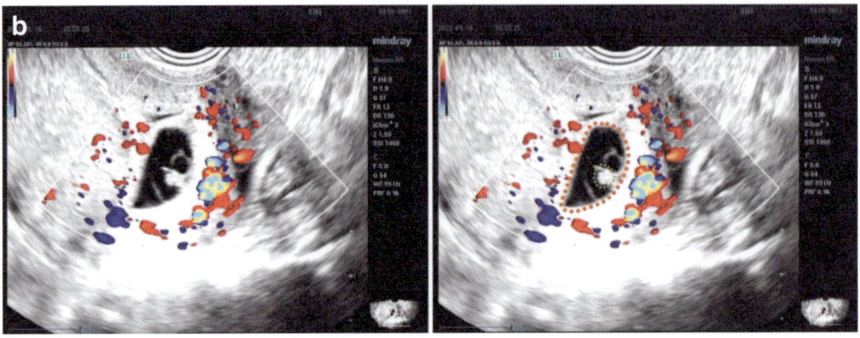

Fig. 8.7 (continued)

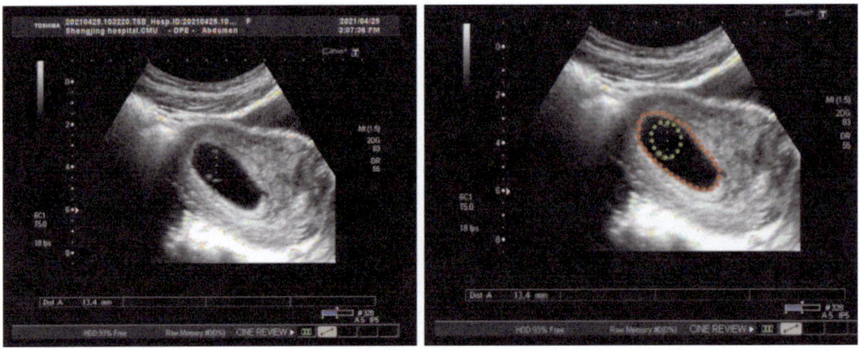

Fig. 8.8 The gestational sac with an enlarged yolk sac visible in the uterine cavity. The gestational sac is circled in orange; the enlarged yolk sac is circled in green

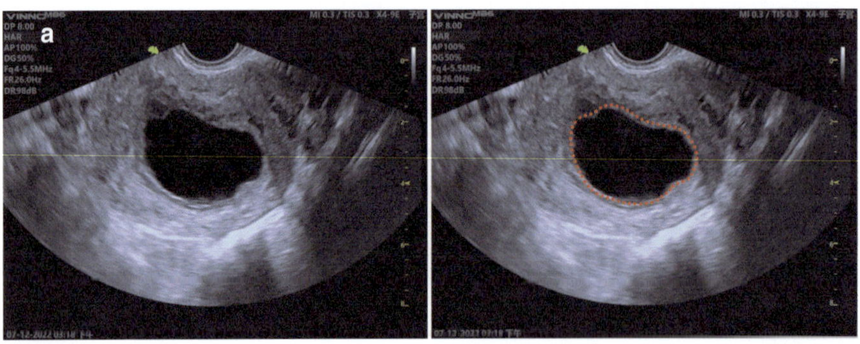

Fig. 8.9 (**a**) Early embryonic (fetal) demise (transverse section): The gestational sac in the uterine cavity is irregularly shaped, with no yolk sac and no embryonic structure. The gestational sac is outlined in orange. (**b**) Early embryonic (fetal) demise (longitudinal section): No blood flow in the gestational sac. The gestational sac is circled in orange

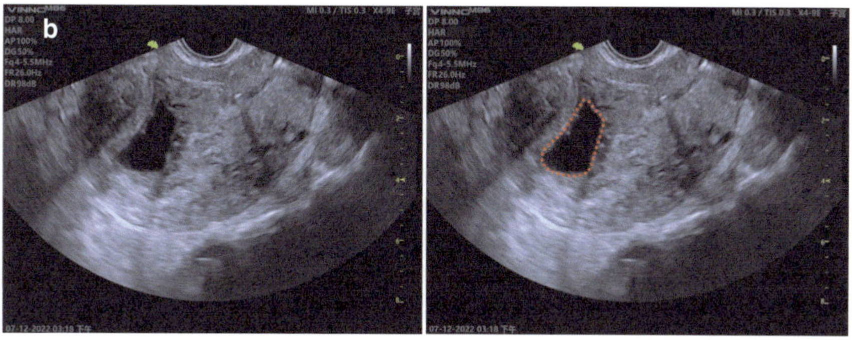

Fig. 8.9 (continued)

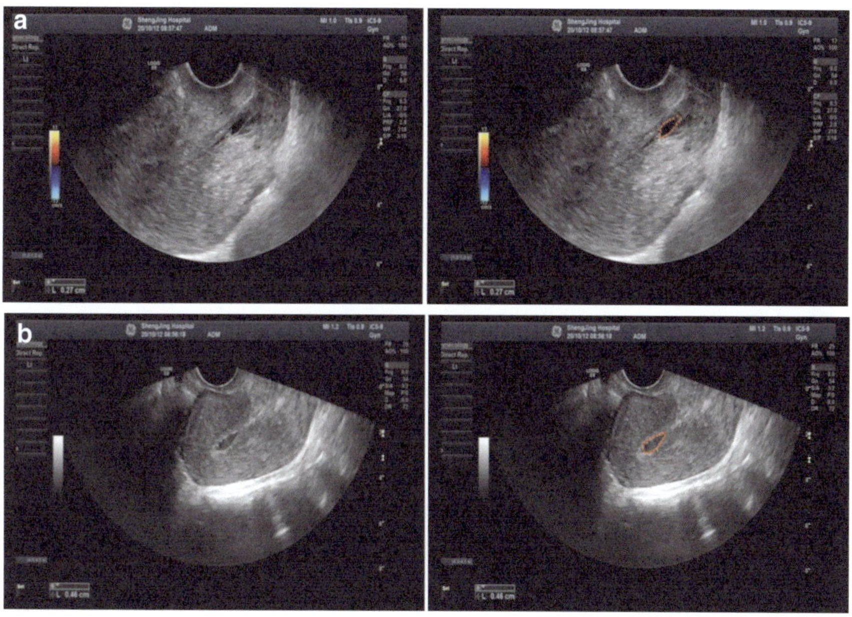

Fig. 8.10 (**a**) Early embryonic (fetal) demise: The gestational sac is located in the lower segment of the uterus, with irregular morphology and poor tonicity. The embryo is about 3 mm long, and CDFI shows no blood flow within the embryo. The gestational sac is circled in orange. (**b**) Early embryonic (fetal) demise: Fluid accumulation with punctate echoes observed in the upper segment of the uterus. The fluid area is circled in orange

Key clinical features include the following:

Symptoms:

- Increased vaginal bleeding
- Intensified abdominal pain

Uterine size:

- Typically smaller than expected for the gestational age.
- However, in cases where the uterus is filled with blood clots, its size may match or exceed the gestational age.

Gynecologic examination:

- Dilated cervical opening with visible blood flow.
- Pregnancy tissue may block the cervical canal or be partially expelled into the vagina, with remaining tissue (and blood clots) in the uterus.

2. Typical ultrasonic features

General findings:

- The uterus is typically smaller than expected for the gestational age.
- Endometrial thickness varies.
- Heterogeneous tissue is seen, with or without a visible gestational sac [13].
- Distorted endometrial echoes (Fig. 8.11a) may represent retained placenta, decidual tissue, or blood within the uterine cavity.
- The cervical canal may appear dilated, with pregnancy tissues partially occluding it.

CDFI and pulsed wave Doppler:

- Blood flow signals are often detected within retained uterine contents (Fig. 8.11b).
- Low-resistance blood flow signals may indicate trophoblastic tissue.
- When residual contents consist only of fetal membranes or decidual tissue, no blood flow signals are observed within these structures.

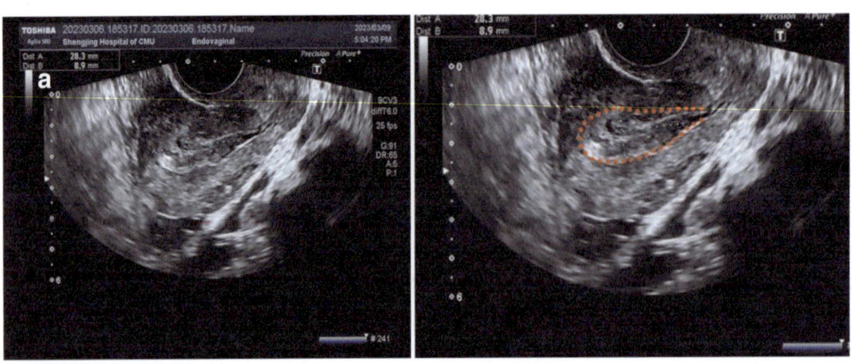

Fig. 8.11 (**a**) Incomplete miscarriage: Irregular hyperechoic masses and fluid detected within the uterine cavity. The remaining conceptus is circled in orange. (**b**) Incomplete miscarriage: CDFI shows a hyperechoic mass with punctate blood flow signals around and within the mass. The hyperechoic mass is circled in orange

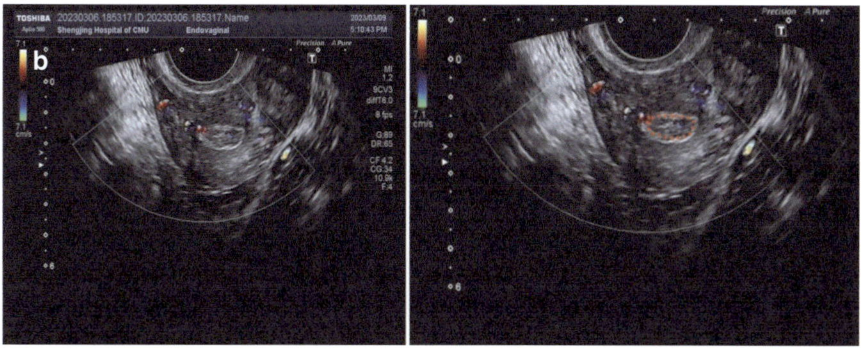

Fig. 8.11 (continued)

3. Differential diagnosis

   An incomplete miscarriage must be differentiated from a pseudogestational sac, which may occur in cases of ectopic pregnancy.

   Irregular vaginal bleeding is often observed in ectopic pregnancies.

   Ultrasonic features of a pseudogestational sac:

   - Appears as an anechoic central area, representing accumulated blood
   - Surrounded by a peripheral hyperechoic pattern, corresponding to the decidua
   - Typically located centrally within the uterus
   - No detectable blood flow signals within the pseudogestational sac, as confirmed by Doppler imaging

   By contrast, an incomplete miscarriage may show heterogeneous retained tissue with associated blood flow signals in the uterus.

8.2.4 Complete Miscarriage

1. Clinical overview

   A complete miscarriage occurs when all pregnancy tissues are expelled from the uterus with the following clinical features:

   - Relief from abdominal pain
   - Closed cervical orifices
   - Well-contracted uterus, returning to near-normal size
   - Minor or no vaginal bleeding
2. Typical ultrasonic features
   - An empty uterine cavity following the initial visualization of an intrauterine gestational sac (with or without an embryo).
   - If associated with a positive pregnancy test and a rapid decline in serum hCG levels, this may be termed a failed pregnancy of unknown location until an ectopic pregnancy is excluded [14].
   - The uterus is either normal in size or slightly enlarged.
   - The pregnancy tissue has been completely expelled.

- Endometrium appears thin and thread-like, with possible minor blood accumulation.
- No patchy or clustered echoes are visible within the uterine cavity.

8.3 Ectopic Pregnancy

Ectopic pregnancy occurs when a fertilized egg implants and develops outside the uterine cavity [15]. Approximately 98% of ectopic pregnancies occur in the fallopian tubes, with the most affected region being the oviductal ampulla, followed by the isthmus [16, 17].

Other less common sites include the following:

- Ovarian
- Abdominal
- Cervical
- Heterotopic (co-occurring intrauterine and ectopic pregnancy)
- Cesarean scar [18]

Clinical manifestations include the following:

Key symptoms:

- Bleeding: Vaginal bleeding often occurs after a period of amenorrhea.
- Pain: Lower abdominal pain is a hallmark symptom.
- Shock: Severe cases may present with hypovolemic shock due to ruptured ectopic pregnancy [19].

Laboratory findings:

- Urine pregnancy test: positive result.
- Serum β-hCG levels: elevated, but the rate of increase may be slower than in normal intrauterine pregnancies.

8.3.1 Tubal Pregnancy

1. Clinical overview

   Tubal pregnancy refers to the implantation of a fertilized egg within the fallopian tube.

   (1) Pathophysiology:

   The fallopian tube's thin walls and narrow lumen cannot support a developing fetus. As the embryo grows, the tube may either

   - Miscarry: Resulting in partial expulsion of the pregnancy tissue.
   - Rupture: This leads to significant internal bleeding.

   (2) Clinical presentations:

   Tubal miscarriage:

   - Mild-to-moderate abdominal pain.
   - Vaginal bleeding may be present but is not excessive.

Tubal rupture:

- Severe abdominal pain, often sudden in onset
- Signs of hypovolemia, such as dizziness or fainting, due to internal bleeding
- Accompanied by anemia in many cases

"Old" tubal pregnancy:

- Prolonged history of irregular vaginal bleeding.
- Initial severe abdominal pain, evolving into chronic, insidious discomfort.
- It may mimic other gynecological conditions due to its subtle and persistent nature.

2. Typical ultrasonic features

(1) General findings:

- The uterus appears morphologically plump with thickened endometrium, but no gestational sac is present within the uterine cavity.
- In some cases, a pseudogestational sac may be visible in the uterine cavity.
- In the adnexal region, masses with relative mobility to the ovaries and significant tenderness upon palpation are commonly detected.
- Pelvic effusion may be present, indicating potential rupture or internal bleeding.

(2) Sonographic findings of tubal pregnancy on 2D ultrasound [13, 18, 20, 21]:

(a) Adnexal mass

- An extraovarian mass is observed, which may include a yolk sac and/or a fetal pole, with or without cardiac motion.
- The gestational sac appears as a thick-walled, hyperechogenic sac with an anechoic center, creating the characteristic "bagel sign."
- On CDFI, a "ring of fire" pattern surrounds the gestational sac, representing trophoblastic blood flow.
- At this stage, pelvic and abdominal fluid accumulation is minimal or absent (Fig. 8.12).

In the case of a ruptured gestational sac:

- An irregular, mixed-echoic mass is seen in the adnexal region, making the "bagel sign" difficult to distinguish.
- CDFI shows punctate blood flow signals within the mass, with occasional trophoblastic-like blood flow.
- A significant amount of free fluid is detected in the pelvic and abdominal cavities.
- This fluid often contains dense punctate or cloudy echo patterns, indicative of hemorrhage (Fig. 8.13).

(b) Pseudosac

- A pseudosac (seen in about 20% of ectopic pregnancies) appears as a fluid collection within the endometrial cavity, often mimicking a small gestational sac.
- The pseudosac is heterogeneous, containing blood and debris.
- It lacks the double-ring sign and other definitive features of a true intrauterine gestational sac.

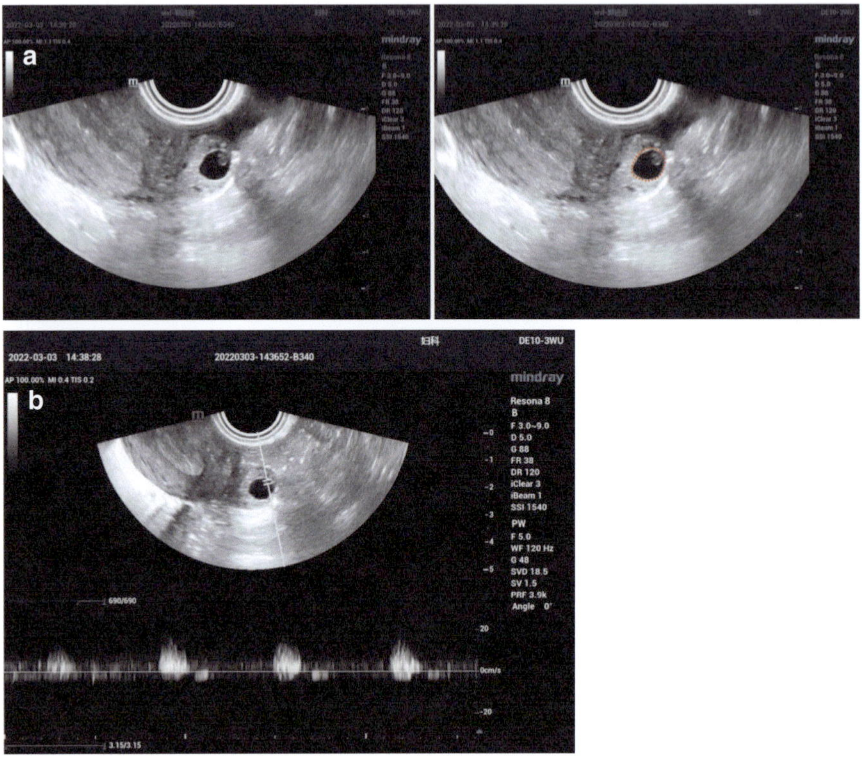

Fig. 8.12 (**a**) Tubal pregnancy: A gestational sac visualized in the adnexal region, containing a visible yolk sac and embryo. The gestational sac is circled in orange. (**b**) Tubal pregnancy: Spectral Doppler showing fetal heartbeats within the fetal pole

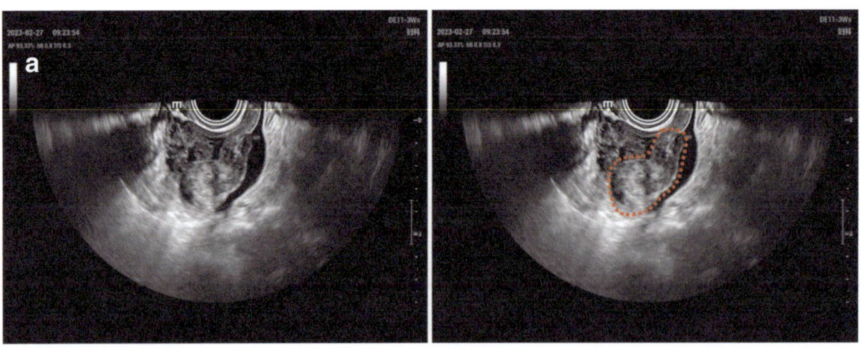

Fig. 8.13 (**a**) Tubal pregnancy: A heterogeneous mass visualized in the adnexal region, large and irregular in shape, with disorganized internal echoes and blurred borders. The heterogeneously echogenic mass is circled in orange. (**b**) Tubal pregnancy: CDFI showing a small amount of colored blood flow signals within the mass. The mass is circled in orange. (**c**) Tubal pregnancy: Free fluid detected in the pelvis. The fluid area is circled in orange

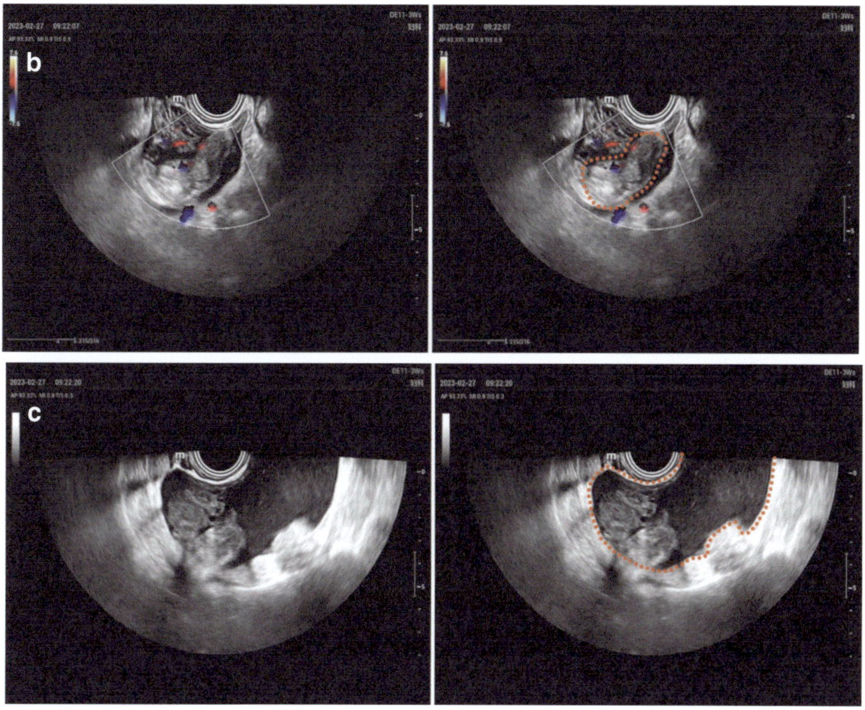

Fig. 8.13 (continued)

3. Differential diagnosis
   (1) Rupture of ectopic pregnancy vs. rupture of the corpus luteum:
   Rupture of corpus luteum features the following:
   It typically occurs late in the menstrual cycle without a history of missed menstruation.
   It often manifests as a sudden onset of abdominal pain with massive internal bleeding.
   Ultrasound findings:
   - The uterus is not significantly enlarged.
   - The affected ovary is enlarged and displays an irregular, mixed echogenic mass.
   - Fluid accumulation (hemoperitoneum) may be seen in the pelvic and abdominal cavities.

   Laboratory findings: Serum β-hCG and urine pregnancy tests are negative.
   (2) Tubal pregnancy with intrauterine blood accumulation vs. incomplete miscarriage: Incomplete miscarriage:
   Ultrasound findings of an incomplete miscarriage:
   - A deformed intrauterine gestational sac or heterogeneous tissue is present.

- The hyperechogenic ring surrounding the gestational sac appears thinned and reduced in echogenicity, resembling the pseudogestational sac seen in tubal pregnancy with intrauterine blood accumulation.
- Key differentiation: No mass is detected in the bilateral adnexal regions, ruling out tubal pregnancy.

8.3.2 Interstitial Pregnancy and Angular Pregnancy

1. Clinical overview
   Interstitial pregnancy:
   - Accounts for 2–4% of ectopic pregnancies [22].
   - Implantation occurs at the origin of the proximal fallopian tube within the myometrium and lateral to the round ligament.
   - The increased expansibility of this region allows progression to later gestations compared to distal tubal pregnancies.
   - Rupture results in significant blood loss and morbidity, with mortality rates up to 2.5% [17].

   Angular pregnancy:
   - This is a rare condition in which the embryo implants in the endometrial cavity at the superior and lateral angle, medial to the utero-tubal junction [22].
   - Often confused with interstitial pregnancy due to proximity to the utero-tubal junction.
   - A potentially viable pregnancy that might be carried to term with a live-born baby [22].
2. Typical ultrasonic features
   Interstitial pregnancy:
   - Thickened endometrium with no gestational sac in the uterine cavity.
   - Mass protruding outward from one side of the uterine fundus containing a structured gestational sac.
   - The gestational sac has minimal surrounding uterine muscle.
   - The endometrial line appears closed at the uterine horn, with no continuity between the endometrium and the mass.
   - A thin echogenic line is visible, extending laterally from the endometrial cavity through the myometrium toward the uterine serosa (Fig. 8.14).

   Angular pregnancy:
   - A gestational sac implanted in the lateral angle of the uterus, possibly protruding slightly.
   - The gestational sac is entirely surrounded by circumferential endometrium [23] (Fig. 8.15).
3. Differential diagnosis
   Interstitial pregnancy vs. angular pregnancy:
   Gestational sac in angular pregnancy:
   - Located within the uterine cavity.
   - Completely surrounded by endometrium.

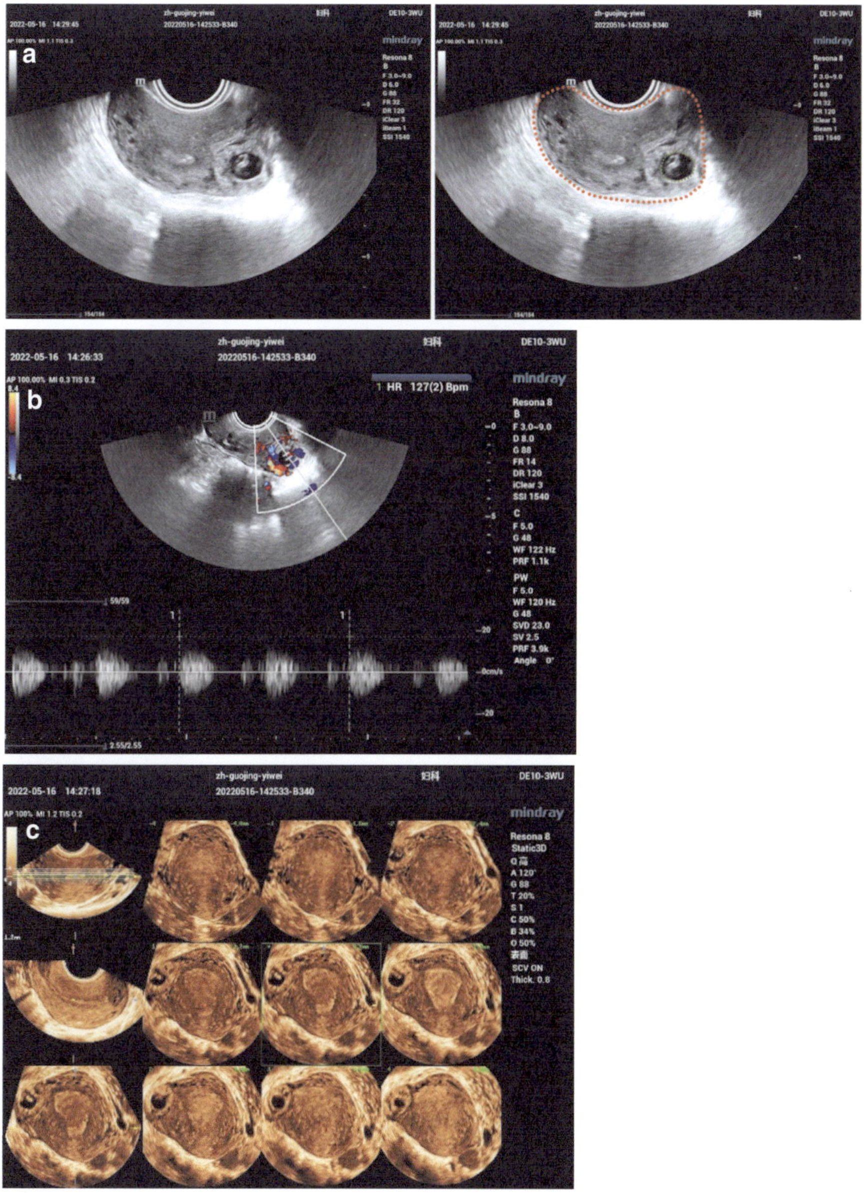

Fig. 8.14 (**a**) Left tubal interstitial pregnancy: The gestational sac is located adjacent to the left uterine horn, with a thin muscular encasing at the periphery. The gestational sac is circled in green; the uterus is circled in orange. (**b**) Left interstitial pregnancy: CDFI shows blood flow signals around the gestational sac, with fetal heartbeats detectable within the embryo. (**c**) Tomographic ultrasound showing the gestational sac protruding out of the uterus. (**d**) Intraoperatively, a gestational sac in the interstitium of the left fallopian tube is identified, partially purplish-black in color

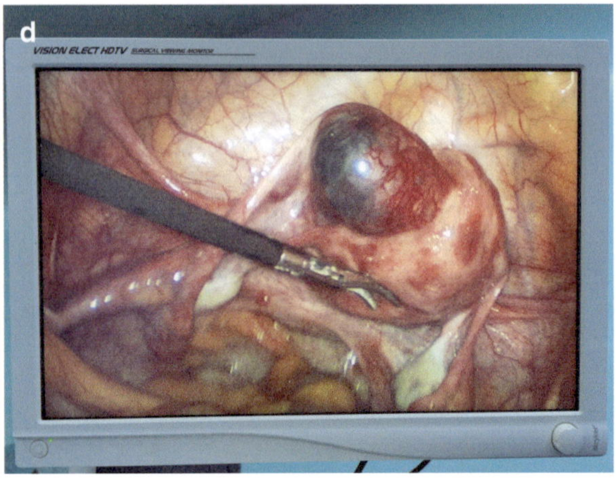

Fig. 8.14 (continued)

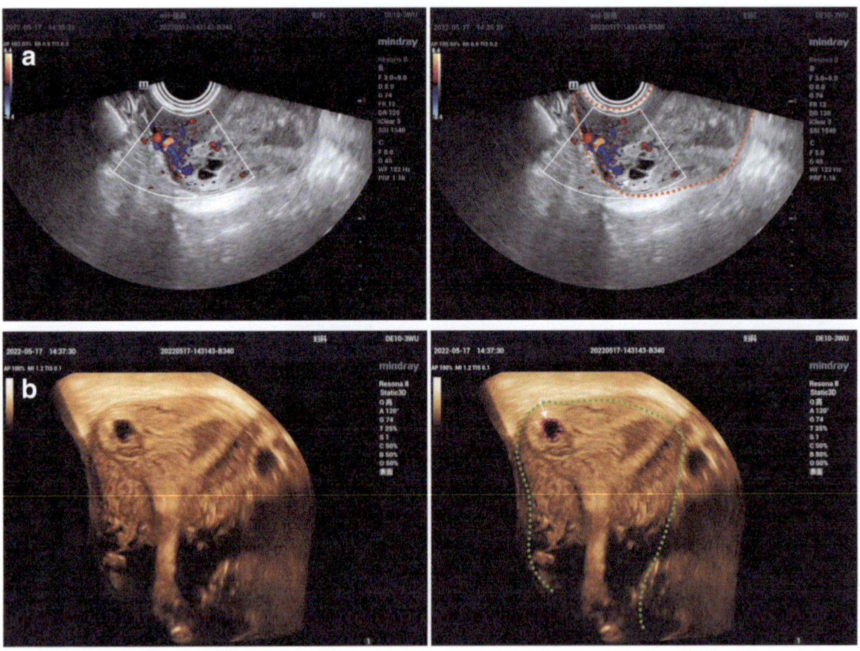

Fig. 8.15 (**a**) Angular pregnancy: The gestational sac is located at the uterotubal junction and encircled by endometrium; CDFI shows blood flow signals around the gestational sac. The uterus is outlined in orange; the white arrow indicates the gestational sac. (**b**) 3D ultrasound showing a gestational sac at the uterotubal junction. The uterus is outlined in green; the gestational sac is circled in pink; the white arrow indicates the uterotubal junction

Gestational sac in interstitial pregnancy:
- Located outside the uterine cavity in the myometrium.
- Surrounded by myometrium, not endometrium.

8.3.3 Cervical Ectopic Pregnancy

1. Clinical overview
   Cervical ectopic pregnancy occurs when the gestational sac implants and develops within the mucosa of the endocervical canal. It represents <1% of all ectopic pregnancies [21].
   Risk factors include the following:
   - Previous uterine surgeries
   - ART
   - Asherman's syndrome [24]

   Clinical manifestations:
   - History of menstrual cessation and early pregnancy signs.
   - Characteristic symptom: painless vaginal bleeding.
   - A gynecologic exam may reveal significant enlargement of the cervix.
2. Typical ultrasonic features
   - Hourglass-shaped uterus with ballooning of the cervical canal.
   - Gestational tissue within the cervix, with no intrauterine gestational tissue [17].
   - "8-shape" pattern: A bridge of the endocervical canal is seen between the empty endometrial canal and the cervical pregnancy.
   - The gestational sac is non-mobile when gentle pressure is applied with the transducer.
   - Color Doppler shows a hypervascular trophoblastic ring around the cervical region, indicating a live cervical ectopic pregnancy (Fig. 8.16).
3. Differential diagnosis
   Cervical ectopic pregnancy vs. miscarriage:
   Cervical pregnancies can be mistaken for miscarriages where the gestational sac has fallen into the cervical canal.
   In the case of a miscarriage:
   - The gestational sac that was originally located within the uterine cavity becomes deformed and moves downward.
   - No fetal heartbeats will be detected in the embryo.
   - The cervix remains of normal size.
   - The endocervical os is open.
   - No low-resistance nourishing blood flow signals are seen in the muscle layer of the cervix.

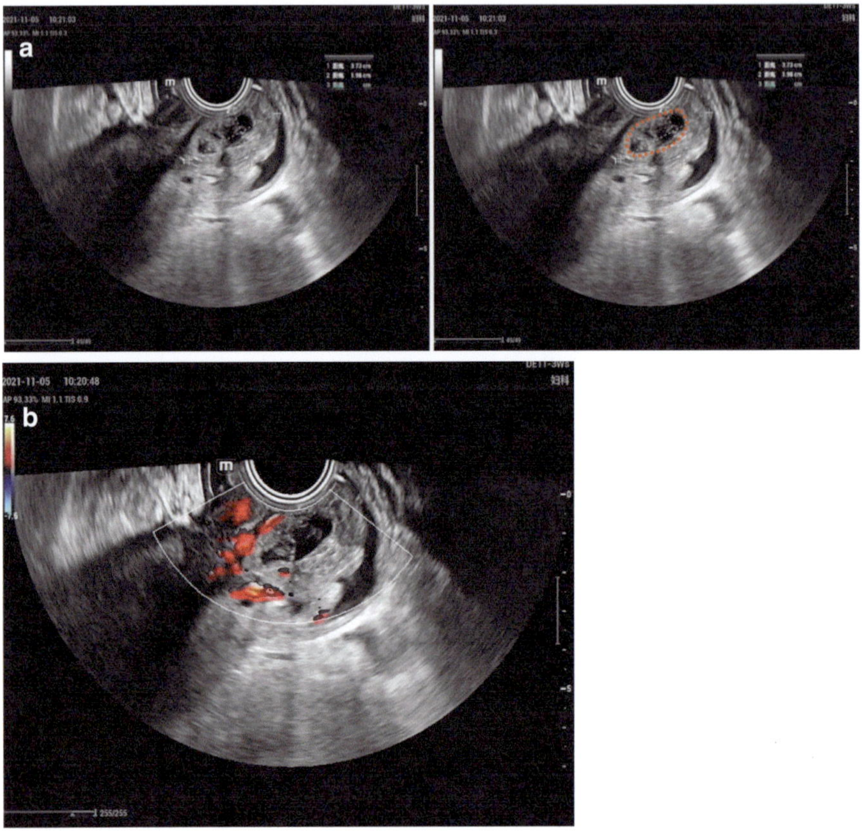

Fig. 8.16 (**a**) Cervical pregnancy: A gestational sac is observed within the cervical canal. The gestational sac is circled in orange. (**b**) Cervical pregnancy: CDFI shows blood flow signals around the gestational sac

8.3.4 Cesarean Scar Pregnancy (CSP)

1. Clinical overview
   Cesarean Scar Pregnancy (CSP) is a rare but serious complication in which an early pregnancy implants in the scar left by a prior cesarean section. CSP can only occur if a niche (a small defect in the scar tissue) is present; it cannot occur in a completely healed cesarean scar [25].
   Clinical manifestations include the following:
   - History of a cesarean section
   - Cessation of menstruation
   - Positive serum and urine pregnancy tests
   - Irregular vaginal bleeding, sometimes with or without lower abdominal pain
2. Typical ultrasonic features
   The first ultrasound to assess for CSP is recommended between 6 and 7 weeks gestation, using transvaginal ultrasound [26]. The diagnosis of CSP is best con-

firmed before 8 weeks gestation, as the gestational sac may grow toward the uterine fundus after this period.

Essential sonographic features to assess include the following:

- Gestational sac size
- Vascularity
- Location in relation to the uterine vessels
- Thickness of the residual myometrium
- Location of the pregnancy in relation to the uterine cavity and serosa

Sonographic criteria include the following [27]:

(1) A uterine cavity that appears empty, with a closed endocervical canal.
(2) The presence of an early gestational sac and/or placenta located near the cesarean scar/niche. This may include the visualization of a fetal or embryonic pole and/or yolk sac, with or without detectable fetal heartbeat, depending on the gestational age. Before 7 weeks of gestation, the gestational sac may adapt to the shape of the niche where it implants.
(3) A reduced or absent myometrial layer between the gestational sac and the anterior uterine wall or bladder.
(4) Doppler ultrasound shows significant blood flow surrounding the gestational sac with rich peritrophoblastic blood flow (Fig. 8.17).

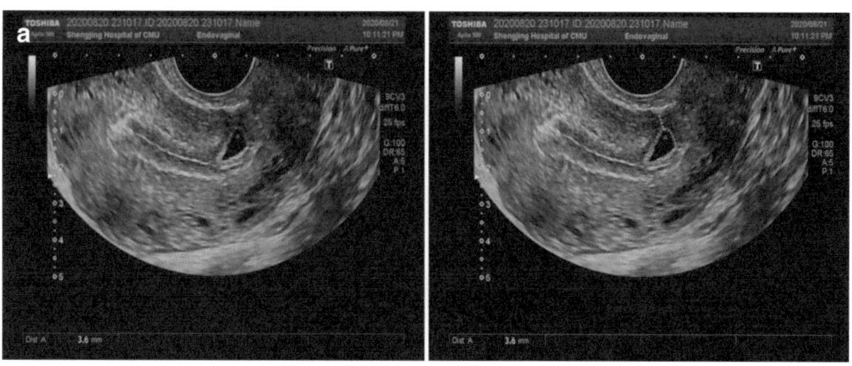

Fig. 8.17 (**a**) Cesarean scar pregnancy: The gestational sac is implanted in the scar, with most of it located in the uterine cavity. The residual myometrial thickness is 3.6 mm. The gestational sac is circled in orange; the residual myometrium is indicated by the green dotted line. (**b**) Cesarean scar pregnancy: The gestational sac is partially implanted in the scar, with most of it located in the uterine cavity. The residual myometrial thickness is 2.3 mm. The gestational sac is circled in orange; the residual myometrium is indicated by the green dotted line. (**c**) Cesarean scar pregnancy: The gestational sac is completely implanted in the myometrium at the uterine scar and protrudes toward the bladder. There is no residual myometrium between the gestational sac and the bladder. The uterus is outlined in orange; the gestational sac is circled in green; the white arrow indicates the protrusion toward the bladder. (**d**) Cesarean scar pregnancy: A mixed echogenic mass in the lower uterine scar is visualized, with irregular morphology and an angular shape in the scar. The mass is circled in orange. (**e**) Cesarean scar pregnancy: A high-velocity, low-resistance arterial flow spectrum is detected around the gestational sac

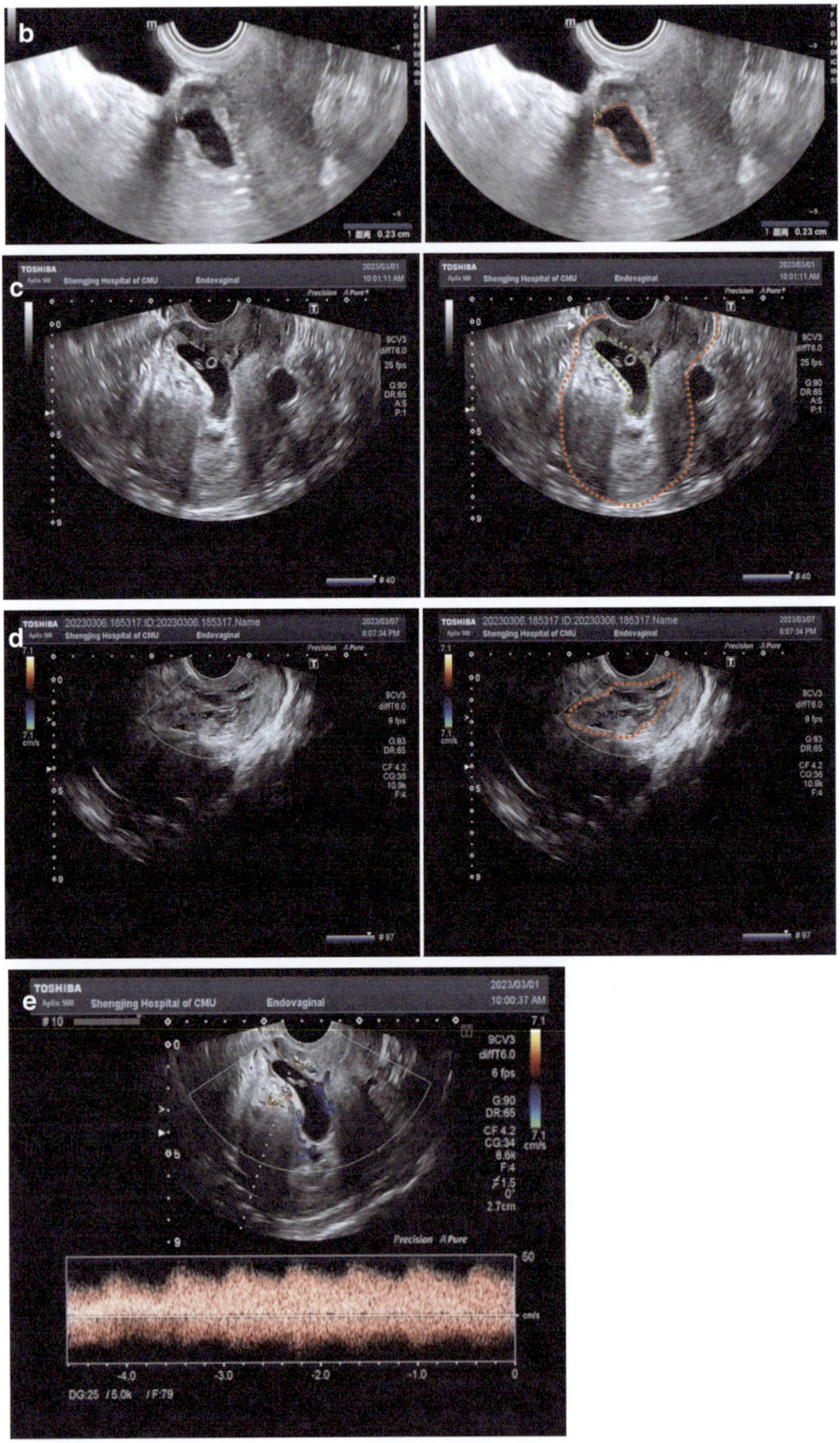

Fig. 8.17 (continued)

3. Differential diagnosis
   A cesarean scar pregnancy should be differentiated from low implantation of a normal pregnancy, cervical ectopic pregnancy, and evolving pregnancy loss. Key factors for differentiation include the patient's clinical history, particularly prior cesarean section, the location of the gestational sac, and its proximity to the cesarean scar.
4. Clinical management
   Treatment options include expectant management, pharmacologic therapy, surgery, and interventional therapy [28]. Methotrexate (MTX) is the drug of choice for pharmacologic therapy. Surgical treatment often involves ultrasound-guided curettage followed by pregnancy removal and uterine scar repair. Uterine artery embolization is another interventional option with unique advantages.

8.3.5 Abdominal Ectopic Pregnancy

1. Clinical overview
   Abdominal ectopic pregnancy refers to the implantation of a pregnancy within the peritoneal cavity, outside the uterine cavity, and fallopian tubes [29]. Unlike tubal ectopic pregnancies, abdominal pregnancies can often remain undetected until a later gestational stage. Diagnostic criteria include the following:
   (1) Normal fallopian tubes and ovaries with no signs of tubal or ovarian pregnancy
   (2) Absence of a utero-peritoneal fistula
   (3) Exclusive location of the pregnancy within the abdominal cavity, ruling out tubal pregnancy

   Secondary abdominal pregnancies typically result from a ruptured or miscarried tubal or ovarian pregnancy. Clinically, patients may present with anemia, sudden and severe abdominal pain, and minimal vaginal bleeding during early pregnancy, often accompanied by a history of missed menstruation. The abnormal placental attachment in abdominal pregnancies leads to poor blood supply, making fetal survival to term unlikely. In rare cases where the fetus reaches term, uterine contours are difficult to palpate, but fetal limbs may be distinctly palpable, often accompanied by detectable fetal heartbeats.
2. Typical ultrasonic features
   These include the following:
   - Absence of a gestational sac in the uterine cavity or difficulty visualizing standard sonographic features in mid-to-late-term pregnancies.
   - In advanced abdominal ectopic pregnancies, the gestational or amniotic sac lacks the characteristic thick, smooth, hypoechoic muscular uterine wall, and the fetus appears to be in direct contact with the maternal abdominal wall.
   - In cases of fetal demise, the fetal body becomes poorly defined on imaging.
   - Due to limited amniotic fluid, the placenta appears as an irregular, heterogeneous echogenic mass with multiple adhesions (Fig. 8.18).

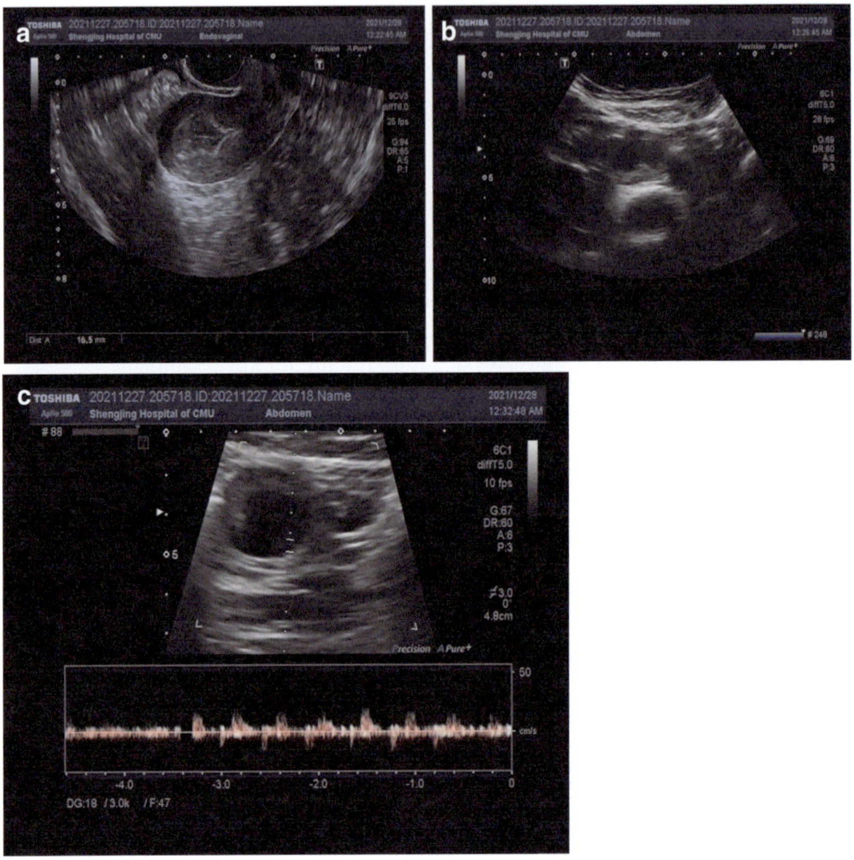

Fig. 8.18 (**a**) Abdominal pregnancy: No gestational sac is present in the uterine cavity. (**b**) Abdominal pregnancy: A gestational sac is visualized in the retroperitoneum. (**c**) Abdominal pregnancy: Fetal heartbeats are detected in the fetal sac

3. Differential diagnosis
   (1) Tubal pregnancy
   Differentiating an early abdominal ectopic pregnancy from a tubal pregnancy is often challenging. However, abdominal ectopic pregnancies located outside the pelvis—such as between the spleen and kidney or between the liver and kidney—are more easily distinguished from a tubal pregnancy.
   (2) Rudimentary horn pregnancy
   At a later gestational age, a rudimentary horn pregnancy can be mistaken for an abdominal pregnancy. This is because the thin hypoechoic muscular layer surrounding the gestational sac in a rudimentary horn pregnancy may resemble the peritoneal and greater omental wrappings of abdominal pregnancy. Multisection scanning, however, can reveal the rudimentary horn's connection to the uterus, a feature absent in abdominal pregnancies.

4. Clinical management
   Surgical intervention is the primary treatment for abdominal ectopic pregnancy. This is crucial information, as removing an abnormally implanted placenta can cause significant bleeding.

8.3.6 Ovarian Pregnancy

1. Clinical overview
   Ovarian pregnancy is a rare form of ectopic pregnancy where the embryo implants within ovarian tissue. Common clinical symptoms include the following:
   - Missed menstruation
   - Abdominal pain
   - Vaginal bleeding

   Due to the limited capacity of the ovary to sustain a growing pregnancy, rupture often occurs at an early stage.
2. Typical ultrasonic features
   In unruptured ovarian pregnancy, the affected ovary appears enlarged and irregularly shaped, with a visible gestational sac that may or may not contain fetal structures. After rupture, ultrasound typically reveals a heterogeneous echogenic mass with irregular morphology and poorly defined borders, making differentiation from a ruptured tubal pregnancy or corpus luteum challenging (Fig. 8.19). A key distinguishing feature is the inability to separate the pregnancy from the ovary on palpation. Color Doppler imaging is essential to identify peritrophoblastic blood flow distinct from the corpus luteum [30]. CDFI highlights abundant low-resistance blood flow signals surrounding the gestational sac within the ovary.
3. Differential diagnosis
   (1) Tubal pregnancy
   Ovarian pregnancy presents as a mass firmly attached to the ovary (no sliding sign), whereas an unruptured tubal pregnancy does not exhibit this feature. Distinguishing between a ruptured ovarian pregnancy and a ruptured tubal pregnancy can be challenging. However, following a ruptured tubal pregnancy, a normal ovary may be visible on transvaginal ultrasound, whereas in a ruptured ovarian pregnancy, the ovary is not identifiable.
   (2) Corpus luteum
   A corpus luteum typically shows circumferential or semicircumferential blood flow signals with a resistive index (RI) of approximately 0.5, while ovarian pregnancies present focal blood flow signals. There is considerable overlap in RI values between the two, so attention should be given to the internal echogenicity of the mass. If the echogenicity of the mass is higher

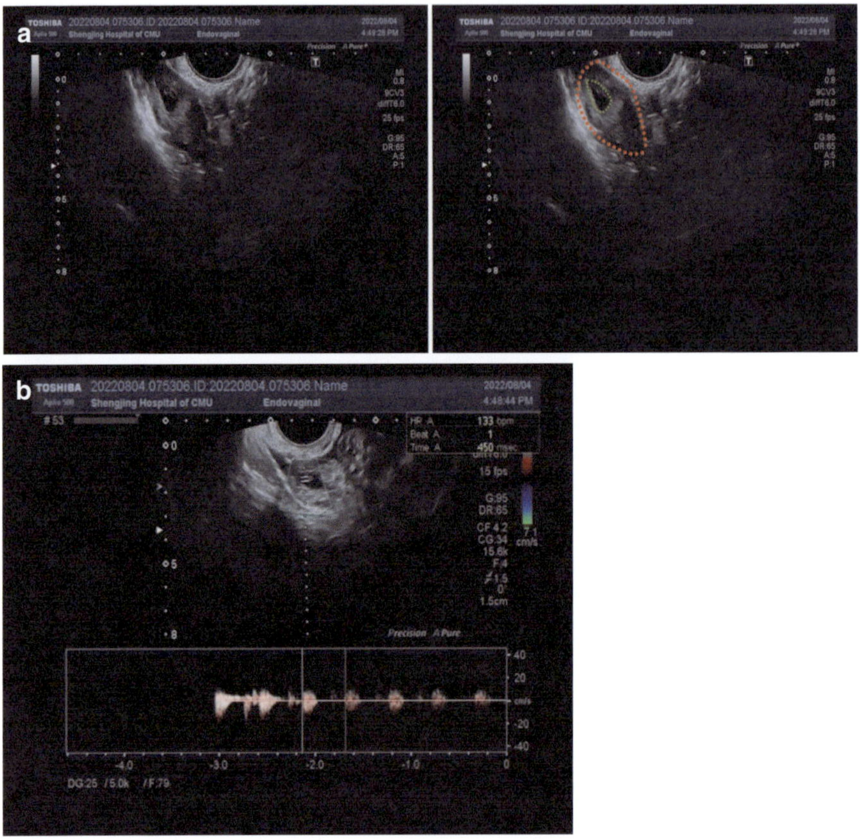

Fig. 8.19 (**a**) Ovarian pregnancy: A gestational sac is visible in the ovary with clear borders, yolk sac, and embryonic structure. The ovary is circled in orange; the gestational sac is circled in green. (**b**) Ovarian pregnancy: Spectral Doppler detects fetal heartbeats within the embryonic structure

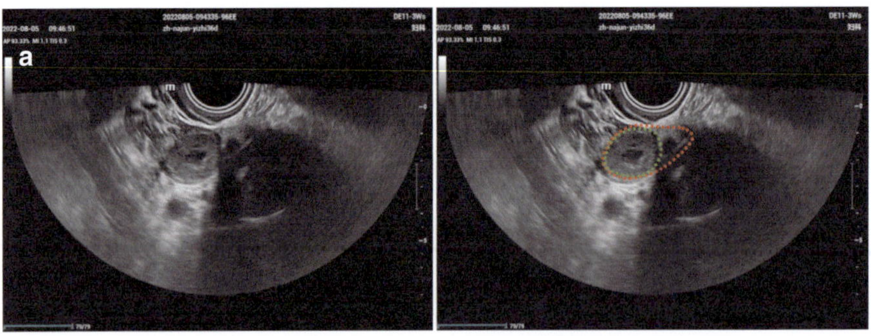

Fig. 8.20 (**a**) Corpus luteum of pregnancy: A roundish mass is visualized in the ovary with well-defined borders, moderate peripheral echogenicity, and a liquid center. The ovary is circled in orange; the mass is circled in green. (**b**) Corpus luteum of pregnancy: Circumferential blood flow signals are detected in the periphery on CDFI

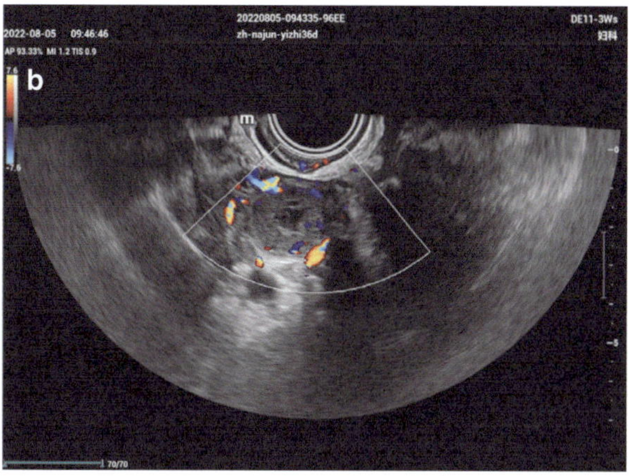

Fig. 8.20 (continued)

than that of the ovarian parenchyma, this suggests an ovarian pregnancy. Conversely, a corpus luteum is usually a hypoechoic mass (Fig. 8.20).

4. Clinical management
   Ovarian pregnancies are typically managed through surgical removal of the affected ovary. In cases of unruptured ovarian pregnancy, conservative treatment with pharmacological therapy may be considered as an alternative.

8.3.7 Heterotopic Pregnancy (HP)

1. Clinical overview
   Heterotopic pregnancy (HP) refers to the coexistence of an intrauterine pregnancy alongside an ectopic pregnancy. In the general population, the incidence of HP is approximately 1 in 30,000 pregnancies [31]. However, in patients who undergo ART, such as drug-induced ovulation or IVF-ET, the prevalence rises to 1–3% [32]. With the increasing use of selective single-embryo transfer strategies, the incidence of HP has decreased [33, 34].
2. Typical ultrasonic features
   HP can involve ectopic pregnancies located in different sites, including the uterine horn, cervix, and cesarean scar, each presenting distinct sonographic features. It is essential to maintain a high level of suspicion for ectopic pregnancy, even when an intrauterine gestational sac is observed. A thorough examination of the uterine horns and adnexal areas is necessary. Additionally, the extrauterine gestational sac development may lag behind the intrauterine sac. In cases where the patient has an ovarian corpus luteum cyst or ovarian hyperstimulation syndrome, the ectopic pregnancy mass may be obscured (Fig. 8.21).

8.4 Ultrasound Evaluation of Twin and Multiple Pregnancies

A multiple pregnancy refers to a pregnancy in which two or more fetuses are conceived simultaneously. Twin pregnancies are the most common type of multiple pregnancies, followed by triplets, with four or more fetuses being quite rare. Twin pregnancies are classified into the following types based on the number of fertilized eggs and the timing of differentiation:

- Dichorionic diamniotic (DCDA) twins (Figs. 8.22, 8.23, and 8.24)
- Monochorionic diamniotic (MCDA) twins
- Monochorionic monoamniotic (MCMA) twins (Fig. 8.25)

The classification of a twin pregnancy on ultrasound depends on the estimated gestational age, as well as the chorionicity and amnionicity of the pregnancy. The determination of chorionicity is most accurate during early gestation, and it is ideally performed in the first or early second trimester [35].

1. Chorionic sac count
   Ultrasound is highly accurate in counting the number of gestational sacs before the 10th week of pregnancy, where each gestational sac corresponds to a chorionic sac. Chorionic sacs appear as round, sonolucent structures with a brightly echogenic rim (chorion) implanted on one side of the cavity within the thick decidua [36].
2. Amniotic sac count
   Amniotic sac differentiation occurs after chorionic sac differentiation. In dichorionic twin pregnancies, there must be two distinct amniotic sacs. The number of amniotic sacs can be determined ultrasonographically by counting the number of fetal heartbeats in each gestational sac by the 6th week of gestation.
   The yolk sac is visible on ultrasound 2 weeks earlier than the amniotic sac. The number of yolk sacs corresponds directly to the number of amniotic sacs [37]. Therefore, in monochorionic twin pregnancies, the number of amniotic sacs can be inferred by counting the yolk sacs before the amniotic sacs become visible.
   If the ultrasound reveals two embryonic buds within one gestational sac, the pregnancy may be either MCDA or MCMA. To make a definitive diagnosis, the number of amniotic sacs must be confirmed. A transabdominal ultrasound scan can typically detect the amniotic sac between the 7th and 8th week of gestation. Transvaginal ultrasound offers a better view of the amniotic cavity, often providing a clear image of two separate amniotic sacs, thereby confirming a diagnosis of MCDA. If no amniotic membrane is seen separating the two embryonic structures, MCMA should be considered. However, careful examination is required later in pregnancy to look for a septal membrane between the twin fetuses to rule out MCDA.

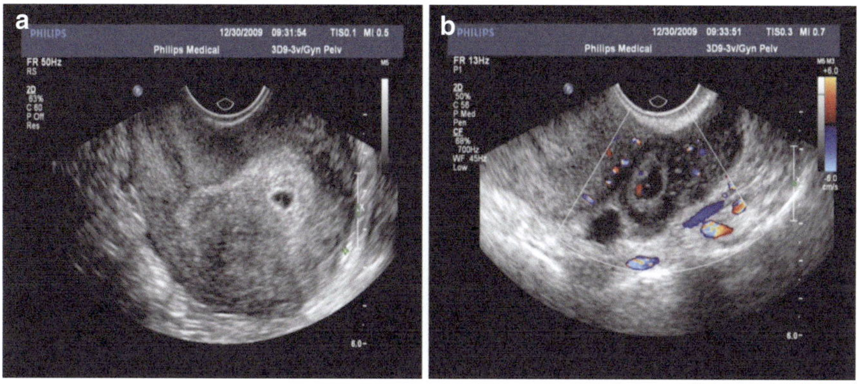

Fig. 8.21 (**a**) After IVF, a gestational sac is visualized in the uterine cavity, with a yolk sac visible within the gestational sac. (**b**) A tubal ectopic pregnancy is present in the left adnexa, with detectable fetal heartbeats

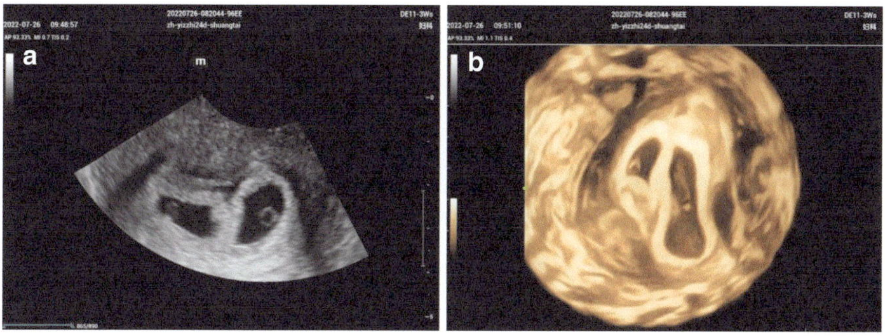

Fig. 8.22 (**a**) DCDA twin pregnancy, 24 days post transplantation: two gestational sacs are visible in the uterine cavity, with a yolk sac visible in each sac. (**b**) 3D ultrasound showing two gestational sacs

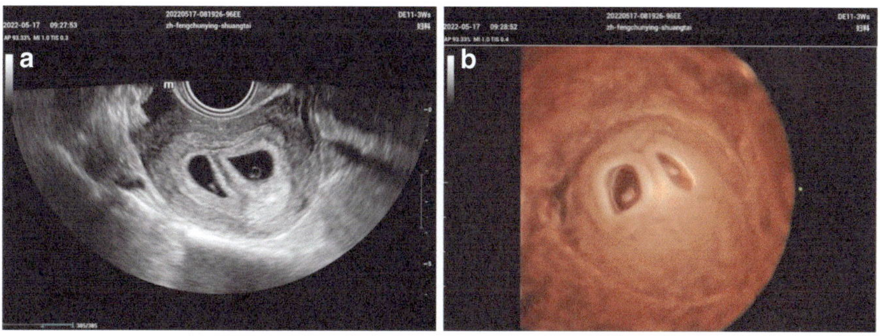

Fig. 8.23 (**a**) A case of DCDA twin pregnancy, 40 days into natural gestation: two gestational sacs are visible in the uterine cavity, with a yolk sac present in each sac. (**b**) 3D ultrasound showing two gestational sacs

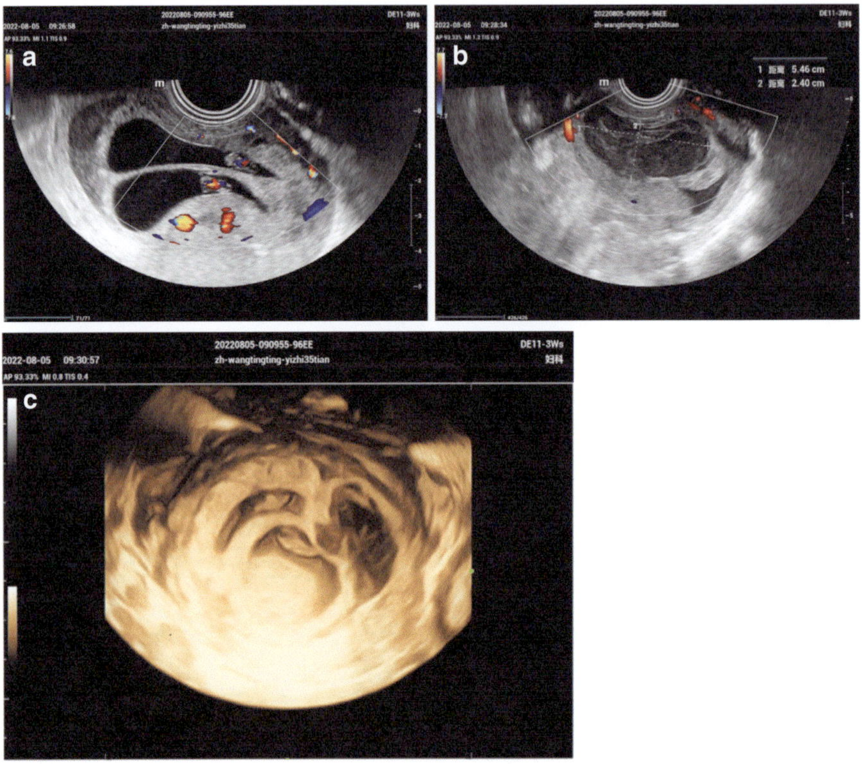

Fig. 8.24 (**a**) DCDA twin pregnancy with intrauterine hemorrhage, 35 days post transplantation: two gestational sacs are visible in the uterine cavity, each containing an embryonic structure. Fetal heartbeats are detected on CDFI. (**b**) Intrauterine fluid is observed within the uterine cavity, with punctate and flocculent echoes. No blood flow signals are detected on CDFI. (**c**) 3D ultrasound showing two gestational sacs and fluid in the uterine cavity

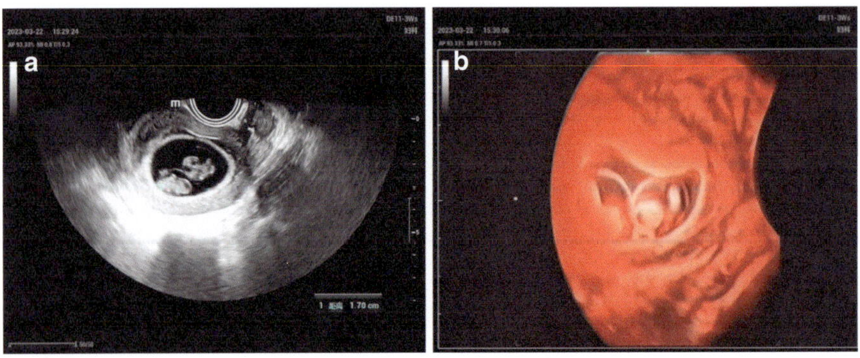

Fig. 8.25 (**a**) MCDA twin pregnancy: One gestational sac is visible in the uterine cavity, with two amniotic sacs, each containing an embryonic bud. (**b**) MCDA twin pregnancy: 3D ultrasound shows one gestational sac in the uterine cavity, with two amniotic sacs visible within it

References

1. Richardson A, Gallos I, Dobson S, et al. Accuracy of first-trimester ultrasound in diagnosis of intrauterine pregnancy prior to visualization of the yolk sac: a systematic review and meta-analysis. Ultrasound Obstet Gynecol. 2015;46(2):142–9.
2. Marin M, Pătru CL, Manolea MM, et al. Can ultrasound analysis of the yolk sac be a predictor of pregnancy outcome? Curr Health Sci J. 2021;47(4):547–52.
3. Kurjak A, Kupesic S, Banovic I, et al. The study of morphology and circulation of early embryo by three-dimensional ultrasound and power Doppler. J Perinat Med. 1999;27(3):145–57.
4. Salomon LJ, Alfirevic Z, Bilardo CM, et al. ISUOG practice guidelines: performance of first-trimester fetal ultrasound scan. Ultrasound Obstet Gynecol. 2013;41(1):102–13.
5. Doubilet PM. Ultrasound evaluation of the first trimester. Radiol Clin North Am. 2014;52(6):1191–9.
6. Napolitano R, Dhami J, Ohuma EO, et al. Pregnancy dating by fetal crown-rump length: a systematic review of charts. BJOG. 2014;121(5):556–65.
7. Quenby S, Gallos ID, Dhillon-Smith RK, et al. Miscarriage matters: the epidemiological, physical, psychological, and economic costs of early pregnancy loss. Lancet. 2021;397(10285):1658–67.
8. Newbatt E, Beckles Z, Ullman R, et al. Ectopic pregnancy and miscarriage: summary of NICE guidance. BMJ. 2012;345:e8136.
9. Pillai RN, Konje JC, Richardson M, et al. Prediction of miscarriage in women with viable intrauterine pregnancy: a systematic review and diagnostic accuracy meta-analysis. Eur J Obstet Gynecol Reprod Biol. 2018;220:122–31.
10. Knez J, Day A, Jurkovic D. Ultrasound imaging in the management of bleeding and pain in early pregnancy. Best Pract Res Clin Obstet Gynaecol. 2014;28(5):621–36.
11. Jauniaux E, Johns J, Burton GJ. The role of ultrasound imaging in diagnosing and investigating early pregnancy failure. Ultrasound Obstet Gynecol. 2005;25(6):613–24.
12. Jurkovic D, Overton C, Bender-Atik R. Diagnosis and management of first trimester miscarriage. BMJ. 2013;346:f3676.
13. Perriera L, Reeves MF. Ultrasound criteria for diagnosis of early pregnancy failure and ectopic pregnancy. Semin Reprod Med. 2008;26(5):373–82.
14. Bottomley C, Bourne T. Diagnosing miscarriage. Best Pract Res Clin Obstet Gynaecol. 2009;23(4):463–77.
15. ESHRE Working Group on Ectopic Pregnancy, Kirk E, Ankum P, et al. Terminology for describing normally sited and ectopic pregnancies on ultrasound: ESHRE recommendations for good practice. Hum Reprod Open. 2020;2020(4):hoaa055.
16. Al Wattar BH, Solangon SA, de Braud LV, et al. Effectiveness of treatment options for tubal ectopic pregnancy: a systematic review and network meta-analysis. BJOG. 2024;131(1):5–14.
17. Scibetta EW, Han CS. Ultrasound in early pregnancy: viability, unknown locations, and ectopic pregnancies. Obstet Gynecol Clin N Am. 2019;46(4):783–95.
18. Houser M, Kandalaft N, Khati NJ. Ectopic pregnancy: a resident's guide to imaging findings and diagnostic pitfalls. Emerg Radiol. 2022;29(1):161–72.
19. Farquhar CM. Ectopic pregnancy. Lancet. 2005;366(9485):583–91.
20. Richardson A, Gallos I, Dobson S, et al. Accuracy of first-trimester ultrasound in diagnosis of tubal ectopic pregnancy in the absence of an obvious extrauterine embryo: systematic review and meta-analysis. Ultrasound Obstet Gynecol. 2016;47(1):28–37.
21. Levine D. Ectopic pregnancy. Radiology. 2007;245(2):385–97.
22. Durand YG, Capoccia-Brugger R, Vial Y, et al. Diagnostic dilemma between angular and interstitial ectopic pregnancy: 3D ultrasound features. J Ultrasound. 2022;25(4):989–94.
23. Bollig KJ, Schust DJ. Refining angular pregnancy diagnosis in the first trimester: a case series of expectant management. Obstet Gynecol. 2020;135(1):175–84.
24. Köninger A, Nguyen BP, Schwenk U, et al. Cervical ectopic pregnancy – the first case of live birth and uterus-conserving management. BMC Pregnancy Childbirth. 2023;23(1):664.

25. Jordans IPM, Verberkt C, De Leeuw RA, et al. Definition and sonographic reporting system for Cesarean scar pregnancy in early gestation: modified Delphi method. Ultrasound Obstet Gynecol. 2022;59(4):437–49.
26. Kennedy A, Debbink M, Griffith A, et al. Cesarean scar ectopic pregnancy: a do-not-miss diagnosis. Radiographics. 2024;44(7):e230199.
27. Timor-Tritsch IE, Monteagudo A, Calì G, et al. Cesarean scar pregnancy: diagnosis and pathogenesis. Obstet Gynecol Clin N Am. 2019;46(4):797–811.
28. Lin R, DiCenzo N, Rosen T. Cesarean scar ectopic pregnancy: nuances in diagnosis and treatment. Fertil Steril. 2023;120(3 Pt 2):563–72.
29. Gorincour G, Boukerrou M. Abdominal ectopic pregnancy. N Engl J Med. 2023;389(24):e51.
30. Solangon SA, Naftalin J, Jurkovic D. Ovarian ectopic pregnancy: clinical characteristics, ultrasound diagnosis and management. Ultrasound Obstet Gynecol. 2024;63(6):815–23.
31. Maleki A, Khalid N, Rajesh Patel C, et al. The rising incidence of heterotopic pregnancy: current perspectives and associations with in-vitro fertilization. Eur J Obstet Gynecol Reprod Biol. 2021;266:138–44.
32. Hewlett K, Howell CM. Heterotopic pregnancy: simultaneous viable and nonviable pregnancies. JAAPA. 2020;33(3):35–8.
33. Clayton HB, Schieve LA, Peterson HB, et al. Ectopic pregnancy risk with assisted reproductive technology procedures. Obstet Gynecol. 2006;107(3):595–604.
34. Perkins KM, Boulet SL, Kissin DM, et al. Risk of ectopic pregnancy associated with assisted reproductive technology in the United States 2001–2011. Obstet Gynecol. 2015;125(1):70–8.
35. Committee on Practice Bulletins. Multifetal gestations: twin, triplet, and higher-order multifetal pregnancies: ACOG practice bulletin, number 231. Obstet Gynecol. 2021;137(6):e145–62.
36. Monteagudo A, Roman AS. Ultrasound in multiple gestations: twins and other multifetal pregnancies. Clin Perinatol. 2005;32(2):329–54.
37. Hirshberg A, Dugoff L. First-trimester ultrasound and aneuploidy screening in multifetal pregnancies. Clin Obstet Gynecol. 2015;58(3):559–73.

MIX
Papier aus verantwortungsvollen Quellen
Paper from responsible sources
FSC® C105338

If you have any concerns about our products,
you can contact us on
ProductSafety@springernature.com

In case Publisher is established outside the EU,
the EU authorized representative is:
Springer Nature Customer Service Center GmbH
Europaplatz 3, 69115 Heidelberg, Germany

Printed by Libri Plureos GmbH
in Hamburg, Germany